Social Scaffol

Applying the Lessons of Contemporary Social Science to Health and Healthcare

Social Scaffolding

Applying the Lessons of Contemporary Social Science to Health and Healthcare

Edited by

Richard Williams
University of South Wales

Verity Kemp
Healthplanning Ltd., UK

S. Alexander Haslam
University of Queensland

Catherine Haslam
University of Queensland

Kamaldeep S. Bhui
Queen Mary University of London

Sue Bailey
Centre for Mental Health, UK

Associate Editor
Daniel Maughan
Oxford Health NHS Foundation Trust

CAMBRIDGE
UNIVERSITY PRESS

CAMBRIDGE
UNIVERSITY PRESS

University Printing House, Cambridge CB2 8BS, United Kingdom

One Liberty Plaza, 20th Floor, New York, NY 10006, USA

477 Williamstown Road, Port Melbourne, VIC 3207, Australia

314–321, 3rd Floor, Plot 3, Splendor Forum, Jasola District Centre, New Delhi – 110025, India

79 Anson Road, #06–04/06, Singapore 079906

Cambridge University Press is part of the University of Cambridge.

It furthers the University's mission by disseminating knowledge in the pursuit of education, learning and research at the highest international levels of excellence.

www.cambridge.org
Information on this title: www.cambridge.org/9781911623045
DOI: 10.1017/9781911623069

First published 2019

Printed and bound in Great Britain by Clays Ltd, Elcograf S.p.A.

A catalogue record for this publication is available from the British Library.

Library of Congress Cataloging-in-Publication Data
Names: Williams, Richard, 1949 February 5– editor.
Title: Social scaffolding : applying the lessons of contemporary social science to health and healthcare / edited by Richard Williams, Verity Kemp, S. Alexander Haslam, Catherine Haslam, Kamaldeep S. Bhui, Sue Bailey ; associate editor, Daniel Maughan.
Description: Cambridge, United Kingdom : Cambridge University Press, 2019. | Includes bibliographical references.
Identifiers: LCCN 2018053754 | ISBN 9781911623045 (pbk.)
Subjects: | MESH: Social Determinants of Health | Social Support | Health Services Needs and Demand | Resilience, Psychological | Social Medicine | Social Identification
Classification: LCC RA418 | NLM WA 30 | DDC 362.1–dc23
LC record available at https://lccn.loc.gov/2018053754

ISBN 978-1-911-62304-5 Paperback

Contents

Section 3: Sourcing

Section 4: Scaffolding

Section 5: Sustaining

Contributors

Dr Peter Aitken MB ChB, MRCGP, FRCPsych, FHEA
Consultant Liaison Psychiatrist, Clinical Director for Individual Patient Placement & Director of Research, Development and Medical Education, Devon Partnership NHS Trust & Honorary Associate Professor, University of Exeter Medical School, UK

Professor, John, Lord Alderdice MB BCh BAO, FRCPsych
Senior Research Fellow and Director of the Centre for the Resolution of Intractable Conflict, Harris Manchester College, University of Oxford, UK & Clinical Professor, Department of Psychiatry, School of Medicine, University of Maryland (Baltimore), USA

Dr Khalifah Alfadhli BA(Hons), MA, PhD
Department of Psychology, King Saud University, Riyadh, Saudi Arabia & School of Psychology, University of Sussex, UK

Dr Hani Alnabulsi BS, MA, PhD
Directorate of Civil Defence, Jeddah, Saudi Arabia

Dame Sue Bailey DSc, FRCPsych
Chair of the Children and Young People's Mental Health Coalition, Chair of the Centre for Mental Health, UK & Bevan Commissioner, Wales, UK

Professor Kamaldeep S. Bhui CBE, MD(Lon), FRCP(Edin), FRCPsych, FRSA, PFHEA
Professor of Cultural Psychiatry and Epidemiology, Barts and the London School of Medicine and Dentistry, Queen Mary University of London & Honorary Consultant Psychiatrist, East London Foundation NHS Trust, UK

Professor Jerome E. Bickenbach PhD, LLB
Leader, Disability Policy Group, Leiter Unit, Schweizer Paraplegiker-Forschung Research (SPF), Nottwil, Switzerland & Professor, Department of Health Sciences and Health Policy, University of Lucerne, Switzerland

Dr Francesca Brady BSc, MSc, DClinPsy
Clinical Psychologist, Helen Bamber Foundation, UK

Dr Holly Carter BSc(Hons), PhD
Behavioural Science Emergency Response Department Science and Technology, Health Protection Directorate, Public Health England, UK

Professor Alarcos Cieza MSc, MPH, PhD
Professor of Medical Psychology, Faculty of Human and Social Sciences, University of Southampton, UK & World Health Organization, Geneva, Switzerland

Dr Tegan Cruwys PhD
Senior Lecturer in Psychology and Australian Research Council DECRA Fellow, Research School of Psychology, Australian National University, Australia

Professor John Drury BA(Hons), MSc, PhD
Professor of Social Psychology, School of Psychology, University of Sussex, UK

Dr Hinemoa Elder PhD, MB ChB, FRANZCP
Professor Indigenous Health Research, Te Whare Wānanga o Awanuiārangi, Māori

Strategic Leader, Brain Research New Zealand, Fellow Australia and New Zealand College of Psychiatrists, Child and Adolescent Psychiatrist, New Zealand Mental Health Review Tribunal

Professor Neil Greenberg BSc(Hons), BM, MMedSc, MFMLM, FHEA, DOccMed, MInstLM, MEWI, MFFLM, MD, FRCPsych
Professor of Defence Mental Health, King's Centre for Military Health Research, Kings College London, UK

Professor Catherine Haslam PhD
Professor of Clinical Psychology, School of Psychology, University of Queensland, Australia

Professor S. Alexander Haslam PhD, FAcSS
Professor of Psychology and Australian Laureate Fellow, School of Psychology, University of Queensland, Australia

Dr Tim Healing MSc, PhD, CBIOL, FZS, FRSB, DipClinMicro, DMCC
Course Director, Conflict and Catastrophe Medicine, Faculty of Conflict and Catastrophe Medicine, Worshipful Society of Apothecaries of London, UK

Dr Peter Hindley MBE, BSc, MB BS, FRCPsych, Dip Cert CBT (children and adolescents)
Retired child and adolescent psychiatrist

Professor Rachel Jenkins MD(Cantab), FRCPsych, FFOHM, MPH
Institute of Psychiatry, Kings College London, UK

Professor Jolanda Jetten PhD, FASSA
Professor of Psychology and Australian Laureate Fellow, School of Psychology, University of Queensland, Australia

Professor Cornelius Katona
Medical Director, Helen Bamber Foundation & Honorary Professor, Division of Psychiatry, University College London, UK

Verity Kemp BA(Hons), DipHSM
Director, Healthplanning Ltd & Associate, Welsh Institute for Health & Social Care, University of South Wales, UK

Dr Daniel Maughan MD, BSc, MB BCh, MRCPsych
Consultant Psychiatrist, Early Intervention Service, Oxford Health NHS Foundation Trust, UK & Associate Registrar in Sustainability for the Royal College of Psychiatrists, UK

Dr Deirdre MacManus BSc(Hons) MBChB MRCPsych MSc PhD
Senior Clinical Lecturer, King's College London, UK

Richard Mills BSc, DipHSM
Director, Healthplanning Ltd & Non-Executive Director, Sheffield Health & Social Care NHS Foundation Trust, UK

Professor Sir Jonathan Montgomery BA, LLM, HonFRCPCH
Professor of Health Care Law, Faculty of Law, University College London. UK & Chair of the Health Research Authority, England, UK

Dr Adrian Neal BA(Hons), MA, MSc, DClinPsych, CPsychol
Consultant Clinical Psychologist and Head of Employee Wellbeing Service, Aneurin Bevan University Health Board, NHS Wales, UK & Chair of the Division of Clinical Psychology (Wales) of the British Psychological Society, UK

Dr Kim Peters PhD
Senior Lecturer in Psychology, School of

Psychology, University of Queensland, Australia

Dr Oliver Quantick BSc, MB BS, MSc, MFPH
Consultant Public Health Physician, Army Medical Services, UK

Professor Anthony D. Redmond OBE, MD, FRCPGlasg, FRCSEd, FRCEM, FIMCRCSEd, HonMFPH, DMCC
Professor of International Emergency Medicine, Head, WHO Collaborating Centre for Emergency Medical Teams and Emergency Capacity Building & Deputy Director of the Humanitarian and Conflict Response Institute, University of Manchester, UK

Professor Stephen Reicher PhD, FBA, FRSE, FAcSS
Wardlaw Professor of Psychology, School of Psychology and Neuroscience, University of St. Andrews, Scotland, UK

Professor David Ross QHP, MSc, MRCGP, FRCPCH, FFPH, FFTM RCPS(Glasg) FRCP(Glasg)
Parkes Professor of Preventative Medicine, Army Medical Services, UK

Professor Steven R. Smith PhD, MSc, CQSW, BA
Professor of Political Philosophy and Social Policy, School of Humanities and Social Sciences, Faculty of Business and Society, University of South Wales, UK

Dr Niklas K. Steffens PhD
Lecturer in Psychology and Australian Research Council DECRA Fellow, School of Psychology, University of Queensland, Australia

Anna F. Taylor BSc(Hons), MSc
Research Associate, Kings College London, UK

Professor Richard Williams OBE, TD, MB ChB, FRCPsych, FRCPCH, DPM, DMCC
Emeritus Professor of Mental Health Strategy, Welsh Institute for Health and Social Care, University of South Wales, UK & Director of PROJECT CARE for the Faculty of Pre-Hospital Care of the Royal College of Surgeons of Edinburgh, UK

Foreword

Psychiatry is one of the major specialties in medicine and carries with it clear imperatives on the role of social factors in the genesis and perpetuation of mental illnesses. There is clear evidence that geopolitical factors influence social determinants which in turn affect rates of psychiatric disorders. It is well known that rates of psychiatric illnesses are higher among homeless, unemployed and other vulnerable groups. Poor housing, overcrowding and lack of access to green spaces have been shown to be related to high rates of psychiatric disorders. The use of occupational and social therapies is often ignored in many settings. Recent acknowledgement of the role of social prescribing has been shown to alleviate stress and distress. Social prescribing has been used at a number of levels and in multiple ways. Social structures are changing, and inter-generational shifts are more prominent than ever. In parallel, the rise of channels of communication means that, although we may be better connected, we are still socially isolated and lonelier than ever. For people with psychiatric disorders, the sense of loneliness and isolation can further contribute a spiral of abandonment by the system and the people.

Social scaffolding as a concept has its value in improving engagement and helping build resilience. As societies change under the influence of globalisation, personal, social and ethnic identities change, and these changes may bring with them material gains, but there are winners and losers. The traditional social resources of help such as churches and religious institutions are also changing and shifting. The traditional high streets are disappearing, being replaced by more cafés where people may congregate and often work, thereby creating different places of work. Human beings are social animals and at all levels social structures and strictures define us in a number of ways. Human beings interact and flourish together and are interconnected in a number of ways. However, these avenues of connections change as societies change from traditional to more modern cultures. Sociocentric cultures emphasise close-connectedness and kinship-based responsibilities. Studies have shown that rates of many psychiatric disorders, along with those of divorce and crime, are much higher in ego-centric societies thereby indicating that human interactions do play a role in the genesis of psychiatric disorders as well as help-seeking.

There is little doubt that social factors are critical in managing mental illnesses. Social capital is not static and waxes and wanes throughout one's life, and these patterns are also affected by other factors. A person's identity, as well as social or ethnic identity, play a major role in the creation of 'the other' which contributes further to stigma, prejudice and discrimination. Therefore, healthcare professionals need to be cognisant of the role social factors can play in the protection, as well as deterioration, of each person's functioning. Not all social relationships are positive, so the challenge for each clinician is to explore and understand the roles and expectations of family members and other social contacts in any individual patient's orbit.

This volume comes at an appropriate time. The editors have brought together a wealth of expertise, enabling us to explore and understand the relationship between health and social connectedness. Shared social identities can facilitate flourishing at an individual and neighbourhood level. As has been highlighted across this volume, healthcare professionals need to be aware and be trained in using new social models of supporting and helping to build social connections in order for patients and communities to thrive. Scaffolding has to be built from the bottom-up rather than being imposed by policies from the top. People with a vision can bring this about and this volume provides a strong theoretical background. The socially informed approach to diagnosis, management, research and policy development is an absolute must, and this volume provides a very welcome addition.

Dinesh Bhugra, CBE
MA, MSc, MBBS, PhD, FRCP, FRCPE, FRCPsych, FFPHM, FRCPsych(Hon), FHKCPsych (Hon), FACPsych(Hon), FAMS(Singapore), FKCL, MPhil, FAcadME, FRSA, DIFAPA

Emeritus Professor Mental Health & Cultural Diversity, IoPPN, Kings College, London

Past-President, Royal College of Psychiatrists (2008–2011)
Past president, World Psychiatric Association (2014–2017)
President, British Medical Association (2018–2019)

Note

Some chapters contain vignettes regarding named people. Most of these vignettes are based upon the stories of several members of the public but have been adapted and altered to highlight the content of the book chapter and do not pertain to any specific person. Chapter 20 includes two case studies that are about real events. The information presented there concerning the people involved is in the public domain.

Section 1 **Schooling**

Chapter 1

Health and Society: Contributions to Improving Healthcare from the Social Sciences

Richard Williams

Setting the Scene

This book's roots are in an impactful seminar series hosted by the Royal College of Psychiatrists in which practitioners and scientists from a wide array of disciplines came together in 2014 to explore the social influences on our health and recovery from ill health. This volume echoes the evocative conversations in that College and is intended to rehearse research of potentially great impact. It presents practitioners, researchers, policymakers and students of a wide array of disciplines and roles with the material to support them in better harnessing what we now know about the impact of social factors on health. Thereby, the editors hope to influence how practitioners and the responsible authorities work together with members of the public and communities to design and deliver services. Our aspiration is to contribute to creating better-targeted approaches to promoting health and mental health and more effective and integrated interventions for people who have health problems or disorders. Importantly, we set the task in the context of current world dilemmas.

While writing this book, there were and remain in the UK widespread and powerful concerns about funding services that promote health and deliver healthcare for people who are unwell that are able to keep pace with advances in science and practice and the expectations of the public. This evokes concerns about the values that underpin public services. The UK is by no means alone in experiencing these tensions. There are contemporary challenges in providing mental healthcare that meets the needs of populations in ways that match the provisions for physical healthcare in their funding, esteem and acceptability. Chapter 8 picks up this matter of parity of esteem for physical and mental healthcare services.

Worldwide, there are determined efforts to base policy, funding and practice on robust and rigorously gleaned evidence. Yet, there are also concerns about the balance of evidence employed to inform how services are designed and delivered to reflect the preferences of patients and the nature of their needs. Within evidence-based practice, there are also concerns about the sorts of evidence and scientific methods that we are ready to allow to influence policy and practice (see Chapter 26).

Progress over the last two decades in the brain sciences and, to a lesser extent, in developing healthcare delivery now points to promising lines of intervention within public health, public mental health and personalised healthcare with a view to developing and implementing evidence-based services. But, other considerations, such as those described by Heath (2016) and Abbasi (2016), indicate that, on their own, the contributions from the physical, genetic and neurosciences and study of service need and delivery by epidemiological means may not be sufficient. While what we are learning from research topics in the health sciences is of enormous importance, and they are shifting healthcare hugely, there are also highly relevant developments in the social sciences.

This book looks at the impacts on our health and healthcare services of the social worlds in which we live. The editors do not pretend that taking the social sciences into account will necessarily fill the gaps or answer the questions relating to values and funding public services. Also, we have had to limit the evidence that we can include from the social sciences in this single volume; in particular, we have focused on the social identity approach. Nonetheless, we hope that the contents of this book illustrate the importance of our including research from the social sciences in the evidence that we consider when we plan and deliver health and social care services and think about their patients and clients as human beings. They have many needs, preferences and expectations that interconnect with the physical and brain sciences, the nature of their problems, and their outcomes.

We generate thinking about novel approaches to problem-solving. While readers will find that this book particularly features wellbeing, mental health, mental ill health and mental healthcare in its pages, we also include in this endeavour people's physical health. We see all aspects of health and healthcare as intimately related rather than as representing separate matters. In other words, we stand away from the body–mind dualism on which so many practitioners were reared because we see that approach as having done more harm than good. As Smith and Bhui et al. remind us in Chapters 2 and 6, respectively, there is a tendency to associate the processes of social causation and social construction with mental health, but we see this as representing history rather than essential features. Indeed, these philosophical understandings can and, I think, should be applicable to health generally, and to all of healthcare.

Thus, readers will find in this book a focus on how people experience their health and needs. We see this as a defining part of the vital interface between assisting people to sustain their health and how they may best be advised and assisted when they are ill. We hope that readers will be stimulated to think broadly about how best to interact with people, how to work with them in coproductive relationships in which people and practitioners create a shared social identity, and, thus, how to better design services by taking a wider array of science and patients' and researchers' perspectives into account. Indeed, coproduction is a matter that recurs through this book. I hope that readers also find that the reflection that this book provokes may save scarce resources.

Tensions in Health and Healthcare Services

Equity and Equality in Health and Healthcare

The Chief Medical Officer (CMO) for England (Mehta, 2014) presents six strong arguments for choosing to focus her report for 2013 on population mental health. They include: the huge burden and costs of mental illness; the reduced real-term investment in mental health services; and the significant treatment gaps and unacceptably large premature mortality gap when comparing people who have mental ill health with those who do not. She defines public mental health as consisting of mental health promotion, mental illness prevention, and treatment and rehabilitation. The CMO points out that there is a wealth of robust evidence for public health approaches to mental illness prevention and mental health promotion. She identifies that mental illness is defined by the attributes or diagnosis of people whose problems meet ICD-10 (*International Statistical Classification of Diseases and Related Health Problems*, 10th Revision) or DSM-5 (*Diagnostic and Statistical Manual of Mental Disorders*, Fifth Edition, published by the American Psychiatric Association) criteria for mental disorders. This includes common mental disorders, which affect nearly one in four of the population, and severe mental illness, such as psychosis, which is less common, affecting 0.5–1 per cent of the population.

These findings alone would be sufficient motivation for writing this book, but there are wider considerations. We do not see healthcare and mental healthcare as separate: as we have said, Chapter 8 draws attention to endeavours to promote parity of esteem for mental health since the topic was passed into law in the UK, at a time when there is huge pressure on resources. But, importantly, most of the ideas that readers find in this volume are applicable to healthcare generally. Thus, we do not see public mental health as separated from public health.

The concept of the social determinants of health and mental health, and awareness of their huge impacts, have been established beyond doubt by, for example, the World Health Organization, based on the work of many researchers worldwide. There are powerful ways in which differences in our social relationships and resources influence our health.

First, they may influence our wellbeing and the nature and prevalence of the disorders that we may develop. A past US Surgeon General, Vice Admiral Vivek Murthy (Stone, 2017), has said,

> When I began my tenure as surgeon general, I did not intend to focus on emotional well-being. But it became a priority after I travelled the country listening to people in small towns and big cities. I think of emotional well-being as a resource within each of us that allows us to do more and to perform better [and] to be resilient in the face of adversity … There are tools … They include sleep, physical activity, contemplative practices like gratitude and meditation, and social connection as well.

This book unpacks these themes and focuses on social connection.

Second, we recognise that distribution of services in response to people's healthcare needs is not driven in a linear manner by those needs but is impacted by people's social circumstances. Recognition of the significance of these circumstances to generating and sustaining people's problems and their access to effective services goes back well beyond the origins of the inverse care law that was first described by Julian Tudor Hart in 1971. In part, they drove creation of the National Health Services (NHS) in the UK. Tudor Hart (1971) said then that 'the availability of good medical care tends to vary inversely with the need for it in the population served'. In other words, despite continuing advances, both **inequity** (i.e. failure of health systems to adequately meet the needs of people in the populations they serve) and **inequality** (i.e. failure of health systems to treat people with similar needs in similar ways within and across communities) continue to strongly influence our societies. I draw attention to longitudinal population research on North–South disparities in English mortality from 1965 to 2015 (Buchan et al., 2017). The researchers found that:

> England's northern excess mortality has been consistent among those aged <25 and 45+ for the past five decades but risen alarmingly among those aged 25–44 since the mid-90s, long before the Great Recession.
>
> England has profound and persistent regional divides in economy, society and health [and] The extended period of austerity following the 2008–2009 recession has raised concerns about detrimental impacts on population health, particularly the health of disadvantaged socio-economic groups and more economically precarious regions. [They note

> that, however]... the divergent trends in mortality we noted in the 1990s and early 2000s suggest that inequalities can increase rapidly during periods of sustained economic growth.

While the editors do not pretend that this book provides substantial ways forward in dealing with the enormity of these challenges, we show myriad examples of ways in which social science may be harnessed to improve our understanding of mechanisms that influence problems with equity and equality. We recognise, for example, research showing that low neighbourhood socioeconomic status (SES) predicts worse mental health outcomes and '... perceived neighbourhood quality was the means through which neighbourhood SES affected mental health' (Fong et al., 2018). Also, we recognise vital matters relating to the social determinants of health and mental health that have attracted less attention than has the epidemiology of conditions or the neurosciences. They include drawing together:

- What is known about the power of social determinants of health;
- Evidence about the mechanisms by which the social determinants operate, for good or ill, within the dynamic array of factors that affect people's states of health and their recovery from ill health; and
- Identifying constructive but practical mechanisms for harnessing the positive power of the social influences on good health and mental health.

The achievements of the physical sciences and neuroscience are many, and they are highly likely to have an enormous impact in the future. However, it is arguable that these achievements could be unnecessarily limited in their impacts if the opportunities provided by what we know of the social influences on health and mental health are not grasped at much the same time. Indeed, the science of epigenetics points to powerful ways in which genetics, cultures and social influences are drawn together within and across generations.

Capability, Need, Expectations and Finance

There are many other tensions in health promotion and protection and healthcare. Nearly 15 years ago, Kerfoot, Warner and Williams illustrated one tension, that between the approaches based on public health and personal healthcare and, therefore, between directing existing and new resources towards health promotion or to relief of existing disease and disorder (Warner & Williams, 2005; Williams & Kerfoot, 2005). This debate continues worldwide.

Arguably, it has arisen once more in how the UK has been approaching responses to the healthcare needs of people who were affected by the series of disasters and terrorist events in the UK, from late 2016 to the middle of 2018. It seems to me that both policymakers and practitioners have found it more pressing to focus on how best to meet the needs of people who may go on to develop mental disorders. Less finance and energy has been expended on preventing people who are well from developing disorders or promoting their health. In part, but only in part, this approach is evidence-based and represents the extent of the research that has been conducted to date. But, in this regard, I think that there would be great advantage to policymakers, managers and practitioners in allocating scarce resources to treatments or to prevention and health promotion if there was greater awareness of the topics covered in this book.

Progressive Improvement in Capability, Changes in Need and Limitations of Resource

Health policy and practice throughout the world must contend with the very rapid increases in capability and the ever-widening array of people who are able to influence the health and/

or otherwise of populations and persons. These developments compete for finance, training and staff, and they highlight the importance of better coordination between people, teams and agencies.

Ingenuity and research have driven spectacularly rapid improvements in the potential to deliver healthcare interventions. This has rapidly and substantially increased the financial costs of healthcare. In the UK, it has led to continuing debate about the role of the NHS and whether or not the principle of universality of availability of services in response to need can continue to underpin the roles and responsibilities of the state. Targets of healthcare cannot be static. While the risks of certain diseases have reduced substantially since the NHS was created, and there are now new possibilities for effective intervention with previously intractable conditions and undesirable circumstances, it is also the case that entirely new disorders, unknown in 1948, when the UK's NHS was created, have arisen while 'other' disorders have been defined and recognised.

Furthermore, democratisation of knowledge and rapid improvements in communications have played their part in accelerating public expectations of healthcare services. But, the affluence of societies and their willingness to give priority to health and healthcare have not expanded in parallel with the rise of potential capability. Thus, although increasing volumes of resource have been put into healthcare, the gap between the ability and/or willingness of the state to fund healthcare services and what could be done, if sufficient resources were available, continues to increase.

Rationality versus Humanity

In 2016, Abbasi, executive editor of the *British Medical Journal* (*BMJ*), looked at how the task of improving services in the current financial circumstances might be approached when he asked, 'Is it possible to improve health, improve care, and save money?' His opinion is, 'While we demand more evidence for changes to health services', which an endeavour to reduce the costs might require, there is a risk that 'our obsession with evidence may lessen our humanity' in clinical consultations.

In parallel, Abbasi (2016) observes a rift between evidence-based medicine, which guidelines and protocols ask us to deliver, and the humanity that patients seek in clinical encounters. Heath (2016) demands a new approach and calls on clinicians to bridge the rift between evidence and humanity, to deliver more coherence. Her view is '. . . evidence based medicine tempts us to try to describe people in terms of data from biomedical science: these are not, and will never be, enough. Such evidence is essential but always insufficient for the care of patients'. She continues, 'Each patient has unique values, aspirations, and context', and urges clinicians to ' . . . see and hear each patient in the fullness of his or her humanity in order to minimise fear, to locate hope (however limited), to explain symptoms and diagnoses in language that makes sense to the particular patient, to witness courage and endurance, and to accompany suffering'. These opinions emphasise the position of values in research, in developing and conducting practice and in designing and delivering services.

Nolte (2017) says,

> . . . political and policy declarations now widely acknowledge that the individuals should be at the heart of the health system. A person centred approach has been advocated on political, ethical, and instrumental grounds and is believed to benefit service users, health professionals, and the health system more broadly. The underlying premise is that people

> requiring healthcare should be treated with respect and dignity, and that care should take into account their needs, wants, and preferences.

However, person-centred healthcare does not and should not imply taking an approach based on individualism. Rather it calls for each person to be seen and their needs to be construed in the context of the nexus of their relationships (see Chapter 14), including those with healthcare professionals, and the environments in which they live. Yet Nolte finds that,

> Studies exploring understanding of self-management . . . have shown that many outcomes important to people receiving care are rarely mentioned by health professionals. These include maintaining independence and a desire that the health problem should not define people's lives ('being me').
>
> Even where overlaps occur, outcomes are interpreted differently. For example, knowledge is regarded as important, but health professionals tend to view this as knowledge about the disease process ('knowing that'), whereas people receiving care emphasise knowledge that is personally relevant and tailored to their specific situation ('knowing how'). People place particular value on the quality of their relationship with their healthcare professional, but this understanding is not commonly expressed by providers.

Nolte's recommendation is that, 'This apparent disconnect between people's and health professionals' views and interpretations about what constitutes person centredness highlights a need to adapt the training of health and care professionals to enable them to engage in a true partnership with people receiving care'. She welcomes the person-centred care framework, published by Health Education England, Skills for Health, and Skills for Care (2017). It '. . . places communication and relationship building skills at the centre of all interactions, setting out the necessary underlying values and behaviours, describing desirable (what people receiving care and their carers want to see) and undesirable practices along with the expected learning outcomes from education and training for staff'. Importantly, Nolte says, '. . . the framework recognises that simply developing new skills and knowledge will not be enough to achieve fully person centred health systems. Professionals also need a supportive culture within organisations that encourages and fosters long term behaviour change'.

Working in Healthcare Systems

The contents of this book reflect these values and speak to matters of the kind that I raise here. We consider, for example, the culture aspects for professionals in Chapters 26, 27 and 28. The contents also recognise the stress imposed on people who work in health systems that emerge from:

- Increasing potential capability of the system;
- Finite limitations of resource to fund what could be done; and
- Lack of social care to accompany healthcare and get the best for society from healthcare advances.

Social Connectedness, Relationships, Health and Healthcare

Haslam et al. (2018) have published a paper reporting meta-analytic research indicating that social support and social integration are highly protective against mortality, and that their importance is comparable to, or exceeds, that of many established behavioural risks, such as smoking, high alcohol consumption, lack of exercise and obesity. Their findings suggest that people, generally, underestimate the importance of social factors for health.

Social connectedness and social support lie at the core of this book. They do have substantial impacts on our health, recovery from ill health and coping effectively with adversity, emergencies and other untoward events. Thus, for example, Saeri et al. (2018) report that social connectedness improves public mental health. Miller et al. (2017) report the reciprocal effects between multiple group identifications and mental health in adolescents. However, Saeri et al. also found that social connectedness was a stronger and more consistent predictor of mental health, year-on-year, than mental health was of social connectedness.

Recently, Professor Cath Haslam, a clinical psychologist who was involved in the Royal College of Psychiatrists' Seminars, and one of this book's editors, has developed the 'Five Ss' to encapsulate a programme for intervention. She has allowed us to use her approach to structure this book. Hence, the titles of this book and the five parts in it.

This first section, in which this chapter provides an introduction to the book, is titled Schooling. It introduces social scientific concepts that are central to, or building blocks of, the approach that this book takes. Steve Smith, a social philosopher, examines six dimensions of the human condition that recur through this book. The chapters that follow highlight important approaches to broadening our understanding of people's social connectedness and its importance to their health and meeting their needs.

Section 2, titled Scoping, covers the field in more detail. Its authors summarise an approach to health and healthcare that builds from recognising the social determinants of health through to meeting our core human social needs for belonging that impact on our health, resilience and endeavours to work together.

Section 3, called Sourcing, provides an overview of humans' experiences from a wide variety of perspectives, including crowd science. It examines topics and events that are rare for most people though we note that they are the kinds of matters on which national news bulletins focus daily. Our aspiration is to draw, or source, from these extreme circumstances lessons about how humans might approach more common events. Thus, we examine statistically uncommon, but all too frequent, events to seek evidence for social influences on societies. We consider disasters to show that people are unlikely to panic in the face of disaster and the importance of emergent relationships in these circumstances. We examine the behaviour of crowds to challenge the myth that groups are potentially dangerous.

Importantly, this book looks at the mental health of refugees. We know that psychosocial distress and loss are very common experiences and that a substantial percentage of refugees develop mild to moderate mental disorders (Weissbecker et al., 2019). Psychosocial support is vitally important to their care in humanitarian crisis settings. Also, I note that Morina et al. (2018) identify perceived self-efficacy (SE), which we might term 'agency' in this book, as an important factor that underlies wellbeing. They say that their research findings provide initial evidence that:

- Promoting SE in tortured refugees can assist with managing distress from trauma reminders and promoting greater distress tolerance; and
- Enhancing perceived SE in tortured refugees may increase their capacity to tolerate distress during therapy and may be a useful means to improve treatment response.

These findings recur in Chapter 18 in which Katona and Brady offer a commentary on the breadth of the programme of interventions that are required by people who have been through highly traumatic experiences, including torture.

We also examine radicalisation and how it might be that people are drawn to extreme movements. Thus, social connectedness and identity do not always have a positive valency and it is important to study the circumstances in which connectedness is a force for good rather than problems. This is a matter on which Reicher touches in Chapter 23. Chapter 21, in the final part of Section 3, examines the nature of the leadership that is required to help populations of people escape from intractable conflict.

In Section 4, we draw into a process, which we call social scaffolding, ideas from the preceding three parts with a view to synthesising a way forward and identifying approaches to solving persisting problems and, thereby, effect change. The messages have much wider resonance to promoting health and delivering effective health and social care more generally. Finally, in Section 5, we consider the challenges to the process of whole system change that is required, and how these approaches might be sustained.

Each section has been written on the back of the ones that precede it with a view to achieving a resonant, iterative approach. Thus, we have included a chapter at the end of each section in which we have invited several authors to draw together their personal accounts of the themes and ideas that stand out for them in the authors' contributions. In Section 4, that chapter describes a mythical town, which we are calling Smithtown, and links its many problems with the approaches we describe in Section 4. Thus, we see social scaffolding as applying to families, small groups of people, communities, towns and cities.

Concluding Comments

This book is intended to develop and present an approach to advancing our understanding in these arenas that is based on selected contributions from social science. Much of the content focuses on people coming together in groups and the potential power of what happens in the space between people. Chapters in it examine these matters in a novel way.

Harford (2016) draws attention to 'the unexpected connection between creativity and mess'. He argues that 'we often succumb to the temptation of a tidy-minded approach when we would be better served by embracing a degree of mess' (p. 4). He provides many examples to show that, perhaps unexpectedly, '... creativity, excitement, and humanity lie in the messy parts of life' (p. 264) and others that help us to '... understand why unexpected changes of plans, unfamiliar people, and unforeseen events can help generate new ideas and opportunities even as they [make us] anxious and angry ...' (cover).

Put in a different language, I think that Harford is also talking about certain conditions that encourage our social connectedness and agency. Thus, he argues that good jobs, good buildings and good relationships are open and adaptable (p. 265).

These are powerful themes that run through this book on social scaffolding. All the contributions in it are built on the best of emerging science, hard-won experience and careful review. This book encourages openness to exploring new ideas, viewing established ones from new perspectives and expanding our adaptability in seeking solutions to some age-old, as well as new, and complicated, problems in promoting health and improving healthcare.

References

Abbasi, K. (2016). We need more humanity as well as better evidence. British Medical Journal, 355: i5907; doi: 10.1136/bmj.i5907.

Buchan, I. E., Kontopantelis, E., Sperrin, M., Chandola, T. & Doran, T. (2017). North–South disparities in English mortality 1965–2015: longitudinal population study. Journal of Epidemiology and Community Health; doi: 10.1136/jech-2017-209195. Published online 7 August 2017.

Fong, P., Cruwys, T., Haslam, C. et al. (2018). Neighbourhood identification and mental health: how social identification moderates the relationship between socioeconomic disadvantage and health. Journal of Environmental Psychology; doi: org/10.1016/j.jenvp.2018.12.006.

Harford, T. (2016). Messy: The Power of Disorder to Transform Our Lives. New York, NY: Riverhead Books.

Haslam, S. A., McMahon, C., Cruwys, T. et al. (2018). Social cure, what social cure? The propensity to underestimate the importance of social factors for health. Social Science and Medicine, **198**, 14–21; https://doi.org/10.1016/j.socscimed.2017.12.020.

Health Education England, Skills for Health, and Skill for Care Person-Centred Approaches (2017). Empowering People in their Lives and Communities to Enable an Upgrade in Prevention, Wellbeing, Health, Care and Support. London: Health Education England, Skills for Health, and Skill for Care.

Heath, I. (2016). How medicine has exploited rationality at the expense of humanity. British Medical Journal, **355**: i5705; doi: 10.1136/bmj.i5705.

Mehta, N. (2014). Annual Report of the Chief Medical Officer 2013, Public Mental Health Priorities: Investing in the Evidence. London: Department of Health for England.

Miller, K., Wakefield, J. R. H. & Sani, F. (2017). On the reciprocal effects between multiple group identifications and mental health: A longitudinal study of Scottish adolescents. British Journal of Clinical Psychologists, **56**: 357–371; doi: 10.1111/bjc.12143.

Morina, N., Bryant, R. A., Doolan, E. L. et al. (2018). The impact of enhancing perceived self-efficacy in torture survivors. Depression and Anxiety, **35**: 58–64.

Nolte, E. (2017). Editorial: Implementing person centred approaches. British Medical Journal, **358**: j4126; doi: 10.1136/bmj.j4126.

Saeri, A. K., Cruwys, T., Barlow, F. K., Stronge, S. & Sibley, C. G. (2018). Social connectedness improves public mental health: Investigating bidirectional relationships in the New Zealand attitudes and values survey. Australian & New Zealand Journal of Psychiatry, **52**: 365–374; doi: 10.1177/0004867417723990.

Stone, D. (2017). 3 Questions – Vivek Murthy – former Surgeon General: I'm worried about America's stress. National Geographic, September 2017: 8.

Tudor Hart, J. (1971). The inverse care law. The Lancet, **297**: 405–412.

Warner, M. & Williams, R. (2005). The nature of strategy and its application in statutory and non-statutory services. In Williams, R. & Kerfoot, M., editors, Child and Adolescent Mental Health Services: Strategy, Planning, Delivery and Evaluation. Oxford: Oxford University Press, pp. 39–62.

Weissbecker, I., Hanna, F., El Shazly, M., Gao, J. & Ventevogel, P. (2019). Integrative mental health and psychosocial support interventions for refugees in humanitarian crisis settings. In Wenzel, T. & Droždek, B., editors, An Uncertain Safety: Integrative Health Care for the 21st Century Refugees. Heidelberg: Springer, pp. 117–153.

Williams R. & Kerfoot, M. (2005). Setting the scene: Perspectives on the history of and policy for child and adolescent mental health services in the UK. In Williams, R. & Kerfoot, M., editors, Child and Adolescent Mental Health Services: Strategy, Planning, Delivery and Evaluation. Oxford: Oxford University Press, pp. 3–38.

Chapter 2

Six Features of the Human Condition: The Social Causation and Social Construction of Mental Health

Steven R. Smith

Introduction

In this chapter, I consider the social causation and social construction of mental health. To do this, I draw on sociology and social philosophy, and key findings from this book, to put forward an argument in three parts. I begin by summarising them and then explore each part in greater depth. I also provide footnotes that expand on the core content.

Social Causation and Social Construction

First, when considering the social determinants of mental health, we should not only uncover the processes of **social causation**, by focussing on the social epidemiology of mental illness and mental health, but also those processes of **social construction** that affect how notions of illness, health and care are defined within professional contexts and wider society. Identifying these social processes as distinct helps us to clarify two principal social dimensions of mental health. There are those social determinants that give rise to the phenomena of mental illness and mental health and there are the ways in which these phenomena are variously conceptualised. The second dimension affects how people are viewed in society and this includes whether they are defined as mentally ill by caring professionals, family members and broader communities. This influences how they are treated by society and within it, by health and social care systems.

Six Features of the Human Condition

Second, whatever social conceptions of wellbeing and mental health are used and developed, all must accommodate six features of the human condition that I describe in this chapter. Moreover, the precise relationship between these features varies. It depends on the philosophical meanings of wellbeing and their relationship to our understanding of 'positive' and 'negative' mental health outcomes, and also on how these meanings are, in turn, socially constructed. Therefore, social construction affects the ways in which health and illness are defined, explained and addressed across different social contexts.

Agency, Cognition and Evaluation

Third, the roles that personal agency, cognition and evaluation play in people's lives should be accommodated when explanations of mental health, which are derived from both medical and social causation and/or construction, are used as social conceptions. That is, defending a broadly non-determinist account of wellbeing and mental health, which I argue here, should be central to developing mental healthcare. This accommodation also allows scope for personal choice and agency. This opens up new possibilities for both viewing and treating those persons who are defined as mentally ill. In short, patients, clients or service-users are not seen as passive recipients of circumstances beyond their control. They are seen as active participants or coproducers in how their care is defined, managed and implemented, and how their mental illness and mental health is subjectively defined and given meaning in their lives.

The Social Causation and Social Construction of Mental Health

There is a distinction made in sociology between social causation and social construction (Burr, 2003; Clarke and Cochrane, 1998; Gergen & Gergen, 2003). Simply described, the former concept significantly underpinned the origins of sociology in the late nineteenth and early twentieth centuries, when academic enquiry began to systematically identify social determinants of human characteristics and behaviour. For example, although its methodology has since been criticised, Emile Durkheim's seminal study on suicide identified how social as well as individual factors affect suicide rates (Durkheim, 2006; first published in 1897). By comparing social statistics between countries, Durkheim found that people of Catholic faith, especially in southern Europe, women, and married persons with children are least likely to commit suicide. Therefore, he concluded that what seems to be a highly individual decision to take one's life, reflecting individual personality, personal circumstances and so on, is a decision with causal factors relating to membership of social groups. Reflecting the themes explored throughout this book, it can be claimed, then, that there are many social causes of mental illness and mental health rates, which reflect the social groups a person belongs to, and affect the individual decisions she makes and the kinds of experiences she has concerning her mental illness and mental health.

However, the notion of social construction is differently orientated and comes from later sociological and social philosophical analysis. This analysis was developed particularly, but not exclusively, in the second half of the twentieth century and has had a profound influence on the study of social policy, sociology and branches of psychology and social psychology (Burr, 2003; Clarke & Cochrane, 1998; Gergen & Gergen, 2003; Horwitz, 2012). It was influenced by, for example, the philosophy of Ludwig Wittgenstein (1998, 2000) and of Martin Heidegger (1962), Peter Berger and Thomas Luckmann[1] (Berger & Luckmann, 1967) and Michel Foucault (1954, 1988). The work included the study of how our use of language affects how we view certain forms of behaviour or personal characteristics, define them and treat them within these contexts (Clarke & Cochrane, 1998; Walker, 2006; Busfield, 2008). According to this analysis, the social construction process is socially caused. However, social causation, as interpreted traditionally in sociology, does not take account of how social factors also contribute to the various meanings attributed to individual people's and/or group's behaviour or characteristics.

Moreover, for social constructionists, these socially attributed meanings are mediated through exercising institutional power, which changes over time and between cultures, resulting in the same behaviour and characteristics being viewed differently depending on the social context. Foucault, for example, explored how the very term 'mental illness' was

[1] Berger and Luckmann were the first to use the term social construction. However, their central treatise concerning the sociology of knowledge and how public or shared meaning is socially created is also traceable to the other primary sources referenced here, and more besides.

Table 2.1 Six features of the human condition, summarised

1. Embodiment	We have the physical and/or biological characteristics that enable us to relate and connect to the world
2. Finiteness	We are linked by beginnings and ends
3. Sociability	We are members of social groups that produce rules of behaviour
4. Cognition	We have our mind-oriented processes that: exercise logic; gather information and evidence; and engage imagination
5. Evaluation	We engage in complex processes of evaluation
6. Free will or agency	We have capacity as individual people and groups to plan and set goals

created by an European Enlightenment discourse, which defined this condition as symptomatic of cognitive dysfunctions that are to be remedied, if possible, through medical institutional practices (Foucault, 1954, 1988). Whereas, within mediaeval Europe, the behaviour and characteristics associated with what we now call mental illness were viewed as symptomatic of satanic possession to be remedied, if possible, through religious institutional practices (and see Busfield, 2008; Horwitz, 2012; Walker, 2006).

To summarise so far, the epidemiology of mental illness and mental health does not only have social causes. The concepts of wellbeing, mental health and mental illness are socially constructed in ways that shape how wider society views and responds to behaviours and characteristics, associated with what is socially defined as 'mental illness' and 'mental health'. It is this social construction process which determines how 'mental health' and 'mental illness' are variously viewed, which in turn influences both the perspectives and practices of health professionals. The social constructionist explains this variance as a product of how language is used socially and created through public discourses. In turn, these reflect powerful institutional practices that shape how the social world we live in is defined or 'given meaning'.[2]

Six Features of the Human Condition and Competing Conceptions of Wellbeing

This section identifies six features of the human condition and it explores how they relate to competing conceptions of wellbeing and mental health. The main contention is that the relationship between these features varies depending on which philosophical position is taken regarding the meanings of wellbeing and mental health, and how these meanings are socially constructed. In turn, these meanings affect how both the medical and the social causation factors for mental health and illness are identified and defined. Table 2.1 summarises the six features of the human condition.

[2] The relationship between exercising power and public discourse is a moot point and is not explored in detail here (for example, see Lukes, 2005; Mackenzie, 2004; Rabinow 1984). Suffice it to say, that, in whatever way this relationship is understood, the claim here is that exercising power and the social production of discourse and shared meaning has a profound effect on those people who are defined as mentally ill and the professionals engaged in working with this group.

Embodiment

The first feature is our embodiment. Simply put, we have physical and/or biological characteristics that enable us to relate and connect with the world through, in part, bodily sensations and experiences. These connections include: our senses of touch, sight, hearing and taste; our experiences of pain and pleasure; our physical needs for food, water, shelter, rest and warmth; our wants, desires and aversions; our emotions of joy, happiness, anger, sadness and fear; and our emotional feelings towards others, such as pity, compassion, disgust, love and hate[3] (Haybron, 2011; Smith, 2014; Tiberius, 2008).

My contention is that conceptions of wellbeing and mental health must acknowledge embodiment and reflect these biological and physical characteristics. Arguably, some conceptions of wellbeing and mental health may over-stress embodiment and so fetishise our physicality and biological experiences. Chapters 3 and 4, for example, offer critiques of medicalised understandings of health, which, it is claimed, often fail to sufficiently acknowledge the part that social factors play in influencing our health, thereby exaggerating the role that biology plays in our lives. Attention is, instead, directed to how mental illness and mental health, and other health problems, are often caused by or accompanied by social factors that occur outside an individual person's physical or biological experiences. However, it would be a mistake if our understandings of wellbeing and mental health did not accommodate at all these facts about the biologically embodied or medicalised features of the human condition. My claim is that there exist fixed 'universal facts' about our embodiment, which in some sense, at least, transcend[4] the social worlds we inhabit, although the precise way in which we both view and experience this embodiment is also socially mediated via social construction and social causation processes, as I explore them in this chapter.

Finiteness

The second feature is our finiteness. Put abstractly, we are limited by beginnings and ends. Less abstractly, we are bound by: our biology or embodiment; our limited capabilities, constrained by physical and social environments; our inability to have full control over our circumstances; and by incomplete and/or over-complex information when we make reflective decisions. These constraints make us vulnerable to harm, disappointment, failure, conflicting choices and error, when calculating what is best to pursue for our wellbeing

[3] This is not implying that our emotions are entirely caused by these biological and/or physical characteristics, merely that some or part of our emotional responses can be caused by these characteristics, reflecting our embodiment. Precisely how our physical bodies and experiences are interpreted and viewed by us as members of social groups is highly debated, especially within the social constructionist literature (see Rabinow, 1984; Lechte, 1994; Joseph, 2003; Lloyd, 2004; MacKenzie, 2004; and footnote 4 below).

[4] This raises questions about the meaning of transcendence here. So, underpinning the arguments in this chapter is the assumption that none of the six features of the human condition outlined here can occur *independently* of social context. Nevertheless, insofar as these features of the human condition are universal, and so are shared across time and between cultures, they transcend social contexts. Once this, admittedly controversial, move is made, it is possible to accommodate the social constructionist account of mental health, but without reducing explanations about what human beings experience *solely* to use of language (and see footnote 3 above). This move can also be found in my arguments concerning disability issues more widely, exploring how the medical and social models of disability can coherently relate and be interpreted (see Smith, 2009, pp. 15–29, 2011, pp. 107–132).

and mental health (Brink, 2003; Haybron, 2011, pp. 177–198; Sobel, 1994; Tiberius, 2008, pp. 23–64).

However, being limited in these respects also gives shape and form to our experiences. Our finiteness means that we cannot avoid being committed to certain objects of attachment, which we care for, but not to others, and only at any one time. Paradoxically, perhaps, our finiteness allows us to choose these attachments meaningfully, and with purpose (Heidegger, 1962; Tiberius, 2008, pp. 65–88). In so doing, this commitment enables us to enjoy our lives by becoming immersed in the moment (Sumner, 1999, pp. 26–44; Tiberius, 2008, pp. 74–75), and to become attuned to our lives (Haybron, 2011, pp. 116–120). Nevertheless, it is important to acknowledge that this individual immersion and attuning is worked out within wider social contexts.

So, personal ambitions, as one type of attachment, are, for example, often shaped by dominant social values and ideologies, which, according to the arguments presented here, are socially constructed or 'given meaning' through socially embedded institutional practices (Clarke & Cochrane, 1998; Lukes, 2005; Raz, 1988). Likewise, our capacities to implement our personal ambitions are influenced by social causation factors, which either diminish or expand opportunities for their fulfilment, depending upon social contexts (and see Clayton & Williams, 2004; Sen, 1985). Nevertheless, even if personal commitments are mediated through these wider social processes, I have argued elsewhere that acknowledging our finiteness regarding what we pursue or matters to which we are committed allows us to better accept and value ourselves as we are and in terms of what we can do, rather than remain frustrated with what we cannot be or do (Smith, 2011, pp. 48–58, 2012; and see also Tiberius, 2008, pp. 104–105).

Sociability

The third feature is our sociability. We, for example, learn language and communicate with others, and we are members of social groups. These groups produce social rules of behaviour that also delineate private and public arenas of wellbeing and mental health. Chapters 3 and 4 explore how maintaining social identities and social capital are important social factors that enhance wellbeing and mental health. In addition, different ways of 'being' and 'doing' are created and reproduced through acts of social cooperation (Rawls, 1973, pp. 548–554; Sen, 1985), and often follow dominant social norms which, again, are defined and embedded within various institutional practices (Clarke & Cochrane, 1998).

Thus, what is defined or socially constructed as meaningful social relationships with others – with friends, lovers, family members, work colleagues, employers, service-users, carers and so on – prompts our pursuit of collective projects and endeavours (Kittay, 1999; Mackenzie & Stoljar, 2000). Chapters 3, 4, 22 and 23 also explore evidence that forming certain kinds of social identities and social relationships enhances our mental health and wellbeing. Moreover, being members of these social groupings leads to the possibility of reciprocal exchanges taking place between individual people and within groups, based on shared understandings of what is defined as socially valuable.[5] Another way of putting this is that we acquire 'value meanings' through these social contexts and the processes of social

[5] The possibility for reciprocity is also central to the practice of coproduction in which patients, clients or service-users are defined as active participants or coproducers in: (i) how their care is conceptualised, managed and implemented; and (ii) how their mental health/illness is given meaning in relation to their lives.

construction (Smith, 2001a, 2001b, 2002). The contents of Chapter 24 are also relevant to applying these value meanings.

Cognition

The fourth feature is the human capacity for cognition. This capability is mind-orientated, and involves exercising logic, gathering information and evidence, and engaging in creative and self-reflexive imagination. Through imagination and self-reflection we can, for example, picture new possibilities for our futures, and remember our pasts (Braddon-Mitchell & West, 2001; Kopf, 2002). We can also understand our experiences, rationally calculate, and be reasonable towards others (Rawls, 1973, pp. 108–117; Scanlon, 1998, pp. 1–77).

Cultivating these abilities is often regarded as crucial to how wellbeing and mental health are best promoted, most notably over lifetimes. For example, cognition facilitates our having a wider perspective on our lives, in which we can critically reflect on our own subjective viewpoint from a more objective perspective (Nagel, 1991, pp. 10–20; Tiberius, 2008, pp. 78–83). That is, we can assess and view the subjective position we interpret and experience from a certain distance, and recognise the existence and perspectives of others as important, including our future selves, while acknowledging the legitimate claims often made against us as a result (Griffin, 1988, pp. 127–312; Tiberius, 2008, pp. 89–108, pp. 161–181).

Moreover, cognition permeates the attitudes or dispositions we have to our present, past and future experiences – of, say, optimism or pessimism, and our critical reflection on our lives as a whole (Tiberius, 2008, pp. 137–160). 'Life-course accounts'[6] of wellbeing and mental health include this capacity for cognition. Consequently, we are cognitively self-aware, and that allows us to make judgements about our wellbeing as we compare our lives with the lives of others. However, an important point is that these judgements are shaped, in part, by social construction processes that attribute social meanings to these judgements, and with these meanings being embedded within institutional practices. In addition, processes of social causation can either facilitate or debilitate our capacity for effective cognition, which then affects our ability to both assess and implement personal life-plans and ambitions.

Evaluation

The fifth feature is that we engage in complex processes of evaluation.[7] It matters to our wellbeing and mental health, for example, not only that we successfully accomplish goals and ambitions, but also that these goals and ambitions are defined as worthwhile (and see

[6] For a discussion concerning our future selves and promoting wellbeing over a whole life, see my arguments in Smith (2018). I identify how *inter*personal comparisons of wellbeing are notoriously problematic as the levels and quality of wellbeing are hard to meaningfully measure between persons. However, I also explore how these problems are apparent with *intra*personal comparisons of wellbeing if plural identities occur over time for one person, which I claim they often do. I argue that these latter problems have important implications for social policy debates about enhancing wellbeing across time and between generations.

[7] Strictly speaking, evaluation is a form of cognition, insofar as evaluation is a mental process, culminating in a value judgement, in the ways described previously. I am grateful to one of the editors of this book for pointing this out. However, the contention here is that evaluation has such a significant effect on wellbeing – and in how people evaluate their own lives – that it should be treated separately to this person's more general capacity for cognition.

Raz, 1988, pp. 288–320). Therefore, we do not just count our successes, we also evaluate them. Thus, what is valued is not created ex-nihilo, but the value attached to goals is formed within social arenas that determine how these evaluations occur, and the kinds of judgements that are made as a result.

Value can be understood as what is worthwhile to pursue, including pastimes, career options, lifestyle choices and so on. These values are pursued individually and/or in social groups, as is explored in Chapters 3 and 4. Moreover, value can also refer to moral or ethical principles, what is considered right or wrong, just or unjust (Griffin, 1988, pp. 127–312; Tiberius, 2008, pp. 161–181). Chapters 12 and 24 return to these matters of value and ethics and their importance in making 'good' decisions, which are regarded as fair. Consequently, if we successfully pursue what we socially define as valuable, and that enhances our wellbeing and mental health, as much of the empirical evidence confirms (Diener & Diener, 2008; Ryff, 1989; Ryff & Keyes, 1995; Seligman, 2002), then identifying those social causation factors that assist in this process is also an essential part of developing effective mental healthcare. This assertion is supported by the work on horizontal epidemiology that is reported in Chapter 7.

In addition, what we value is also derived from exercising self-knowledge and this enables us to be true to ourselves, or authentic, as it is sometimes called (Sumner, 1999, pp. 156–170; Tiberius, 2008, pp. 109–111). Therefore, when we commit to valuable goals, however they are socially constructed or defined, they should reflect our genuine desires, personal characteristics, ideals and so on. Otherwise, these goals become disconnected from our lives (Parfit, 1987; Sumner, 1999, pp. 26–44).

Regarding wellbeing and mental health, if we evaluate our lives within the social world we inhabit as a reflection of what is genuine or authentic about us, then we can say that we 'own' or 'identify' with these shared evaluations, which gives coherence to the way we judge our lives as being successful or not. Subsequently, many people argue that facilitating wellbeing and mental health involves comprehending what is 'true' about the social world we inhabit. We can then make accurate judgements about what individual people and groups seek to accomplish and whether or not that is genuinely valuable. Often, the resulting claim made is that deception, therefore, undermines personal wellbeing and mental health, even if believing the deceit makes us happier (Griffin, 1988; Rawls, 1973, pp. 548–544; Raz, 1988, pp. 288–320; Sumner, 1999; Tiberius, 2008).

The further point here is that our ability to accomplish what we genuinely value is also affected by social causation factors that can either undermine or enhance our capacities for accomplishment. In addition, social construction processes, which are apparent as notions of what is valuable, vary considerably across time and between cultures. Therefore, focussing on the potential deceit concerning the factual mismatch between what we believe and what we have actually accomplished can risk disguising a further social fact, namely, that the values we authentically hold dear are not entirely of our own making, but arise from particular social contexts, and so are shared.

Agency

Finally, the sixth feature is our human capacity for free will or agency. As individual people and/or as members of social groups, we set ourselves goals and have plans and ambitions that are considered valuable or worthwhile to pursue. For many people,[8] this capacity is underpinned by individual agency. This means that, to lesser or greater degrees, we choose from alternatives, and so become authors of our own actions and life-plans (Kagan, 1986; Nozick, 1974; Shoemaker, 1996). These alternatives are restricted by our biological and/or social environments, but, despite these restrictions, the broad claim here is that we all have options, however limited they might be. Moreover, these choices reflect our desires, which are shaped by information concerning these desires, and so become 'informed' (Griffin, 1988, pp. 7–39). And, if we are genuinely successful in pursuing these informed desires, then our lives are said to be going well, and our wellbeing and mental health is enhanced.

In various liberal philosophies of wellbeing, this view of agency has, unsurprisingly, been prominent, with arguments often focussing on how accomplishing individual goals is properly understood and measured, reflecting our evaluations, life-plans, and creative endeavours (Mill, 1991; Raz, 1988; and my arguments in Smith, 2012).

These liberal philosophies also raise questions concerning the value of wellbeing, whether it should be valued substantively, even as the dominant end of all values, or as an inclusive or transparent value, with the latter leaving room for other values, sitting independently of promoting wellbeing, such as freedom, justice and aesthetic creation (Rawls, 1973, pp. 548–544; Scanlon, 1998, pp. 108–143; Sen, 1985). However, despite the important contribution made by these liberal theories to the philosophy and practice of wellbeing, our ability to fulfil our informed desires is also profoundly influenced by social causation factors, which either restrict or augment our capacities to pursue these goals and ambitions. In addition, what is viewed or socially constructed as valuable coheres with wider social understandings of what are 'best' or 'important', which then affects which goals and ambitions we choose.

Conclusion: Some Implications for Coproduction in Mental Healthcare

Six Features of the Human Condition as Dynamic and Interrelated Characteristics

Whatever specific conception of wellbeing and mental health is defended, my claim in this chapter is that the six features of the human condition are both dynamic and interrelated. Furthermore, these characteristics have an important bearing on how mental health is subsequently viewed and promoted. For example, and as evidenced throughout this book, the social determinants of wellbeing and mental health, within and across social groupings, relate in complex ways to the embodied, medicalised or biological constitution of individual people. This complexity derives, in part, from how embodiment and sociability, as features of the human condition, are dynamically

[8] Biological and/or social determinists argue that human beings exercise little or no agency or free will, as human lives are shaped or determined by their natural and/or nurtured environments (for a recent defence of this determinist view see Miles, 2015). The question of agency is also debated extensively within the social constructionist literature explored here, with various positions being taken as to whether, or the extent to which, human beings can exercise agency, given the influence of public discourse and language in shaping how we view and experience our lives (for example, see Rabinow, 1984; Mackenzie, 2004).

related and often changing, leading to large variances both in people's experiences and in the social and medical causes of their mental health. The implication for mental healthcare is that we should not assume that one type of intervention strategy is likely to suit all people, because the complex and dynamic character of the relationship between these features is bound to produce an array of idiosyncrasies between people as these features variously interrelate.

When the social determinants of mental health are properly considered, it has been argued throughout this chapter that we must not only uncover the social processes of social causation concerning the epidemiology of mental illness and mental health, but also those processes of social construction that affect how notions of illness, health and wellbeing are defined or given meaning within social contexts. The latter processes include, for example, how some minority groups are defined as 'other' and 'different' by more dominant groups, including those minority groups defined as 'mentally ill' by dominant groups defined as 'healthy'. These processes affect how these minority groups are both viewed and treated. Notions of functional personhood, for example, are given meaning within social contexts that often make rigid distinctions between 'normality' and 'abnormality', which affect how individual people and groups of people are defined and treated as either mentally 'ill' or 'healthy'.

My recommendation is that we should be attentive to how these social construction processes are embedded in healthcare practice. That is, to equip practitioners with the ability to critically reflect on their practice, fully recognising that this practice is an expression of dominant institutional 'norms', sanctioned by socially constructed notions of medical expertise, and so on, which legitimate the exercise of professional power. One of the main points is that these socially constructed notions of medical expertise, and the subsequent exercise of professional power, often disguise or underestimate the role that social causation can play in the epidemiology of mental health.

This chapter highlights the argument that most accounts of wellbeing and mental health should include reference to agency as a central feature of care; that is, the capacity to formulate and implement life-plans that are considered by the agent as valuable and worthwhile to pursue. Chapter 22 considers agency from the perspective of its potential loss in many disadvantageous or extreme circumstances that are surveyed in Section 3. Conversely, restoring people's opportunities for expressing agency has been shown to produce better outcomes.

Moreover, from many philosophical perspectives, other features of the human condition also come into play when agency is exercised. So, our physical and biological make-up count, when we, for example, explain motivation concerning the choices and plans we make for ourselves. In addition, sociability also counts in exercising agency, as social groups not only socially construct or define the parameters in which choices are defined as valuable, but they allow us to focus on social causation factors that facilitate the degree to which these choices can be exercised (and see Chapters 3 and 4). Our cognitive features have an important role to play if these choices are to be properly informed by rational reflection, self-reflection and by collecting information and evidence prior to decision-making (Griffin, 1988, pp. 11–20; Sobel, 1994; Tiberius, 2008, pp. 109–36). Similarly, our evaluations also affect our choices, as we can also judge that our choices and actions are worthwhile and valuable, again, recognising that these judgements are also influenced and shaped within social contexts.

This chapter highlights how agency is exercised when the various human features dynamically interrelate, which then contributes to what is a complex multilayered decision-making process for people who inhabit various social worlds. This complex process leads to each person devising and implementing authentically held personal life-plans, which they and wider society understand as valuable. It is a process that also includes acknowledging the importance of each person exercising their agency, albeit while recognising the presence of dominant norms and values that help to define what is seen as authentically owned, valuable, personal life-plans. Nevertheless, the capacity for responsible decision-making is then given a relatively free rein under this conception. This capacity acts as an alternative to more determinist accounts of wellbeing and mental health, that is, whether these determining factors are in our embodied biological make-up, our social environments or a mixture of both.

We can see that the implications for mental healthcare are profound and far-reaching. Exercising agency means, by definition, that it is impossible to entirely predict outcomes for individual people and groups when intervention strategies are put in place. Nevertheless, what becomes centrally important when recognising a person's agency is that institutional mechanisms are established on the assumption that patients, clients or service-users are not passively engaged with circumstances that are beyond their control; but are, instead, defined, or socially constructed, as active and participant coproducers in how their care is managed and implemented. Coproduction includes participating equally and reciprocally in how people's conditions are defined or given meaning in relation to their lives (Davies et al., 2014; Raffay et al., 2016; Spencer et al., 2013). The principle of coproduction takes seriously service-users' subjective experiences and perspectives and how they define or give meaning to their lives, with people who are diagnosed as ill being viewed as equal participants and experts on their conditions, and who are able to work alongside practitioners in developing their care.

The arguments presented in this chapter provide coproduction with a social philosophical justification that is derived from identifying six features of the human condition, understood as universal. It is important to acknowledge both social causation and construction processes because they define and promote mental health within particular social contexts, and they impact variously upon these universal features.

Tensions in Coproduction and Social Policy Development

Finally, acknowledging that these complex and multilayered understandings of wellbeing should be promoted in mental health and welfare practice leads to tensions within social policy development, which also need to be addressed. More specifically, aspects of the six features of the human condition described here can be in sharp conflict depending on how they are defined and relate. This has implications for how coproduction is viewed in policy and practice.

There is, for example, considerable philosophical disagreement over how rational capacities concerning a person's agency should be understood and facilitated. So, is someone acting rationally when she takes a bird's-eye-view of her life and tries to make decisions without any perspectival bias toward time (past, present or future)? Or, is she being more rational when she has a perspectival bias toward her present and near future, over the past and distant future (Braddon-Mitchell & West, 2001; Brink, 2003; Parfit, 1987, pp. 152–186; Persson, 1988; Shoemaker, 1996; Smith, 2018; Yeager, 2008)? The point here is that, whatever way this question is answered, capacities for cognition, including critical self-reflection and exercising self-knowledge, may be construed as problems within these philosophical accounts because matters concerning the nature of time, our place, and attitudes toward it, are highly contested.

As a result, other difficult questions concerning how we understand and promote coproduction in healthcare are also thrown into sharp relief. To what degree should mental health practitioners accommodate for the present cognitive perspectives of the persons in their care, based on a certain bias toward this perspective, given that it is held by the service-user who has been defined (or socially constructed) by others as mentally ill? Or, to what degree should practitioners assume a so-called bird's-eye-view of this present perspective – this view being derived from their socially constructed medical expertise, and so on?

With regard to issues of agency, wellbeing and mental health may be enhanced if we accept, and become attuned to, the limits of the human condition as explored previously, which may include accepting the social and other limitations of persons who have mental ill health. We should also recognise that a presently orientated 'self-acceptance', being conducive to presently occurring subjective wellbeing, may conflict with the desire for change and enhanced objective capacities for the future, which, if implemented, would also enhance a person's future wellbeing and mental health, however they are conceptualised (Clifton et al., 2013).

Managing these tensions and conflicts in the coproduction process, among others, is integral to how wellbeing, mental health and mental healthcare are properly understood and practised across various social contexts, and which trajectories, actual and potential, of a person's life over time are managed and facilitated.

References

Berger, P. & Luckmann, T. (1967). The Social Construction of Reality: A Treatise on the Sociology of Knowledge. New York, NY: Anchor Books.

Braddon-Mitchell, D. & West, C. (2001). Temporal phase pluralism. Philosophy and Phenomenological Research, **62**: 59–83.

Brink, D. O. (2003). Prudence and authenticity: Intrapersonal conflicts and values. The Philosophical Review, **112**: 215–245.

Burr, V. (2003). Social Constructionism, 2nd edition. Brighton: Routledge.

Busfield, J. (2008). Mental illness as social product or social construct: A contradiction in feminists' arguments? Sociology of Health and Illness, **10**: 521–542.

Clarke, J. & Cochrane, A. (1998). The social construction of social problems. In Saraga, E., editor, Embodying the Social: Constructions of Difference. London: Routledge, pp. 3–42.

Clayton, M. & Williams, A., editors (2004). Social Justice. Oxford: Blackwell.

Clifton, A. Repper, J. Banks, D. & Remnant, J. (2013). Co-producing social inclusion: The structure/agency conundrum. Journal of Psychiatric and Mental Health Nursing, **20**: 514–524.

Davies, J. Sampson, M. Beesley, F. Smith, D. & Baldwin, V. (2014). An evaluation of knowledge and understanding framework personality disorder awareness training: Can a co-production model be effective in a local NHS mental health trust? Personality and Mental Health, **8**: 161–168.

Diener, E. & Diener, R. (2008). Happiness: Unlocking the Mysteries of Psychological Wealth. Oxford: Blackwell.

Durkheim, E. (2006). On Suicide. London: Penguin Classics (first published in 1897).

Foucault, M. (1954). Mental Illness and Psychology. Paris: Presses Universitaires.

Foucault, M. (1988). Madness and Civilization: A History of Insanity in the Age of Reason. New York, NY: Vintage Books.

Gergen, M. & Gergen, K. J. (2003). Social Construction: A Reader. London: Sage Publications.

Griffin, J. (1988). Well-Being: Its Meaning, Measurement, and Moral Importance. Oxford: Oxford University Press.

Haybron, D. M. (2011). The Pursuit of Unhappiness: The Elusive Psychology of Well-Being. Oxford: Oxford University Press.

Heidegger, M. (1962). Being and Time. Oxford: Blackwell Publishers (original publication (1927), Sein and Zeit. Tubingen: Max Niemeyer Verlag).

Horwitz, A. (2012). Social constructions of mental illness. In Kincaid, H., editor, The Oxford Handbook of Philosophy of Social Science. Oxford: Oxford University Press.

Joseph, J. (2003). Social Theory: Conflict, Cohesion and Consent. Edinburgh: Edinburgh University Press.

Kagan, S. (1986). The present-aim theory of rationality. Ethics, **96**: 746–759.

Kittay, E. F. (1999). Love's Labour: Essays on Women, Equality, and Dependency. New York, NY: Routledge.

Kopf, G. (2002). Temporality and personal identity in the thoughts of Nishida Kitaro. Philosophy East and West, **52**: 224–245.

Lechte, J. (1994). Fifty Key Contemporary Thinkers: From Structuralism to Postmodernity. London: Routledge.

Lloyd, M. (2004). The body. In Ashe, F., Finlayson, A., Lloyd, M. et al., editors, Contemporary Social and Political Theory: An Introduction. Maidenhead: Open University Press.

Lukes, S. (2005). Power: A Radical View, 2nd edition. Basingstoke: Palgrave MacMillan.

Mackenzie, C. & Stoljar, N., editors (2000). Relational Autonomy: Feminist Perspectives on Autonomy. New York, NY: Oxford University Press.

Mackenzie, I. (2004). Power. In Ashe, F., Finlayson, A., Lloyd, M., et al., editors, Contemporary Social and Political Theory: An Introduction. Maidenhead: Open University Press.

Miles, J. B. (2015). The Free-Will Delusion. Leicester: Matador.

Mill, J. S. (1991). On Liberty and Other Essays. Oxford: Oxford University Press.

Nagel, T. (1991). Equality and Partiality. New York, NY: Oxford University Press.

Nozick, R. (1974). Anarchy, State and Utopia. Oxford: Blackwell.

Parfit, D. (1987). Reasons and Persons. Oxford: Clarendon Press.

Persson, I. (1988). Rationality and maximization of satisfaction. Nous, **22**: 537–554.

Rabinow, P., editor (1984). The Foucault Reader. New York: Pantheon Books.

Raffay, J. Wood, E. & Todd, A. (2016). Service user views of spiritual and pastoral care (chaplaincy) in NHS mental health services: A co-produced constructivist grounded theory investigation. Bio-Med Central Psychiatry, published online; doi 10.1186/s12888-016–0903-9, pp. 1–11.

Rawls, J. (1973). A Theory of Justice. Oxford: Oxford University Press.

Raz, J. (1988). The Morality of Freedom. Oxford: Oxford University Press.

Ryff, C. (1989). Happiness is everything, or is it? Explorations on the meaning of psychological well-being. Journal of Personality and Social Psychology, **57**: 1069–1081.

Ryff, C. & Keyes, C. (1995). The structure of the psychology of well-being revisited. Journal of Personality and Social Psychology, **69**: 719–727.

Scanlon, T. M. (1998). What We Owe to Each Other. Cambridge, MA: Harvard University Press.

Seligman, M. (2002). Authentic Happiness: Using the New Positive Psychology to Realize Your Potential for Lasting Fulfillment. New York, NY: Free Press/Simon and Schuster.

Sen, A. (1985). Well-being, agency and freedom. The Dewey lectures 1984. Journal of Philosophy, **82**: 169–221.

Shoemaker, D. W. (1996). Theoretical persons and practical agents. Philosophy and Public Affairs, **25**: 318–332.

Smith, S. R. (2001a). Distorted ideals: The 'problems of dependency' and the mythology of independent living. Social Theory and Practice, **27**: 579–598.

Smith, S. R. (2001b). The social construction of talent: A defence of justice as reciprocity. Journal of Political Philosophy, **9**: 19–37.

Smith, S. R. (2002). Defending Justice as Reciprocity: An Essay on Political Philosophy and Social Policy. Lampeter: Edwin Mellen.

Smith, S. R. (2009). Social justice and disability: Competing interpretations of the medical and social models. In Kristiansen, K. Vehmas, S. & Shakespeare,T. editors, Arguing About Disability. Abingdon: Routledge.

Smith, S. R. (2011). Equality and Diversity: Value Incommensurability and the Politics of Recognition. Bristol: Policy Press.

Smith, S. R. (2012). Liberal ethics and well-being promotion in the disability rights movement, disability policy, and welfare practice. Ethics and Social Welfare, April issue.

Smith, S. R. (2014). Melancholy and happiness. South African Journal of Philosophy, **33**: 1–12.

Smith, S. R. (2018). Well-being and self-interest: Personal identity, parfit, and conflicting attitudes to time in liberal theory, social policy and practice. In Galvin, K., editor, A Handbook of Well-Being. London: Routledge.

Sobel, D. (1994). Full information accounts of well-being. Ethics, **104**: 784–810.

Spencer,M. Dineen, R. & Phillips, A. (2013). Tools for Improvement 8 – Co-Producing Services: Co-Creating Health. Cardiff: NHS Wales 1000 Lives Improvement.

Sumner, W. L. (1999). Welfare, Happiness and Ethics. Oxford: Clarendon Press.

Tiberius, V. (2008). The Reflective Life: Living Wisely With Our Limits. New York: Oxford University Press.

Walker, M. T. (2006). The social construction of mental illness and its implications for the recovery model. International Journal of Psychosocial Rehabilitation, **10**: 71–87.

Wittgenstein, L. (1998). Culture and Value. Oxford: Blackwell.

Wittgenstein, L. (2000). Philosophical Investigations. Oxford: Blackwell.

Yeager, D. M. (2008). The deliberate holding of unproven beliefs: Judgment post – critically considered. Political Science Reviewer, **37**: 96–121.

Chapter 3

Social Sciences and Health: A Framework for Building and Strengthening Social Connectedness

Catherine Haslam and S. Alexander Haslam

Social Relationships and Health

Social relationships affect health. Of that we are certain. People who are more strongly connected live longer (e.g. Holt-Lunstad et al., 2010), are in better health (e.g. Boden-Albala et al., 2005) and experience better wellbeing (e.g. Helliwell & Putnam, 2004). None of us is immune to these effects although, clearly, poverty, inequality and age, among other factors, contribute to, and exacerbate the consequences of, social disconnection.

What is more remarkable, in the context of the evidence-base showing the profound impact of these effects, is the relatively limited investment in efforts to build and preserve the social capital of vulnerable communities, on health grounds. Recognising the potential benefits that social resources bring and the mechanisms through which they can emerge is important, but not enough. What is needed is a coherent approach to embed these resources in communities to ensure that the products of social connectedness can be sustained in the longer term. In this chapter, we identify these factors and introduce the '5S' framework, comprising *schooling, scoping, sourcing, scaffolding* and *sustaining*, as a general approach to developing and embedding the social capital needed to support and maintain the health of communities that are at risk.

Social Capital, Connectedness and Health

Social capital refers to the network of relationships and ties between people who work together for mutual benefit, whether in the context of our families, neighbourhoods or wider society. It is often reflected in a community's sense of social cohesion, which can be observed and measured in different ways, through trust, cooperation, norms of reciprocity, civic engagement and openness to giving and receiving support. Critical here is the idea that social capital is the product of communal assets. Personal human capital contributes to these assets, but they come to be realised through collectives of people, for example, members of families, neighbourhoods and communities.

Promoting social capital is recognised as a key mechanism through which disadvantage and poverty, which results in ill health, might be tackled. However, while it is more likely to be lacking in communities where such disadvantage exists, it is important to note that this is not inevitable. Cattell (2011) illustrates this point in her case study involving people living in two estates who had similar experiences of poverty, deprivation and unemployment, but marked differences in their health. More positive outcomes were observed in the group in which there were greater opportunities for casual interaction, participation in clubs and other associations, and for neighbours to be relocated together where housing was no longer fit for purpose.

But what is the evidence that social connectedness and social capital protect health? The trail-blazing research in this field was Berkman and Syme's (1979) prospective study of 6,928 residents, aged between 30 to 69, in Almeda County, California. This showed that, compared to women who were well connected, women who lacked social contacts were 2.8 times more likely to die over the nine-year course of study. This multiplier was 2.3 for men. Importantly too, this effect was independent of differences in baseline physical health and in health-risk behaviour such as, for example, smoking or lack of physical exercise.

Many subsequent studies have highlighted the importance of active engagement and participation in social networks as a key factor, not merely their availability (e.g. Bennet, 2002; Giles et al., 2012; Glass et al., 1999; House et al., 1982). In his book, *Bowling Alone: The Collapse and Revival of American Community*, Putnam attempts to quantify these effects. His analysis led him to conclude that 'if you belong to no groups and decide to join one, you cut your risk of dying in the next year in half' (Putnam, 2000, p. 331). Along similar lines, and echoing Berkman and Syme's earlier findings, results from meta-analysis show that the effects of social connectedness are comparable to those for quitting smoking and exceed those for obesity, high blood pressure and physical inactivity (Holt-Lunstad et al., 2010).

But it is not only in the domain of life expectancy that social connections wield their power. They also make our lives worth living as is evident in their profound impact on our mental health and wellbeing. These observations stem back to Durkheim's analysis, originally published in 1897, (Durkheim, 1951) of the causes of suicide, which showed the vital role that social integration had on enhancing community wellbeing. Along related lines, more recent data show that people with a diverse range of social networks, typically involving interaction with families, friendships, religious and other more informal networks, report fewer depressive symptoms (Fiori et al., 2006).

Also notable in this regard are longitudinal data showing that social group networks have an important role to play in protecting against our developing depression and reducing the risk of relapse among those people with a history of depression (Cruwys et al., 2013). Interestingly too, these effects of group ties are incremental. So, while relapse was reduced by 24 per cent among people who had acquired one group membership, it was reduced by 63 per cent among those who had acquired three groups.

As these and other studies attest, the association between social connectedness and health is not in question. All too often, though, it has been used to leap to the conclusion that any form of social participation is good for health. However, not all social ties are good for us (Haslam et al., 2012), and some social ties seem to be more effective than others (Haslam et al., 2014). Accordingly, there is clearly more to the social-connectedness story that requires explanation. In line with a growing body of research on what is now termed the social identity approach to health (Haslam et al., 2009; Jetten et al., 2012; see Chapter 4 in this volume), we argue that people's sense of belonging and strength of connectedness with others is what drives health behaviour and health outcomes, for good and for ill. Without a meaningful sense of shared identification with others, there is no basis for any of the recognised products of social capital, trust, reciprocity, mutual support and civil engagement to emerge.

Mechanisms for the Effects of Social Connectedness: beyond the Usual Suspects

The main accounts used to explain the powerful effects of social connectedness on health have tended to emphasise the role of physiological and psychological factors. Accounts of the physiological mechanisms that are implicated in the stress process typically focus on biological pathways. In this regard, social isolation and disadvantage are recognised as ongoing causes of stress, all of which can have damaging effects on the body, releasing neurotransmitters that put pressure on immune and other physiological systems (McEwan & Gianaris, 2010; Seeman et al, 2010). In the absence of factors to buffer the stress response, such as, for example, supportive networks, recovery to heightened arousal is slowed, causing neurodegeneration and increasing the risk of mortality.

Psychological explanations tend to focus on the role of social support and social influence in buffering stress (Berkman et al., 2000; Cohen, 2004; Cohen & Wills, 1985). Here, the negative impact of stressful life events is attenuated by access to support or, more particularly, by a sense that such support could be available, which is not the same thing. The support can take a number of forms, for example, emotional, information, instrumental. Active participation in social networks also makes us more open to their influence.

Clearly, these physiological and psychological processes do not operate independently. The psychological experience of stress, for example, produces physiological changes, and these changes feed back into our appraisal and response to that stress. Thus, the pathways through which social connectedness enhances health are multiple and interactive. Nevertheless, still missing from these discussions of mechanism is an explanation of why only particular ties might be perceived as supportive in particular contexts, and why only certain ties might have a positive influence on behaviour. Addressing this gap, researchers in the social identity tradition (after Turner, 1982) argue that identification with groups of others is what makes social participation not only meaningful, but also possible. People need both reason and motivation to connect, and these features are more likely to be present when people perceive themselves as sharing a common bond with groups of others as, for example, members of a family, a neighbourhood, an organisation or a community.

This reasoning has underpinned development of the social identity approach to health and informed a body of work that seeks to account more forensically for the conditions under which social connectedness enhances health. Fundamental to this framework is the idea that social groups of multiple forms provide an important and distinctive basis for self-understanding and self-definition. They frame and inform our beliefs and values, drive our thoughts, influence our emotions and shape our behaviour, but only when, and to the extent that, they get under our skin and are internalised as part of our sense of self, as 'us' rather than 'them'.

This sense of social identification with others is a key mechanism that underpins production and maintenance of our social capital. In particular, this is because it provides a basis and motivation for people not only to promote their own health and wellbeing, but also for them to advance the interests and the health of other ingroup members, through providing social support. As explained further in Chapter 4 (see also Haslam et al., 2012), shared social identity is a basis both for people to provide others with support and for those who receive it to construe and respond to that support constructively, seeing it as kindness, not dominance; as generous, not patronising; as enabling, not humiliating. In this way, a social identity analysis explains the dynamics of support and helps us to understand not only when it is offered, but also why, when it is offered, it is not always beneficial for health. Indeed, in the absence of shared identification, proffered support and social contact is likely to be suboptimal and to impose further strain, and efforts to build social capital can easily backfire.

Social identification also accounts for the effects of social influence. When we internalise group memberships and see others in the group as part of 'us', then we are more likely to engage with the norms of those groups, irrespective of whether they promote behaviours that are good or bad for health. On the one hand, this means that our identification with social networks that encourage positive health norms, for example, good eating habits or regular exercise, are likely to rub off, increasing our willingness to engage in those same productive behaviours. But, on the other hand, we are also likely to be guided by ingroups whose members model negative behaviours, that is, those that harm ourselves or others. Like a badge of honour, whatever its form and valency, such behaviour is a demonstration of the value we place on ingroup ties and of our commitment to living out valued social identities.

Put simply, then, social identification and shared social identity are what make the various products of social capital possible. They account for the helpful effects of social group relationships, both existing and newly developed, the dynamics of support and influence, the development of trust and the motivation for civil engagement and reciprocity. Yet, at the same time, we see that social identity processes also have a hand to play in the erosion of social capital, for example, where one's sense of belonging to a community might be undermined through externally imposed, and not community-driven, urban regeneration. Accordingly, if we want to build social capital, then, more than anything else, it is important for us to get these social identity dynamics 'right'.

A Framework for Building Social Connectedness

If we accept these arguments, as do many of the contributors to this volume, the question that arises is how we can translate the social identity approach into practical forms of social intervention. We outline the 5S framework in the sections of this chapter that follow. It is one broad framework that we have devised as a means of mobilising social identities in ways that serve to build and maintain social group capital. Importantly, too, as we saw in Chapter 1, its five components also inform the structure of this book as well as its title.

As we set out on this task, it is worth observing at the outset that the pursuit of individual-level intervention in healthcare contexts is often at odds with the notion that health has social dimensions. Clearly, single-person-orientated interventions are essential in acute medical settings, but, nevertheless, we still doggedly pursue individual treatments for most health problems. While we acknowledge the growing interest in group-based interventions, we also note that their use is often justified primarily on economic grounds. Of course, this can infuse intervention with a social flavour, but rarely is there any recognition of the therapeutic role that groups play in the success of the intervention, let alone a theory-informed understanding of the dynamics of social connectedness that structure health outcomes. So, this is a meta-theoretical and practical prejudice that we need to tackle head-on if we are really interested in building social capital.

In many cases, it makes sense to start by targeting interventions at the level of groups, for example, families, communities etc., so as to allow the products of social connectedness to do their work in supporting health outcomes. This has always been

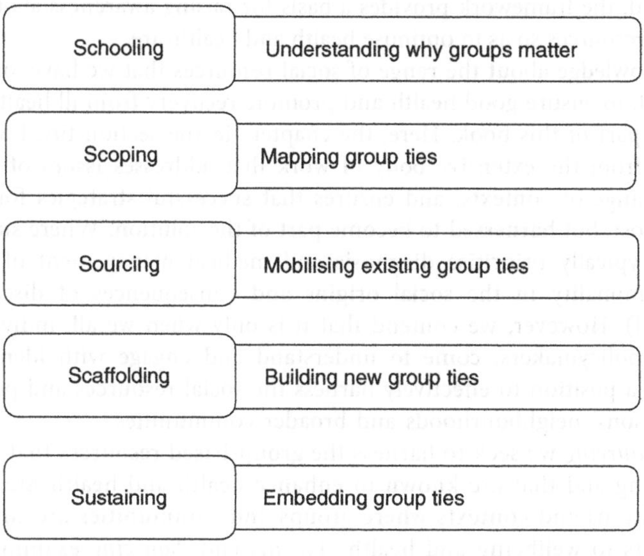

Figure 3.1 Modules in GROUPS 4 HEALTH

the mission of policymakers and practitioners who have a social capital agenda (e.g. after Putnam, 2000), but we argue that their efforts have often fallen short, due largely to an inadequate understanding of when and why social connectedness succeeds and fails. As we have seen, the social identity framework fills this gap in theory, but how might it work in practice?

The primary aim of this book is to answer this question by outlining strategies that serve to promote sustainable forms of social connectedness. As specified in Figure 3.1, we propose five stages through which to do this. As well as lending structure to this volume, these are also the modules of a new social-identity-derived intervention, GROUPS 4 HEALTH (Haslam et al., 2016), which aims to help people who are suffering from the effects of social isolation by providing them with knowledge and skills that allow them to manage their social group memberships, and the identities that underpin them, more effectively. Essentially, then, this is a structure to promote and manage social connectedness that has relevance not only for people who experience disconnection, but also for those who work with them.

In GROUPS 4 HEALTH, *Schooling* is used to raise awareness of the beneficial effects that social group memberships have for health, benefits which, as we have seen, are usually taken for granted. This is a major issue in healthcare, in which practitioners and policymakers tend to prioritise interventions that are biological and pharmaceutical over those that are social, despite an abundance of evidence that the latter can be highly effective, not least in enhancing the efficacy of the former. All too often, then, best practice in healthcare is framed primarily as a problem of coming to terms with the latest developments in epidemiology or neuroscience. Yet we ignore the social dimensions of health at our peril, literally; and failing to use all the resources at our disposal, not only medical but also social, can only ever result in suboptimal outcomes. Schooling targets this problem in two ways. First, it provides the knowledge and theoretical framing needed to appreciate the nature of the problems we confront by drawing on theorising about social identity along the lines of this chapter. Second, the framework provides a basis for raising awareness about how best to harness social resources so as to optimise health and healthcare.

Further knowledge about the range of social resources that we have, or should have, at our disposal, to ensure good health and promote recovery from ill health, is the focus of the second part of this book. Here, the chapters in the section titled *Scoping* engage with findings from the extensive body of work that addresses issues of social disconnection in a range of contexts, and ensures that successful strategies for dealing with these are not lost, but harnessed to become part of the solution. Where such efforts fail, practitioners typically prioritise diagnosis and medical management of the problem, ignoring commonality in the social origins and consequences of disease (Bailey & Williams, 2014). However, we contend that it is only when we all, individual persons, practitioners, policymakers, come to understand and engage with identity dynamics that we are in a position to effectively harness the social resources and potentialities of individual persons, neighbourhoods and broader communities.

Through *Sourcing* we seek to harness the group-based resources that have emerged through scoping and that are known to enhance health and healthcare. This matters most in conditions and contexts where groups and communities are confronted with extreme threats to wellbeing and health. To this end, *Sourcing* examines events and circumstances that, although not commonplace in everyone's experiences, do frame the contents of national and local news programmes and bulletins. Our intention is to draw on people's experience in more extreme situations in which groups of people can use existing resources and knowledge to build attachments and a common sense of belonging. In turn, this allows them to respond to challenge and adversity, overcome social exclusion and realise constructive shared goals. They include people who: experience emergencies and disasters; deal with the trauma of conflict and asylum-seeking; and confront radicalisation. Isolation is a common feature of the landscape here, both as a determinant of the problem and as its consequence, and is a recognised source of ill health and harm. As our analysis throughout this volume shows, overcoming adversity requires knowledge of how best to utilise existing social resources so as to promote constructive forms of collective behaviour.

But in a range of contexts, and particularly among communities confronting severe challenge, it is also naïve to imagine that people can rely only on existing resources. Not least, this is because their lack or inadequacy is likely to have contributed to their problems in the first place. Accordingly, it is important to map out supplementary pathways for intervention. This is the value of *Scaffolding*, which aims to draw on the experience of groups that have (or had) modelled identification and mobilisation of positive social resources, as a basis to build and strengthen new social resources. This also speaks to the importance of developing multiple-group networks, often some that involve sourcing, some that involve scaffolding, in order to provide more opportunities to access forms of support that are right for the situation at hand. Along these lines, Section 4 of this volume focuses on ways we can help people to construct a viable social scaffold in the process of empowering and building the community confidence that is ultimately required for people to manage their social resources independently.

Ultimately, though, these various principles must be embedded into community structures and maintained if interventions based on them are to have enduring benefit. This is the aim of *Sustaining*, which provides an agenda for the future in which the insights gained through schooling, scoping, sourcing and scaffolding are translated into policy, strategy, service design and modes of operation, which ensure that the social foundations identified and developed in the preceding four phases are maintained in the long term.

Conclusion

Contrary to the famous pronouncement of Margaret Thatcher, one of the most important facts to come out of social capital discourse is a recognition that there is such a thing as society and that, providing it is harnessed appropriately, it can be the source of profound health benefit. Our challenge is to identify how best to develop and mobilise social resources to optimise health and healthcare. Over the years, there have been multiple attempts to build social capital through pioneering healthcare and social policy initiatives, but increasing evidence of the grave consequences of social disconnection highlight the fact that more, much more, remains to be done.

Wakefield and Poland (2005), among others, argue that this reflects inadequate theorising and framing around the notion of social capital. This has meant that, while we recognise this as a hugely important phenomenon and construct, we have limited practical understanding of how to develop and maintain it. Providing this understanding is the key challenge for the social and health sciences and a central goal of this book. Armed with insights from the social identity approach and the cognate literatures that inform it, our sense is that we can approach this task afresh and with renewed and realistic hope of success.

References

Bailey, S. & Williams, R. (2014). Towards partnerships in mental healthcare. Advances in Psychiatric Treatment, **20**: 48–51.

Bennett, K. M. (2002). Low level social engagement as a precursor of mortality among people in later life. Age and Ageing, **31**: 165–168.

Berkman, L. F. & Syme, S. L. (1979). Social networks, host resistance, and mortality: A nine-year follow-up study of Alameda County residents. American Journal of Epidemiology, **109**: 186–204.

Berkman, L. F., Glass, T., Brisette, I. & Seeman, T. E. (2000). From social integration to health: Durkheim in the new millennium. Social Science and Medicine, **51**, 843–857.

Boden-Albala, B. Litwak, E., Elkind, M. S. V., Rundek, T. & Sacco, R. L. (2005). Social isolation and outcomes post stroke. Neurology, **14**: 1888–1892.

Cattell, V. (2011). Poor people, poor places, and poor health: The mediating role of social networks and social capital. Social Science and Medicine, **52**: 1501–1516.

Cohen, S. (2004). Social relationships and health. American Psychologist, **59**: 676–684.

Cohen, S. & Wills, T. A. (1985). Stress, social support, and the buffering hypothesis. Psychological Bulletin, **98**: 310–357.

Cruwys, T., Dingle, G., Haslam, C. et al. (2013). Social group memberships protect against future depression, alleviate depression symptoms and prevent depression relapse. Social Science and Medicine, **98**: 179–186.

Durkheim, E. (1951) Suicide. New York: Free Press (originally published 1897).

Fiori, K. L., Antonucci, A. & Cortina, K.S. (2006). Social network typologies and mental health among older adults. Journal of Gerontology B: Psychological Sciences and Social Sciences, **61**: 25–32.

Giles, L. C., Anstey, K. J., Walker, R. B. & Luszcz, M. A. (2012). Social networks and memory over 15 years of follow-up in a cohort of older Australians: Results from the Australian Longitudinal Study of Ageing. Journal of Aging Research, Article ID 856048: 1–7.

Glass, T. A., Mendes de Leon, C., Marottoli, R. A. & Berkham, L. F. (1999). Population based study of social and productive activities as predicators of survival among elderly Americans. British Medical Journal, **319**: 478–483.

Haslam, C., Cruwys, T. & Haslam, S. A. (2014). “The we's have it”: Evidence for the distinctive benefits of social ties in enhancing cognitive health in ageing. Social Science and Medicine, **120**: 57–66.

Haslam, C., Cruwys, T., Haslam, S. A., Dingle, G. A. & Chang, M. X-L. (2016). Groups 4 Health: Evidence that a social-identity intervention that builds and strengthens social group membership improves health. Journal of Affective Disorders, **194**: 188–195.

Haslam, S. A., Jetten, J., Postmes, T. & Haslam, C. (2009). Social identity, health and well-being: An emerging agenda for applied psychology. Applied Psychology: An International Review, **58**: 1–23.

Haslam, S. A., Reicher, S. D. & Levine, M. (2012). When other people are heaven, when other people are hell: How social identity determines the nature and impact of social support. In Jetten, J. Haslam, C. & Haslam, S. A., editors, The Social Cure: Identity, Health and Well-Being. Hove: Psychology Press, pp. 157–174.

Helliwell, J. F. & Putnam, R. D. (2004). The social context of well-being. Philosophical Transactions of the Royal Society of London, B: Biological Sciences, **359**: 1435–1446.

Holt-Lunstad, J., Smith, T. B. & Layton, J. B. (2010). Social relationships and mortality risk: A meta-analytic review. PLoS Medicine, **7**: e1000316.

House, J. S., Robbins, C. & Metzner, H. L. (1982). The associations of social relationships and activities with mortality: Prospective evidence from the Tecumseh community health study. American Journal of Epidemiology, **116**: 123–140.

Jetten, J., Haslam, C. & Haslam, S. A., editors (2012). The Social Cure: Identity, Health and Well-Being. Hove: Psychology Press.

McEwen, B. S. & Gianaris, P. J. (2010). Central role of the brain in stress and adaptation: Links to socioeconomic status, health, and disease. Annals of the New York Academy of Sciences, **1186**: 190–222.

Putnam, R. D. (2000). Bowling Alone: The Collapse and Revival of American Community. New York, NY: Simon and Schuster.

Seeman, T., Epel, E., Gruenewald, T., Karlamangla, A. & McEwen, B. S. (2010). Socio-economic differentials in peripheral biology: Cumulative allostatic load. Annals of the New York Academy of Science, **1186**: 223–239.

Turner, J. C. (1982). Towards a redefinition of the social group. In H. Tajfel, editor, Social Identity and Intergroup Relations. Cambridge: Cambridge University Press, pp. 15–40.

Wakefield, S. E. L. & Poland, B. (2005). Family, friend or foe? Critical reflections on the relevance and role of social capital in health promotion and community development. Social Science and Medicine, **60**: 2819–2832.

Chapter 4

The Social Identity Approach to Health

S. Alexander Haslam, Jolanda Jetten and Catherine Haslam

Introduction

One of the central ideas that is explored throughout this book is that people's social lives and the social worlds they inhabit have a critical bearing on their health. At one level this message is uncontroversial. There is, after all, plenty of evidence both that social contact, social connections and a rich social life are good for one's wellbeing (House et al., 1988) and, that those people who are disadvantaged in this respect as a result, for example, of poverty, prejudice or other forms of social exclusion suffer from relatively poor health outcomes (Wilkinson & Marmot, 2003). In this chapter, though, we present a rather more nuanced analysis, which suggests that *particular forms* of social interaction have an especially important role to play in these dynamics. They are those forms that are grounded in shared *social identity*, an internalised sense of shared group membership, and an associated sense that one is part of a bigger 'us'.

This argument lies at the heart of the *social identity approach to health* that was introduced in Chapter 3: a theoretical perspective on health and wellbeing that has become increasingly influential in recent years and that underpins many of the contributions to this book. In what follows, we set out the core tenets of this approach and explain why its ideas are so central to the various issues that are addressed in the chapters that follow.

Social Identity as a Basis for Group Behaviour

When people refer to 'the self', they are typically referring to something singular about a person. A person who is self-confident, for example, is understood to be assured of their personal place in the world. Importantly, though, we also talk about the self in the first-person plural, *in terms our social identities* as 'us' and 'we'. Accordingly, we can define ourselves as 'us Australians', 'us psychiatrists', 'us men' and so on, and understand ourselves to be self-confident as members of these groups. The fact that we do this speaks to the capacity for the self to be defined not only in unique terms but also in terms of *attributes and qualities we share with other people*.

The significance of this point for psychology was first illustrated in a famous series of experiments conducted by Henri Tajfel and his colleagues, which came to be known as the *minimal group studies* (Tajfel, 1972; Tajfel et al, 1971). In them, schoolboys were assigned to essentially meaningless groups, supposedly on the basis of their liking for abstract paintings by either Klee or Kandinsky, which had to assign rewards to other members of both their own group, their *ingroup*, and another group, the *outgroup*. What the studies found was that even these most minimal of conditions were sufficient to encourage ingroup favouritism, such that the boys awarded more points to ingroup members than to those in the outgroup.

Seeking to make sense of these findings, what Tajfel came to understand was that they reflected the fact that, for the boys who participated in the studies, the process of acting in terms of their group membership was a way of making an otherwise meaningless situation *meaningful*. In particular, the actions they engaged in gave them a positive and distinctive social identity, for example, as 'us in the Klee group' as opposed to 'them in the Kandinsky group'.

Extending analysis of the minimal group studies further, John Turner subsequently noted that they involved the production of a distinctive form of *group behaviour*, and, most critically, that it was the participants' capacity to act in terms of social identity that made this behaviour *possible* (Turner, 1982). In other words, it was only because the boys could see themselves as 'us in the Klee group' that they were able to act as members of the Klee group. This, he argued, is true of all other groups too. So, it is only because, and to the extent that, Welsh people can define themselves in terms of a social identity, *as Welsh*, that they are able to behave as an organised, coordinated national entity. And the same is true for all other groups; teams, clubs, societies, unions, churches and so on.

Social Identity as a Basis for Health

The foregoing observation is clearly important when it comes to understanding the psychology of group behaviour, for example, when wanting to explain why people sometimes engage in social conflict. But why is social identity important for health? The core reason is that humans are social animals who live, and have evolved to live, in social groups. In short, group life makes us human and is a key source of personal meaning, purpose and worth. Among other things, this means that, like hunger and thirst, physical and psychological isolation are inimical to our make-up and design. And in this regard, the fundamental significance of social identity is that, without it, as Turner (1982) argued, group behaviour is impossible.

If one considers a choir, for example, it is the fact that its members share social identity that allows them to sing from the same song sheet, both literally and metaphorically, and that therefore allows the choir to function as a meaningful entity. Shared social identity allows its members to access the benefits of this, and this, at least partly, explains why being in a choir is good for health and wellbeing (Dingle et al., 2013). Moreover, the more that choir members define themselves in terms of shared identity, that is, the higher their *social identification*, the more true this will be.

Of course, this point is not restricted to choirs, but is true of all other collectives be they recreational, religious, occupational, political or community groups. The general point here, then, is that social identities and social identifications allow us to fulfil our potential as humans and, hence, generally have positive implications for health; although, for reasons we discuss below, this is not always the case. Consistent with this point, a recent meta-analysis by Tegan Cruwys and her colleagues found that people's social identification with a broad range of groups was negatively and reliably associated with depression ($r = -.25$; Cruwys et al., 2014), while a meta-analysis led by Nik Steffens found that employees' social identification with workteams was positively and reliably associated with both psychological wellbeing and the absence of stress ($r = 0.27, 0.18$, respectively; Steffens et al., 2016).

Further support for this proposition comes from forensic research by the third author (CH) and her colleagues that used data from the English Longitudinal Survey on Ageing (ELSA) to examine the power of different types of social connection to predict the cognitive health of more than 3,000 English adults over time (Haslam et al., 2014). Contrary to the idea that all forms of social connection are equally protective of health, what this research found was that social group ties proved far more beneficial than individual ties. Indeed, *only* group engagement made a significant and sustained contribution to subsequent cognitive function, and this contribution became more pronounced as people became more vulnerable, that is, with increasing age. Similarly, a study of over 800 Australian high-school students by the second author and her colleagues showed that psychological health, in the form of personal self-esteem, was predicted *only* by the quality of the students' group-based ties (Jetten et al., 2015).

Stated slightly differently, our argument is that social identities are beneficial to health because they are the basis for meaningful forms of group life and hence give us access to important social and psychological *resources* (Jetten et al., 2012, 2014). Indeed, consistent with this notion of social identities as a resource, evidence from a large number of studies supports the argument that the more social identities a person has access to, that is, the more group memberships they have internalised as part of their self, the better their physical, mental and cognitive health. This prediction is confirmed by studies of multiple populations, including high-school students (Jetten et al., 2012), university undergraduates (Iyer et al., 2009), sportspeople recovering from physical exertion (Jones & Jetten, 2011), and people recovering from a stroke (Haslam et al., 2008) or staving off depression (Cruwys et al., 2013; Seymour-Smith et al., 2016).

However, it also follows from this analysis that, if our capacity to form meaningful social connections is compromised because, for example, we lose or lack social identities or because our social identities are stigmatised, then this is likely to limit our access to these same social and psychological resources and hence constitutes a significant threat to our psychological and social functioning. This can also be true if, as a function of their particular nature, groups exert a negative influence on our lives because the *content* of a given social identity, 'us depressives', 'us heroin users', is harmful in some way, because it has, for example, negative connotations or prescribes toxic behaviour. A key point here, then, is that much of the power of the social identity approach to health derives from its capacity to understand the ways in which social identities are implicated in negative health-related dynamics as well as those that are more positive (Haslam et al., 2018).

Social Identity as a Health-Enhancing Resource

These ideas can be fleshed out further by drawing on the full suite of ideas that are contained within *social identity theory* (Tajfel & Turner, 1979) and *self-categorization theory* (Turner, 1982, 1991; Turner et al., 1987, 1994). They are the two key theories that together comprise what has come to be known as the *social identity approach* (Haslam, 2004) and they explore the determinants of social identity and social identification as well as its consequences for social behaviour. This, in turn, allows us to better understand both the origins and the precise nature of health-related social identity resources.

Social Connection

One of the primary consequences of coming to see ourselves as sharing social identity with others is that it draws them closer to us psychologically. As spelled out within *self-categorization theory*, a key reason for this is that shared social identity transforms people who, as individuals, are *different from the self*, that is, are 'others', into people who, as group members, are *part of the self* (Turner et al., 1987).

By way of illustration, as individuals, passengers on the London Underground have no connection to each other and treat each other as strangers, with indifference and disregard. However, if circumstances lead them to see themselves as sharing social identity then they are likely to see themselves as having much more in common and their psychological orientation to each other will become much more positive. This point was confirmed by Drury et al. (2009) in research that documented the sense of solidarity and shared resolve that emerged among passengers who were survivors of the London bombings in 2005. It has also been documented in work by David Novelli and colleagues, which examines passengers' experiences of sharing train carriages with football supporters when those passengers are supporters of the same team, a different team or no team at all (Novelli et al., 2013). More prosaically, a range of controlled experimental studies, including those that involve minimal groups, show that manipulations to make salient a social identity that is shared with another person, for example, as Australians, team members, or Klee-likers, serve to make that person appear more similar to the perceiver.

Furthermore, as well as changing abstract perceptions of similarity and connectedness, manipulations such as these also change our openness and receptivity to others, as evidenced in perceptions of liking and trust. Not only do we understand others to be more yoked to us in such circumstances, but, once we relate to them as ingroup members, we also embrace them more enthusiastically.

The significance of this point for health is that an abundance of research points to the negative consequences of social isolation for a range of health indicators. Indeed, as noted in Chapter 3, meta-analytic reviews show that social isolation places a person at greater risk of death than a range of risks that are far more widely publicised (Holt-Lunstad et al., 2010). Moreover, research also shows that it is the *psychological sense*, rather than the fact, of being alone that is critical here (Cacioppo & Patrick, 2008; Sani, 2012). One key reason why social identity and social identification tend to have positive implications for health is that they serve to counteract, and indeed, are inherently antithetical to a sense of psychological isolation (Cruwys et al., 2014).

Effective Support

As people come to define themselves in terms of shared group membership, it is not simply their perceptions of each other that change. So too does their behaviour. Not least, this is because social identity provides group members with the motivation to engage with each other in ways that advance the identity they share. One obvious way they can do this is by helping each other out by providing social support when it is perceived to be needed (Haslam, 2004). This support can take an emotional, intellectual or material form and again flows from the fact that shared social identity transforms 'other' into 'self'.

Another large body of empirical work supports this claim (Haslam et al., 2012). For example, studies by Mark Levine and colleagues show that, when a football fan trips and falls, a passer-by is far more likely to stop and help them if the person appears to be a fan of the same team rather than of a rival one. However, if the observer's social identity as a football fan has been made salient, rather than their identity as a supporter of a specific team, then they are more likely to help the fan of the rival team than someone who appears not to support any team (Levine et al., 2005).

On a larger scale, studies of international aid show that charitable giving also follows the contours of shared identity. But by the same token, a person's status as an ingroup or outgroup member, and hence the amount of support they receive, varies as a function of the specific identity lens through which they are viewed. Studies have shown, for example, that British people donate more money to Italian earthquake victims if they are encouraged to define themselves as European, in which case they share identity with Italians, rather than as living in a country where the potential beneficiaries do not (Levine & Thompson, 2004).

Importantly, though, effective support is not just a matter of aid provision; it also depends on recipients being receptive to such charity. And this receptiveness is also structured by shared social identity. Studies show that people are more positively oriented to support when it is offered by ingroup rather than outgroup members and, in large part, this is because they are more trusting of the motives that lie behind it (Haslam et al., 2012).

Together then, these two sides of the support equation combine to mean that support tends to be both more forthcoming and more effective when it occurs within, rather than across, the boundaries of social identity. The same is true for the process of *social influence* that is implicated in cognitive forms of support. In particular, whether or not people give advice, and whether or not they take it on board, depends very much on the degree to which they see themselves as sharing social identity. This too is a point that has broad relevance for health. For example, it helps us understand the *therapeutic alliance* between practitioners and clients as something that is predicated on social identity. And it also helps us to understand why clinical treatment tends to be less successful when it occurs across identity fault-lines such as those of ethnicity, culture and class.

Meaning and Worth

We noted above that, within the minimal groups studies, Tajfel observed that it was the process of acting as group members, in terms of social identity, that allowed participants to make an otherwise meaningless task meaningful. At the time, he did not make too much of this, but it turns out that this is largely true of most other forms of social behaviour. It is not an accident that people routinely quip that talking to yourself is a sign of madness. For what makes talking meaningful, and enjoyable, is the process of doing it with someone else. The same goes for singing an operatic aria, kicking a football or writing medical notes. Although these things can be meaningful when done alone, this is generally only true to the extent that a person's behaviour anticipates opportunities to engage with others.

In this regard too, it is obviously the case that what people do in groups, and as individual group members, is largely informed by the *content* of their identity and the degree of their social identification. Choir members sing, football teams play football, doctors practise medicine. And even when they are not doing these things, their members are often preparing for them in various ways, either individually or together by, say, rehearsing, practising, socialising, studying. The significance of this observation for health and wellbeing is that, in this way, social identities lend meaning, direction and purpose to actions that would otherwise be pointless. Not to put too fine a point on it, they give us something apparently useful to do. This point was brought home forcefully in Emile Durkheim's classic study of suicide (Durkheim, 1951) in which he noted that people are far less likely to kill themselves during wartime, something that he attributed to the fact that wars had the power to 'arouse collective sentiments' that brought people together and focused their energies. At the same time, the process of contributing to shared goals tends to be valued and valourised by other ingroup members and hence it instills in people a sense that they and their efforts are worthy and worthwhile.

Control, Efficacy and Power

Finally, because it provides a basis for people to participate in, and promote, collective projects, it is also the case that shared social identity tends to give people a sense of agency and control. As social identity theory suggests, at a group level, this should furnish them with a sense of being in charge of their own destiny and of having power in the world (Turner, 2005). This was apparent in a simulated prison study that the first author conducted with Steve Reicher where, as prisoners' sense of social identity increased, so too did their sense of agency and power (Reicher & Haslam, 2006). Moreover, as studies of protest groups have shown (and as fans of perennially underperforming sports teams understand), it is not necessary for a group to achieve its aims in order for these benefits to accrue (Cocking & Drury, 2004).

At an individual level, too, shared social identity also furnishes group members with a sense of efficacy and of personal control over their lives. This point has been shown in research led by Katharine Greenaway and colleagues (2015), which shows that people report a greater sense of personal control to the extent that they identify highly with their community, with a political party, with their nation or with humanity as a whole. Again, this pattern is not contingent on group success, being apparent, for example, among highly identified US Republicans immediately after their party had failed to win the 2012 presidential election.

An abundance of work on the importance of a sense of control for health underlines the importance of this observation for the present volume. Indeed, the World Happiness Report identifies this as one of the 'six pillars' of life satisfaction (Helliwell et al., 2013). Yet, while perceived control is generally thought to have personal origins, social identity research suggests that it actually has its basis in group identities and identifications.

Conclusion

The theorising and evidence that supports the social identity approach has been built up forensically over nearly half a century. However, it is only in the past decade that the approach has been applied specifically to the domain of health (Haslam et al., 2018; Haslam et al., 2009; Jetten et al., 2012). Nevertheless, in this comparatively short time, the evidence-base and impact of the approach has increased exponentially, so that there are now well over 400 publications that speak to its utility. Obviously in this short chapter, it is impossible to do justice to this literature. Nevertheless, our goal has been to give readers a sense of the thinking that informs the approach and a flavour of the evidence that backs this up. In simplified terms, the model that this work supports is summarised by Figure 4.1.

The key point to take from this model is that there are important, if complex, interconnections between social identity, group behaviour and health and that the capacity for social identity to deliver positive health outcomes rests on its capacity to give individual persons access to important resources.

These resources are not only psychological but also material. They relate not only to people's *sense of* connection, support, meaning and control, but also to the *social reality* of these things. This is because, as social identity theorists grasped from the outset, groups are not only fundamental to our sense of self, but also to our capacity to *do things* in the world,

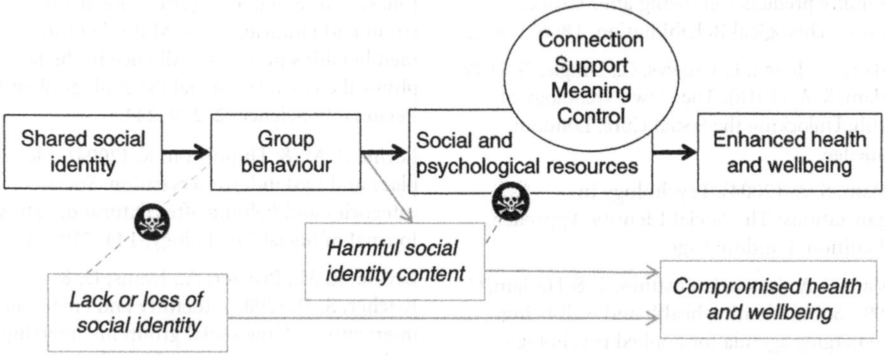

Figure 4.1 Shared social identity and health

in particular, through processes of collective action and social change. Among other things, they provide a basis for us to help those people who are disadvantaged and in need, to build hospitals and care homes, and to make progress in science and society. It is for this reason, then, that social identities are vital not just for the health of individuals but for that of society as a whole.

Acknowledgement

Work on this chapter was supported by Fellowships from the Australian Research Council to the first and second authors (FL110100199, FT110100238).

References

Cacioppo, J. T. & Patrick, W. (2008). Loneliness: Human Nature and the Need for Social Connection. New York, NY: W. W. Norton.

Cocking, C. & Drury, J. (2004). Generalization of efficacy as a function of collective action and intergroup relations: Involvement in an anti-roads struggle. Journal of Applied Social Psychology, **34**, 417–444.

Cruwys, T., Dingle, G., Haslam, S. A. et al. (2013). Social group memberships protect against future depression, alleviate depression symptoms, and prevent depression relapse. Social Science and Medicine, **98**, 179–186.

Cruwys, T., Haslam, S. A., Dingle, G. A., Haslam, C. & Jetten, J. (2014). Depression and social identity: An integrative review. Personality and Social Psychology Review, **18**: 215–238.

Dingle, G. A., Brander, C., Ballantyne, J. & Baker, F. A. (2013). 'To be heard': The social and mental health benefits of choir singing for disadvantaged adults. Psychology of Music, **41**: 405–421.

Drury, J., Cocking, C. & Reicher, S. (2009). The nature of collective resilience: Survivor reactions to the 2005 London bombings. International Journal of Mass Emergencies and Disasters, **27**: 66–95.

Durkheim, E. (1951) Suicide. New York: Free Press (originally published 1897).

Greenaway, K., Haslam, S. A., Branscombe, N. R. et al. (2015). From "we" to "me": Group identification enhances perceived personal control with consequences for health and well-being. Journal of Personality and Social Psychology, **109**: 53–74.

Haslam, C., Cruwys, T. & Haslam, S. A. (2014). "The we's have it": Evidence for the distinctive benefits of group engagement in enhancing cognitive health in ageing. Social Science and Medicine, **120**: 57–66.

Haslam, C., Holme, A., Haslam, S. A. et al. (2008). Maintaining group memberships: Social identity continuity predicts well-being after stroke. Neuropsychological Rehabilitation, **18**: 671–691.

Haslam, C., Jetten, J., Cruwys, C., Dingle, G. D. & Haslam, S. A. (2018). The New Psychology of Health: Unlocking the Social Cure. London: Routledge.

Haslam, S. A. (2004). Psychology in Organizations: The Social Identity Approach, 2nd edition. London: Sage.

Haslam, S. A., Jetten, J., Postmes, T. & Haslam, C. (2009). Social identity, health and well-being: An emerging agenda for applied psychology. Applied Psychology, **58**: 1–23.

Haslam, S. A., Reicher, S. D. & Levine, M. (2012). When other people are heaven, when other people are hell: How social identity determines the nature and impact of social support. In Jetten, J., Haslam, C. & Haslam, S. A., editors, The Social Cure: Identity, Health, and Well-Being. Hove: Psychology Press, pp. 157–174.

Helliwell, J. F., Layard, R. & Sachs, J. (2013). World Happiness Report. See www.earth.columbia.edu/sitefiles/file/Sachs%20Writing/2012/World%20Happiness%20Report.pdf.

Holt-Lunstad, J., Smith, T. B. & Layton, J. B. (2010). Social relationships and mortality risk: A meta-analytic review. PLoS Medicine, **7**; doi: 10.1371/journal.pmed.1000316.

House, J. S., Landis, K. R. & Umberson, D. (1988). Social relationships and health. Science, **241**: 540–545.

Iyer, A., Jetten, J., Tsivrikos, D., Postmes, T. & Haslam, S. A. (2009). The more (and the more compatible) the merrier: Multiple group memberships and identity compatibility as predictors of adjustment after life transitions. British Journal of Social Psychology, **48**, 707–733.

Jetten, J., Branscombe, N. R., Haslam, S. A. et al. (2015). Having a lot of a good thing: Multiple important group memberships as a source of self-esteem. PLoS One, **10**: e0131035.

Jetten, J., Haslam, C. & Haslam, S. A., editors (2012). The Social Cure: Identity, Health and Well-Being. Hove: Psychology Press.

Jetten, J., Haslam, C., Haslam, S. A., Dingle, G. & Jones, J. M. (2014). How groups affect our health and well-being: The path from theory to policy. Social Issues and Policy Review, **8**: 103–130.

Jones, J. M. & Jetten, J. (2011). Recovering from strain and enduring pain: Multiple group memberships promote resilience in the face of physical challenges. Social Psychological and Personality Science, **2**, 239–244.

Levine R. M. & Thompson, K. (2004). Identity, place and bystander intervention: Social categories and helping after natural disasters. Journal of Social Psychology, **144**: 229–245.

Levine, R. M., Prosser, A., Evans, D. & Reicher, S. D. (2005). Identity and emergency intervention: How social group membership and inclusiveness of group boundaries shapes helping behaviour. Personality and Social Psychology Bulletin, **31**: 443–453.

Novelli, D., Drury, J., Reicher, S. & Stott, C. (2013). Crowdedness mediates the effect of social identification on positive emotion in a crowd: A survey of two crowd events. PLoS One, **8**: e78983.

Reicher, S. D. & Haslam, S. A. (2006). Rethinking the psychology of tyranny: The BBC Prison Study. British Journal of Social Psychology, **45**: 1–40.

Sani, F. (2012). Group identification, social relationships, and health. In Jetten, J., Haslam, C. & Haslam, S. A., editors, The Social Cure: Identity, Health, and Well-Being. Hove: Psychology Press, pp. 21–37.

Seymour-Smith, M., Cruwys, T., Haslam, S. A. & Brodribb, W. (2017). Loss of group memberships predicts depression in postpartum mothers. Social Psychiatry and Psychiatric Epidemiology, **52**: 201–210; doi: 10.1007/s00127-016-1315-3.

Steffens, N. K., Haslam, S. A., Schuh, S., Jetten, J. & van Dick, R. (2016). A meta-analytic review of social identification and health in organizational contexts. Personality and Social Psychology Review, **21**: 303–335; doi: 10.1177/1088868316656701.

Tajfel, H. (1972). La catégorisation sociale (English trans.). In Moscovici, S., editor, Introduction à la psychologie sociale. Paris: Larousse, vol. **1**, pp. 272–302.

Tajfel, H. & Turner, J. C. (1979). An integrative theory of intergroup conflict. In Austin, W. G. & Worchel, S., editors, The Social Psychology of Intergroup Relations. Monterey, CA: Brooks/Cole, pp. 33–47.

Tajfel, H., Flament, C., Billig, M. G. & Bundy, R. F. (1971). Social categorization and intergroup behaviour. European Journal of Social Psychology, **1**: 149–177.

Turner, J. C. (1982). Towards a redefinition of the social group. In Tajfel, H., editor, Social Identity and Intergroup Relations. Cambridge: Cambridge University Press, pp. 15–40.

Turner, J. C. (1991). Social Influence. Milton Keynes: Open University Press.

Turner, J. C (2005). Explaining the nature of power: A three-process theory. European Journal of Social Psychology, **35**: 1–22.

Turner, J. C., Hogg, M. A., Oakes, P. J., Reicher, S. D. & Wetherell, M. S. (1987). Rediscovering the Social Group: A Self-Categorization Theory. Cambridge, MA: Basil Blackwell.

Turner, J. C., Oakes, P. J., Haslam, S. A. & McGarty, C. (1994). Self and collective: Cognition and social context. Personality and Social Psychology Bulletin, **20**: 454–463.

Wilkinson, R. G. & Marmot, M. G., editors. (2003). Social Determinants of Health: The Solid Facts. New York, NY: World Health Organization.

Chapter 5

The Relevance of Social Science to Improving Health and Healthcare

Daniel Maughan, Sue Bailey and Richard Williams

The Relevance of Social Science to Improving Health and Healthcare

Reading the first part of this book presents a striking contrast between current preoccupations in healthcare systems and the science presented here. In other words, between extant public concerns about entitlement to, funding of, and delivering healthcare in the second decade of the twenty-first century and the contents of Chapters 2, 3 and 4.

Healthcare systems and the people who fund, run and deliver them are, arguably, necessarily acutely sensitive to the socio-economic environment in which countries sit. The potential capabilities of healthcare continue to develop at increasingly rapid rates. By contrast, we live in a world in which the resources available are affected by austerity and in which the spread of affluence between the most advantaged people and the least affluent continues to grow. This is contributing to an increasing gap between potential capability and actual capacity, which appears to be expanding rapidly. In this context, it is not surprising that funders, managers and practitioners appear to be preoccupied with regulation, measurement and gaining, albeit inconsistently, understanding of what might seem to be the basics of human interactions, openness, transparency and accountability. These approaches are seen to be means to secure healthcare of rising quality in austere financial circumstances. So, is this book irrelevant to these all-too-real challenges that face healthcare systems?

Of course, more finance is definitely required by health and healthcare systems. But we do not deny the reality that healthcare is unlikely to be, and cannot be allowed to be, a bottomless pit into which money is poured: it is a pit full of leaks that cause waste, and, to date, little thought has been given to what sustainability could look like. We are struck that, instead, this pit must become a reservoir for rich reserves that are fundamental to success. They include a healthcare workforce that is valued and sustained and developing emotional intelligence in health systems in ways that understand and deliver values-based practice services.

Clearly, this book is intended to challenge readers to think within a different frame, set by current events and circumstances, and to enquire about whether or not we are delivering healthcare that is as informed by the social sciences sitting alongside the biological sciences, as well as they might. Might meeting current challenges in prevention at all ages, and keeping people well, equitably and with equality of access to services throughout their lives, and, crucially, into extending late life, be eased if we could harness evidence from the social sciences? Might this approach not increase costs but, instead assist us in using what new resources there may be in more effective ways? Might the contents of this book assist us to meet the challenges posed by Heath and Abassi that are summarised in Chapter 1?

The Scope of Section 1

To this end, Section 1 of this book introduces a social philosophical view of people's experience of life and their health, mental health and mental ill health. It outlines an approach to improving people's physical and mental health that is based on social connectedness and social identity.

The second chapter in this section (Chapter 2) takes a novel social philosophical approach to introduce the concepts of social causation and social construction. It identifies six features of the human condition that impact how we view health and ill health. The feature of embodiment, in other words, that our behaviours are affected both by the biology of our brains, and vice versa, sits alongside and contrasts with other features, such as agency, sociability and evaluation. Smith asserts that social groups generate rules and different ways of 'being' and 'doing' that are then attributed with social value. People use these group norms to evaluate their own and other people's behaviours and characteristics and to review their needs for change, development, learning and giving. Managing tensions between these different features of the human condition, for instance between embodiment (a person's biology), sociability (e.g. their conforming or otherwise to group norms) and agency, is what Smith argues is integral to mental health.

The next two chapters (3 and 4) build on this view by asserting that social groups 'frame and inform our beliefs and values, drive our thoughts, influence our emotions and shape our behaviour'. The authors define the impact that social group networks have on mental illness and health, and they put forward a social identity approach to health. This approach suggests that group identities, when internalised and recognised as part of each person, influence health behaviour and outcomes, whether good or bad. They commend the '5S' model, which encourages persons to fully engage with their existing social groups and discover and engage with new networks, with the ultimate aim of improving their health. The authors argue that improved connectedness and socialisation reduces psychosocial isolation and provides meaning, direction and purpose to people's life choices as well as access to psychosocial and material resources, thereby improving both agency and control. Engagement with social groups is clearly a fundamental part of living a mentally healthy life, and developing multiple social identities, through engaging with multiple groups, provides each person with a safety net, to guard against the prevailing psychosocial stressors that exist throughout life.

The Challenge

These topics are relevant in opening this book. Care systems that believe they have no time to reflect and instead function in ways that deal ineffectively with ever-increasing demands are arguably demonstrating learned helplessness and/or frozen watchfulness. In this projection, each layer experiences a sense of being relentlessly ground down in a slow-motion version of the film, *Groundhog Day*. However, what has been squeezed out of the system is emotional intelligence and resilience. We think that these qualities are, in essence, what concern Heath.

We believe that, if most people were given time for reflective thinking, they would adopt a values-based approach to equitably delivered health and social care, which, if nurtured, would work together across agencies, ages and geography. Services informed by these approaches would make sense to patients, clients and carers and help them be better able to understand and use, and choose wisely, from an open-all-hours service.

Services and the Public Working Together on Disease Prevention and Empowering Patients

How then can the authors of this book expect policymakers, the public and practitioners to take a leap of faith into an approach to healthcare that embraces social connectedness and partnerships that are built on shared social identity?

The challenge to the authors of the rest of this book, and which is set for them by this first section is how to bring practical meaning to what is known to many of us who think and work in groups. What happens in the space between groups and persons? And how do we build a social scaffolding approach to health and social care that looks to animal models of group behaviour (geese are a favourite) rather than production-line mentalities?

We hope that contributing the knowledge that derives from social science may assist funders, managers and practitioners to wrestle more successfully with what appear to be, and may indeed be, impossible tasks. In parts of the UK, these challenges, and our current approaches to managing them, have overflowed into tense industrial relationships between the staff who discharge services and the people who are responsible for policy and funding, and there is a growing sense of disrespect. Avoiding these pitfalls is no small task. More positively, we hope that drawing together the knowledge, experience and skill that this book represents will contribute to solving intractable problems.

Chapter 6

The Social Determinants of Mental Health

Kamaldeep S. Bhui, Oliver Quantick and David Ross

Summary

This chapter connects the everyday experience of poor mental health and mental illness with the complex social nexus in which these problems arise. Prevention and recovery might be improved if we assert that social justice, equality and equity are worthy values and essential for a functional and successful society as well as a healthy society. Inequalities, inequity and injustice are drivers of poor health. Some groups, especially those that carry stigmatised social identity or with multiple social disadvantage, are especially affected. Divisions in the social construction of wellness and illness along mind and body lines are unhelpful and serve to fragment efforts for healthy societies and better healthcare. Public health intervention is population-based, universal and engages communities; people are empowered as active citizens who have responsibility for their own and societal health. Ensuring parity of esteem and better mind–body interventions are needed; the spatial and social clustering of illness requires us to revise our models of mind and health.

Introduction

Public health is defined by the UK's Faculty of Public Health as 'The science and art of promoting and protecting health and well being, preventing ill health and prolonging life through the organised efforts of society'.

This definition locates the causes of ill health and the remedies in the realms of personal and societal agency, and not only in the remit of health practitioners. Although the latter have a role as members of society to make prevention a reality for themselves, families and communities, they play a special part in preventing further ill health for people who suffer mental illness and are seeking help for it.

Other chapters in this book attend to the relational and social fabric that enables people to flourish; it is made of good and trusting relationships, and material conditions that permit thought about purpose and meaning beyond survival. Personal agency and unique and collective contributions to society contribute to one's own sense of purpose and well-being (see Chapters 3, 4 and 23). Although public health interventions are intended to be population-based and delivered in partnership with the public, this does not preclude the societal place of health and social care agencies and the necessary partnerships with local government, transport hubs and agencies, law enforcement, housing agencies, schools or the organisations responsible for green space and clean air.

The social determinants of ill health, including mental illness, are well established and have been known of since the early 1980s when the Black Report was first published

(Gray, 1982). Despite the clear links between inequalities and poor health, and between social causes of sickness and shortened and blighted lives, little progress has been made (Sim & Mackie, 2006; Smith et al., 1990). Social determinants of inequalities remain of great importance for health. Marmot's recent work, for example, highlights how almost all health indices in the population are subject to the influence of structural disadvantage (Marmot, 2005; Marmot and Bell, 2016). Research shows that mothers of highest socio-economic status, for example, who live in mixed- or high-status rather than low-status neighbourhoods, had a 65 per cent lower risk of having no friends in the neighbourhood, and 41 per cent lower risk of depression or anxiety (Albor et al., 2014).

The fundamental principle is that social justice and fairness are essential values in a society (see Chapter 24 for coverage of public values in greater depth). Being born into social inequalities and being destined to have a shorter life are not fair. Nor is it fair that poverty is so rife, even in high-income countries, and unemployment high, because poverty and unemployment lead to poor nutrition and premature mortality, albeit through the onset of serious illness. The evidence that large income differences have damaging health and social consequences is strong, and inequality is increasing in many countries (Pickett & Wilkinson, 2015). Furthermore, inequality of income appears to produce social stratification and this explains differences in health status between countries (Wilkinson & Pickett, 2007).

Health-risk behaviours, including smoking, low levels of exercise, poor educational progression and excessive drug and alcohol use, are all patterned by social status and poverty. Marmot's work sets that out clearly. However, intervention requires that we better understand mechanisms and that we develop ways of intervening in the real world as compared with in laboratories or in the artificial setting of clinical trials. Just as the safety and security of our society, especially in the high-income countries, may be overestimated, so the fragility and vulnerability of our societies to new social threats are underestimated (Khan et al., 2016). Thus, healthcare is not only about health professionals and agencies, but also about the political economy in which we consider how to tackle illness. Furthermore, the salience that society gives to health, as an embodied biological asset, is important, but so is considering health as representing social possibilities that are strongly influenced by life-course experiences, nurturing and nourishment.

We argue that policy decisions should be evidence-based, rather than driven by prejudice or unfounded fears; and that a focus on building inclusive, cost-effective health services to promote collective health security is important if we are to build healthy societies. The trend towards greater socio-economic inequalities should be acknowledged and fully considered in planning long-term solutions. Furthermore, this approach fosters a progressive, productive and socially resilient society, with greater benefits that help people to flourish.

Personal Illustrations

In this section, we offer two brief vignettes. They are stories about fictitious people and neither describes persons of our acquaintance. However, the dilemmas faced by Mary and Dave are far from uncommon.

Mary is 41 and has not been able to find work for the past decade. She lives alone, is overweight, suffers from type II diabetes and has recently been told that she is in the first stages of kidney failure.

Dave made an error at work, six months ago, that led to a great loss to the small business he has worked in since he left school 18 years ago. Since the incident, he has been experiencing high levels of anxiety and has symptoms of depression. His symptoms have become so severe that he is currently unable to perform his work duties and has been signed off sick by his GP, and this has exacerbated his feelings of guilt.

These are examples of common health problems, which, at one and the same time, are inherently social, political and economic as much as they are personal and idiosyncratic health tragedies. Illness, life events and social adversity require an adaptive response to improve health. But we must also improve the conditions in which people live and work if we are to protect their health, prevent their ill health and facilitate their recovery. A social context of poverty or poor social networks and few resources, whether material and/or interpersonal, means that people living in poorer and less cohesive neighbourhoods are less able to respond in timely and effective ways to overcome physical and psychosocial stressors.

Bramley et al.'s report on poverty (Bramley et al., 2016) and its impacts on health concludes that:

- Healthcare accounts for the largest portion of additional public spending associated with poverty.
- Use of healthcare services and their costs are strongly related to immediate and historical poverty.
- Around a quarter of all spending on acute hospital care and spending on primary care can be attributed to greater use of these services by people who live in poverty.

The evidence suggests that poverty and other social determinants of poor physical and mental health reflect circumstances into which people are born, grow up, live, work and grow old. These circumstances are, in turn, shaped by a wider set of forces, such as economics, social policies and politics. Social determinants deserve particular attention because they are modifiable, influence health outcomes many years later and so might be the most effective targets for preventive interventions. And, if intervention occurs at the earliest point in our life-courses and at a population level, it is likely to yield the greatest benefits, at the lowest cost and for many years and generations later. These principles underlie the public health approach, which offers opportunities to tackle upstream factors and to reduce inequality (Marmot, 2006).

Health: A Multifaceted Phenomenon

The oft-quoted definition of health created during the constitution of the World Health Organization (WHO) in 1948 states that 'health is a state of complete, physical, mental and social well-being and not merely the absence of disease or infirmity' (Callahan, 1973). This definition has been criticised because it would 'leave most of us unhealthy most of the time' (Smith, 2008). Yet, it reflects the time when it was written, when there was an almost unique emphasis on disease and illness, and insufficient awareness of positive states of health and wellbeing.

Implicit in this proposition is that there are many aspects of wellness that are not attended to for patients who are ill and for people who are not ill but are not functioning as well as they would like. There is also a growing societal crisis in that the overall burden of disease is growing, due to a larger ageing population with, proportionately, fewer people in work. The notion of wellbeing has to be a capability, irrespective of illness and disability, and might be better grasped as functionality, and as people having a purposeful and meaningful life. Chapter 2 comments on wellbeing, health and ill health as social contructions.

Indeed, a more recent, alternative definition has been offered, proposing that health is 'the ability to adapt and self-manage in the face of social, physical and emotional challenges' (Jadad & O'Grady, 2008). This definition takes in the notion of agency (see Chapters 2 and 22). It is important because subjective measurement can take place regarding perceived health according to each person's preferences, and this can sit alongside the measurement of illness by structured and professional definitions. Indeed, many risk and protective factors may influence illness and wellness, in similar or different ways, although establishing the evidence-base for this requires much investment in research and interventions.

Public health practice seeks to invoke 'all organised measures (whether public or private) to prevent disease, promote health and prolong life among the population as a whole' (WHO, 2014a). In order to achieve this, the public health approach aims to reduce the burden of disease by focusing on interventions at a population level. This may involve action that changes national legislation and/or policy, such as that to reduce second-hand smoking by banning smoking in public places (Myers et al., 2009), or a more targeted approach for those people who are at higher risk, such as the cross-government suicide prevention strategy (Department of Health, 2012). Population approaches offer universal interventions, which can be scaled up and applied to all, without tailoring; but there are also selective and indicated interventions that target populations at higher risk and those with clear signs of early illness, respectively.

Definitions of mental health, wellness, wellbeing and complete contentment offer philosophical as well as practical challenges. The definition of mental health, according to the World Health Organization, includes 'subjective well-being, perceived self-efficacy, autonomy, competence, intergenerational dependence and self-actualisation of one's intellectual and emotional potential, among others' (WHO, 2001). A state of wellbeing is one in which 'the individual realises his or her own abilities, can cope with the normal stresses of life, can work productively and fruitfully, and is able to make a contribution to his or her community'. Interestingly, this definition comments on a person's level of functioning within their surroundings. Mental health has also been proposed as 'an unstable continuum, where an individual's mental health may have many different possible values' (Keyes, 2002).

Mind and Body Synchrony

As observed in Chapter 1, one of the unhelpful distinctions made in scientific discourse is the notion that mind and body are, somehow, separate entities and that they exist in isolation from one another. Furthermore, they require different interventions. In this approach, medical and physical diseases are not considered to be the same as mental or psychiatric disorders because the latter often lack a clearly detectable biomarker or pathophysiology. The assumption here is that social and psychological markers are insufficient as a basis for defining illness and disease because these categories gain legitimacy from biomarkers to which illnesses are related. At the same time, the social experience and construction of illness and wellness are neglected for medical diseases and disorders that do have biomarkers.

The efforts to better target assessment and treatment bring a concentration of efforts to mental disorders, and their complexity as entities in which social factors are more prominent in the concerns of health professionals has resulted in a split between mental healthcare and the physical medical specialties. In England, but not in Scotland or Wales, this split is visible in the separation of the agencies that are responsible for providing the two groups of services. Not only are the services different in England, but the provider organisations, policy directions and investment sources are distinct and compete with each other for resources. Recently, this unhelpful position has been questioned by the notion that 'parity of esteem' as a principle should challenge discriminatation against people who have mental disorders (Millard & Wessely, 2014). This matter is considered in greater depth in Chapter 8.

There are two consequences of a parity of esteem approach. First, when there are service challenges due to economic pressures, mental health services should not be penalised by financial cuts that are disproportionate to the burden of disease, while protecting disproportionate investment for physical disease, rather than recognising that integrated care will have better outcomes (Limb, 2014). Second, premature mortality among people who have mental illness must not continue unabated (Thornicroft, 2011). Economic and biological consequences of mental illness are mediated, in part, through material deprivation and poverty, nutritional neglect, loss of employability and stigma, which are associated with mental illnesses. We also know that material deprivation and poverty are likely to describe contexts in which there is a higher incidence of serious mental illnesses, and these experiences may be of aetiological significance (Hudson, 2005). When combined, these two forces produce a compelling argument for improving the social scaffolding of a society, for supporting people from birth to death as empowered citizens, consumers and agents in society. They should not be rendered passive recipients of health interventions only at times when their serious disease states become evident, or when they are evidently distressed and they experience the biological consequences of distress, to the extent that a biomarker is found.

Although the Royal College of Psychiatrists' campaign on parity of esteem challenges the stigma and frank discrimination against mental disorders, it also reflects a failure in science and society to discern the interaction between medical disease or illness and the social environment. This is the case for both physical and psychiatric conditions. We know depression and heart disease, and depression and cancer, each show reverse causality of approximately a two- to three-fold higher level in either direction (Charlson et al., 2011; Jiang et al., 2002). The premature mortality associated with mental illness is largely due to heart disease and cancer, lack of active treatment and more unnatural deaths (Thornicroft, 2011). Prescribing antipsychotics contributes to the higher risk of cardiac disease and may cause mortality in patients who have mental illness. Thus, for a long time, obesity and poor glycaemic control were considered to be inevitable and an acceptable adverse effect, given the risks of not treating people with mental illness (Jones et al., 2013). Separating illnesses based on mind and body makes no sense. Segmenting social causation as being only relevant to mental illness is a failure of imagination and of science and is an aspect of social construction (see Smith's account in Chapter 2). The parity of esteem campaign seeks to provide better integration of health interventions with the intention of improving the outcome for people, regardless of their health conditions and whether or not they have these conditions in isolation or comorbidly.

Explanations for why comorbidities occur and what we should do to prevent them still rely on compartmentalised diagnoses, rather than notions of the greater total disease burden that arises in the context of poor environments in which people experience material and social disadvantages. Efforts to address these multiple disadvantages have failed, to date.

Perhaps this circumstance appropriately invokes notions of 'wicked diseases' for which the causes are multiple, persistent and forever changing, and the solutions have also to be equally 'wicked' (Petticrew et al., 2009)?

Singer has constructed a useful way of thinking about these multiple social causes and the multiple disease outcomes, which are all connected through social and biological interactions and vulnerabilities. Singer describes them as 'syndemic' (Singer, 2010). This concept has been applied to better understanding human immunodeficiency virus (HIV), violence and the impacts of discrimination in gay and bisexual men (Egan et al., 2011; Gonzalez-Guarda et al., 2011). The syndemic model suggests that disease and illness are more likely to occur where risky social conditions are present, where social protection is absent and where biological risk factors are triggered. The expression of a particular disease depends on the precise expression of risk factors and ways of coping. Where there is severe and multiple disadvantage, there is likely to be more illness and more comorbid states, leading to a disproportionate burden of illness. This clustering effect is shaped by the geographical space in which material deprivation occurs and in which disease emerges. It provides a potent mixture of an unequal, unhealthy and substantially less resilient or successful locale. The intersection of poor health localities with wealthier urban areas has not improved the health indices of residents. Public health has to be concerned about the margins of society in which excluded people live, in severe and multiply disadvantageous conditions. Therefore, public health practice relates to social policy, politics and societal responsibilities (Campion et al., 2013).

Biosocial Interactions

The difficulties with defining health, and particularly mental health, remain due to the complex interactions between biology and environments that are mediated and moderated by persons and populations of people. People's psychosocial states, their social circumstances and their lifestyle choices all influence their health. This complex interaction is highlighted by the King's Fund, which has stated that health is 'determined by a complex interaction between individual characteristics, lifestyle and the physical, social and economic environment' (The King's Fund, 2015). The King's Fund went as far as arguing that these broader determinants are more important than healthcare in ensuring a healthy population. This claim may appear less challenging to readers when they have read this book because it raises this possibility in a range of different circumstances. They include how particular people perceive their own needs and aspirations for recovery (see Chapters 7, 15, 17, 22 and 23).

Importantly, biosocial interactions emphasise that health and illness are social as well as medical matters. Smoking, obesity and road traffic accidents cause obvious medical problems, such as chronic obstructive pulmonary disease, heart disease, diabetes and trauma respectively. Individually, the medical problems caused by these behaviours all have established evidence-based treatment regimes. Conversely, the personal choice to indulge in certain behaviours and the social environment that permits these choices remain an underutilised pathway for reducing harmful behaviour. That is, the way in which each person chooses to act could be a matter for healthcare and social interventions because their choices also relate to their relationships and social identities. Importantly, greater understanding is required about how the social circumstances in which people live, work and relate influence them in making their decisions. This book enquires into these matters.

The Costs of Ill Health

The definition of health remains important because, if health is the overall aim, it is vital to know what this ideal entails so that the influences upon it can be understood, measured and quantified. The amount of disease at a population level has been quantified in recent years by using the Global Burden of Disease. The unit of measure is DALYs (disability-adjusted life years), which combines years of life lost due to premature mortality and years of life lost due to the amount of time lived in a state of less than full health. The DALY was developed to assess burden of disease consistently across diseases, risk factors and regions (WHO, 2014b). In 2010, mental disorders accounted for 183.9 million DALYs or 7.4 per cent of all DALYs, worldwide (Whiteford et al., 2010). The Health Survey for England has been conducted annually since 1991 and it gives a more localised illustration of the burden of disease (Health Survey for England, 2014).

These resources provide a quantifiable assessment of the burden of disease according to a specific condition and permit comparison over time. They allow assessment of the potential effect of interventions.

If we are interested in achieving a healthier population, it should be a priority for both healthcare services and the government to reduce the increasing burden of disease, and to limit the spiralling costs. The total costs of mental illness to the economy amount to £105 billion a year in the UK, and modelling from economic experts has shown that savings can emerge for every pound spent. But the political wisdom to invest now in health, to prevent future epidemics, is limited; much more is spent in crisis in acute care as compared with, for example, planning for new rail networks (HS2) or airports (another London airport), in which large sums are invested in the anticipation of rewards to society some 20 years ahead. However, there are significant impacts on people living in poverty and in need of welfare, housing and family support. These trade-offs between spend now and gain later appear not to gather traction in the realms of mental health, which further compounds the desolation, isolation and stigma experienced by people who live at the margins. Consequently, the numbers of people in these groups are likely to grow and not diminish. A Royal College of Psychiatrists' statement has suggested that there was less than £2 per annum spent per child, by some commissioning groups, at a time when suicide rates and distress in young people was a growing concern. By not intervening now, we leave children, and their children, to lifetimes of poverty and health disadvantage.

Developing Health Models

It could be argued that policymakers have misunderstood the nature of illness and have neglected or underestimated the ability of society to influence health. Perhaps this has arisen from the previously popular monocausal models of disease, first proposed by Koch and Pasteur (see Vineis, 2003)? Subsequent experience and research have shown that this approach is too simplistic and, in the past, it focused solely on individual pathogens and their eradication. This is not helpful when considering chronic disease or mental health, just as an overemphasis on particular genetic risks overlooks what in the environment turns on or off those genetic risks. Epidemiology has attempted to widen the perspective but still tends to oversimplify (Centers for Disease Control and Prevention, 2015). However, it does allow consideration of factors in society as well as individual factors.

A web of causation (leading to syndemics) demonstrates the interrelationship of multiple risk factors that contribute to the occurrence and expression of diseases, together with social ills. Although this approach has the advantage of being more complete, it is often difficult to design and to quantify. Despite this, using a web of causation that highlights multiple potential causes of ill health can help to fuel ideas about how to target intervention. This should be based on best evidence and, if unknown, should help to build the evidence-base.

A methodically constructed, expansive web can aid visualisation to enable potential intervention at any stage during people's life-courses. This also requires a better approach to understanding how risk factors intersect by age, gender, ethnic group, income, employment etc. (Ghavami et al., 2016). Populations such as, for example, children in care (Vinnerljung et al., 2006), ethnic groups (McKenzie et al., 2008), homeless people (Eynan et al., 2011), offenders (Fazel & Yu, 2011) and LGB (lesbian, gay and bisexual) people (Chakraborty et al., 2011), have been identified as being at higher risk of mental illness. They share exclusion, a lack of social and political agency, and experiences of stigma and vulnerability. It is possible and necessary for interventions to be designed, developed and targeted for these populations of people at primary, secondary and tertiary levels.

Our Life-Course and Its Stages

The life-course approach is a model that takes a holistic view of people's life stories and how the choices impact on their health, either independently or cumulatively, and can be illustrated, for example, by drawing a web of causation, as we have outlined. Thereby, a person's life-course is broken into specific eras that enable policymakers to more easily comprehend these complex interrelationships. Marmot emphasises the need for a life-course approach to understanding and tackling mental and physical health inequalities.

The UK Faculty of Public Health has used the life-course model to promote mental wellbeing, prevent mental illness and assess and increase the current evidence-base. The model used reflects the periods of humans' life-courses, including starting well, developing well, living well, working well and ageing well. Also included in the model is a section called the wider context. This covers all-encompassing interventions and improvements, such as access to green spaces, improving the built environment and asset-based approaches to community development.

The Main Types of Inequality

The main types of inequality are often grouped into social, economic and environmental. Inequality among people in society can influence each and every stage of their life-courses. Inequality and inequity, see Chapter 1, continue to exist and are the basis for the health gradient seen in the UK across socio-economic groups (Marmot et al., 2010).

Social inequality continues to exist across socio-economic groups, with different mortality rates depending on socio-economic group (Marmot et al., 2010). Gender also affects health behaviour and women report a higher burden of mental illness than do men (Kessler, 2003) despite males continuing to account for four of every five suicides in the UK.

Economically, wealth is linked to health, with increased debt resulting in 'increased mental disorder, even after adjustment for income and other sociodemographic variables' (Jenkins et al., 2008). Suicides in England have been linked to the financial crisis of the last 12 years, with regions that experienced the greatest rises in unemployment levels demonstrating the largest increases in suicides (Barr et al., 2012).

The environment in which each person lives has a great impact on their overall health. Living in a safe environment, which is free from discrimination and violence, improves people's mental health (Lindert & Levav, 2015). However, funding interventions to improve the environment is difficult, as 'current evidence is inadequate to inform the development of specific social capital interventions to combat mental illness' (De Silva et al., 2005).

Priorities For, and Possible Approaches to, Tackling Inequalities

Marmot has highlighted the inequality in society and subsequent inequality in health outcomes in the Whitehall studies. His career has focused on this societal division and, in 'Fair Society, Healthy Lives', the main recommendation is that the 'greatest gain is to give every child the best possible start' (Marmot et al., 2010). This means attempting to reduce the increasing social gradient that continues to adversely affect health.

Reducing this inequality is, arguably, a matter of fairness and social justice (see Chapter 24). Difficulties remain in targeting the poorest people in society in order to reduce inequality and inequity, with those people who are better off often benefiting proportionally more from interventions and improved services (Barat et al., 2004). This is the reason why the WHO has recommended a response called proportionate universalism (WHO, 2014c). It recommends making interventions available universally, but in ways that are calibrated proportionately to the level of disadvantage rather than focussing actions purely on the most disadvantaged people who are at greatest risk. Adopting this approach overcomes the limitations of targeted programmes while providing action that is proportionate to people's different levels of need across the socio-economic gradient.

Due to the relative lack of evidence and the complexity of there being multiple risk factors that contribute towards social inequalities and inequity, a recurring difficulty lies in securing funding for potential interventions. This is particularly difficult when negotiating with a central government that is focused on a five-year parliamentary election cycle. This is especially the case when many of the interventions that are proposed require significant investment, with the possibility that benefits might not be seen for decades.

More success might be achieved by using social impact bonds that are based on a commitment from government to use a proportion of the savings that result from improved social outcomes to reward the non-government investors that fund the early intervention activities (Social Finance, 2009). So far in the UK, social finance methods have been used in a range of long-term schemes, such as prisoner rehabilitation, addressing the needs of chronic rough sleepers and, more recently, is being used by the English government's Department for Children, Schools and Families to support early intervention approaches for children and young people (Social Finance, 2014). Intermediaries and providers of technical assistance have been set up as more countries expand these schemes, such as the not-for-profit organisation, Social Finance Ltd. Further use of these bonds could help to encourage both public and private investment in longer-term social improvement schemes and should be considered, given the tendencies of governments toward adopting short-term priorities.

Reducing health inequalities is likely to benefit society in many broader spheres, such as increasing productivity, tax revenue and welfare payments, and reducing treatment costs. Both central and local action is required to achieve this end. Risk factors and protective factors act upon each person differently depending on, for example, how they interact with their families and their communities as well as with the social structures to which their population belongs. Therefore, interventions that attempt to reduce the effects of adverse social determinants on physical and mental health require joined-up, cross-sector working at multiple levels.

Reflections on the Personal Experiences

Mary is 41 and has not been able to find work for the past decade. She lives alone, is overweight, suffers from type II diabetes and has recently been told that she is in the first stages of kidney failure.

Mary's unemployment and her living alone results in her being socially isolated from her peers and community. She does not participate in community or local workplace health promotion schemes and is disengaged from managing her diabetes. As a result, she misses out on regular diabetic screening, has experienced recent kidney failure and, soon, is likely to experience deteriorating eyesight. Her weight limits her mobility and she is increasingly reluctant to leave her flat. Events throughout her life-course, such as her limited educational opportunities, influence her employment prospects and have contributed to her current situation. Despite this, effective interventions that can help Mary to increase her participation in her local community and engage with health services could assist in improving her life and limit the rapid progression of her ill health.

Dave made an error at work, six months ago, that led to a great loss to the small business he has worked in since he left school 18 years ago. Since the incident, he has been experiencing high levels of anxiety and has symptoms of depression. His symptoms have become so severe that he is currently unable to perform his work duties and has been signed off sick by his GP, and this has exacerbated his feelings of guilt.

Comparing Dave's performance now with that prior to his mistake at work shows that he is unable to function effectively. His GP has recognised his symptoms of depression, but Dave is unable to get access to the care he needs due to long waiting times for specialist services. Arguably, his situation is a matter of inequity but, also, inequality also. His lack of work is causing increasing concerns about his reduced income and mounting debt, and this is exacerbating his current feelings of worthlessness. An investment in social bonds and improving mental healthcare provision may help to halt Dave's deterioration. Multiple life-course factors as well as social inequality have influenced the position in which Dave currently finds himself. Cohesive change on local and national levels may help to improve the opportunities available to Dave and others in similar situations. This would provide him with better opportunities for regaining good health and returning to work.

Work Stress

The economic costs of work stress to the British economy are considerable (Chandola, 2010), amounting to 0.9 per cent of UK gross domestic product (GDP) in 2007 (Confederation of British Industry, 2010). Work stress can lead to poor physical health, psychosocial distress and mental ill health (Eskelinen et al., 1991; Nieuwenhuijsen et al., 2010). Work stressors can take different forms depending on the characteristics of people's workplaces, and may be unique to an organisation or an industry (see Chapters 27 and 28; Karasek & Theorell, 1990). Theoretical models of stress consider it to be either related to adverse life events and stressful environments, each person's physiological and psychosocial responses to stressors, or a transactional interaction between persons and their environments (Cahill, 1996; Cooper et al, 2001; Cox, 1993; Cox et al., 2000; Florio et al., 1998).

Cahill (1996), Cooper et al. (2001) and Marine et al. (2006) describe interventions that target people or organisations that are segmented as preventive interventions at primary, secondary or tertiary levels (De Jonge & Dollard, 2002). Bhui et al's systematic review found that interventions that targeted individual persons showed larger effects when compared with the effects of organisational interventions on personal outcomes such as levels of depression and anxiety (Bhui et al., 2012a). However, personal interventions did not improve organisational outcomes such as absenteeism, which is the most important indicator of loss of organisational productivity.

In a qualitative study of the National Health Services (NHS) in the UK, private organisations and non-governmental organisations, adverse working conditions and management practices were common causes of work stress (Bhui et al., 2016). Management practices might be improved, to address unrealistic demands, lack of support, unfair treatment, low levels of latitude for making decisions, lack of appreciation, imbalances between effort made and reward gained, conflicting roles, lack of transparency and poor communication. Organisational interventions were perceived as effective if they improved managers' skills, and included taking exercise and breaks, and ensured adequate time for planning work tasks. Personal interventions used outside work were important to prevent and remedy stress. Tackling work stress is essential given the need for people to continue working into their older ages. Yet this task is challenging in the face of current economic circumstances and organisational pressures to promote workers' performance, given recent shortages of skilled staff. However, meaningful work itself provides health gains for workers. These conditions in which workers can flourish include a balance between their effort and rewards, and the demands of work and the control they have over it.

Public Health Interventions for 'Wicked' Problems

Public health includes an understanding of the relational and social factors that cause illness and which require modification to prevent and reduce the impact of illness. However, social and relational resources are also fundamental to solving the 'wicked' problems of inequalities and inequity. There are many examples that show the potential power of social relations, social action and public engagement in prevention, which go beyond the roles and work of the conventional health agencies.

Suicide on the railways is one such challenge. Although it affects a small number of people who take their lives, it also affects people who attempt to harm themselves, the families and friends of people who kill themselves or attempt harm, members of the public who observe tragic events and train staff. Also, it has major impacts on the economy (Bhui, 2014). Intervening through conventional health services leads to mental health assessments that often conclude, according to police sources, that a person is not detainable and, therefore, is discharged after being removed from the train tracks.

Partnerships between local police and health services are now being tested. Transport hubs might become places for promoting health, at which vigilant passengers can show concern for one another, but also from whence health messages about self-care, nutrition, exercise and the impacts of commuting on people's health might be offered. Healthier and more pleasant transport environments can also benefit train staff.

Similarly, terrorism, might be better understood and prevented if a community participatory approach were taken to reduce extremist thinking and radicalisation (Bhui et al.,

2012b). Without community participation, solutions are not grounded in the daily realities of young people who are at greater risk, and they may make matters worse by stigmatising the very communities that wish to be part of the solution.

Thus, social networks and our shared human capital can all work in favour of healthier societies and as a key mechanism for improving the health and wellbeing of the population in general, for all disease outcomes. This does require us to take a radical re-look at the ways in which we understand poor health and environments and biological risk factors and how they interact. Thereby, the social-relational capital that we possess can be marshalled more effectively and, perhaps, that might alter the risks presented by biological factors and the poorer fabric of society. However, political will to alter these matters is also fundamental to our healthier futures.

References

Albor, C., Uphoff, E. P., Stafford, M. et al. (2014). The effects of socioeconomic incongruity in the neighbourhood on social support, self-esteem and mental health in England. Social Science and Medicine, **111**: 1–9.

Barat, L.Palmer, N. Basu, S. et al. (2004). Do malaria control interventions reach the poor? A view through the equity lens. American Journal of Tropical Medicine and Hygiene, 71: 174–178.

Barr, B. Taylor-Robinson, D. Scott-Samuel, A. McKee, M. & Stuckler, D. (2012). Suicides associated with the 2008–2010 economic recession in England: Time trend analysis. British Medical Journal, **345**: e5142.

Bhui, K. (2014). Preventing the tragedy of railway suicides. Mental Health Today, Mar–Apr: 24–7.

Bhui, K., Dinos, S., Galant-Miecznikowska, M., de Jongh, B. & Stansfeld, S. (2016). Perceptions of work stress causes and effective interventions in employees working in public, private and non-governmental organisations: A qualitative study. The British Journal of Psychiatry Bulletin, **40**, 318–325.

Bhui, K. S., Dinos, S., Stansfeld, S. A. & White, P. D. (2012a). A synthesis of the evidence for managing stress at work: A review of the reviews reporting on anxiety, depression, and absenteeism. Journal of Environmental and Public Health, **2012**: 515874.

Bhui, K. S., Hicks, M. H., Lashley, M. & Jones, E. (2012b). A public health approach to understanding and preventing violent radicalization. BMC Medicine, **10**: 16.

Bramley, G., Hirsch, D., Littlewood, M. & Watkins D. (2016). Counting the cost of UK poverty. See www.jrf.org.uk/report/counting-cost-uk-poverty.

Cahill, J. (1996). Psychosocial aspects of interventions in occupational safety and health. American Journal of Industrial Medicine, **29**: 308–313.

Callahan, D. (1973). The WHO definition of 'Health'. The Hastings Center Studies, **1**: 77–87.

Campion, J., Bhugra, D., Bailey, S. & Marmot, M. (2013). Inequality and mental disorders: Opportunities for action. The Lancet, **382**: 183–184.

Centers for Disease Control and Prevention (2015). The epidemiological triangle. See www.cdc.gov/bam/teachers/documents/epi_1_triangle.pdf.

Chakraborty, A., McManus, S., Brugha, T. S., Bebbington, P. & King, M. (2011). Mental health of the non-heterosexual population of England. The British Journal of Psychiatry, **198**: 143–148.

Chandola T. (2010). Stress at Work. London: The British Academy. See www.thebritishacademy.ac.uk/sites/default/files/Stress%20at%20Work.pdf.

Charlson, F. J., Stapelberg, N. J., Baxter, A. J. & Whiteford, H. A. (2011). Should Global Burden of Disease estimates include depression as a risk factor for coronary heart disease? BMC Medicine, **9**: 47.

Confederation of British Industry. (2010). On the path to recovery: Absence and workplace health survey 2010. See www.mas.org.uk/uploads/articles/CBI-Pfizer%20Absence%20Report%202010.

Cooper, C, Dewe, P. & O'Driscoll, M. (2001). Organizational Interventions. Organisational Stress. A Review and Critique of Theory, Research, and Applications. Thousand Oaks, CA: Sage.

Cox, T. (1993). Stress research and stress management: Putting theory to work (Health and Safety Executive contract research report no 61/1993). See www.hse.gov.uk/research/crr_pdf/1993/crr93061.pdf.

Cox, T., Griffiths, A., Barlow, C, R. R., Thomson, L. & Rial González, E. (2000). Organisational Interventions for Work Stress. Sudbury: HSE Books.

Department of Health (2012). Preventing suicide in England: A cross-government outcomes strategy to save lives. See https://assets.publishing.service.gov.uk/government/uploads/system/uploads/attachment_data/file/430720/Preventing-Suicide-.pdf.

De Jonge, J & Dollard, M. (2002). Stress in the Workplace: Australian Master OHS and Environment Guide. Sydney: CCH Australia Ltd.

De Silva, MJ, McKenzie, K., Harpham, T. & Huttly, S. (2005). Social capital and mental illness: A systematic review. Journal of Epidemiology and Community Health, **59**: 619–627.

Egan, J. E., Frye, V., Kurtz, S. P. et al. (2011). Migration, neighborhoods, and networks: Approaches to understanding how urban environmental conditions affect syndemic adverse health outcomes among gay, bisexual and other men who have sex with men. AIDS and Behavior, **15** (Suppl. 1): S35–50.

Eskelinen, L., Toikkanen, J., Tuomi, K., et al. (1991). Symptoms of mental and physical stress in different categories of municipal work. Scandinavian Journal of Work, Environment and Health, **17** (Suppl. 1): 82–86.

Eynan, R., Langley, J. & Tolomiczenko, G, (2011). The association between homelessness and suicidal ideation and behaviours: Results of a cross-sectional survey. Suicide and Life-Threatening Behaviour, **32**: 418–427.

Fazel, S. & Yu, R. (2011). Psychotic disorders and repeat offending: Systematic review and meta-analysis. Schizophrenia Bulletin, **37**: 800–810.

Florio, G. A., Donnelly, J. P. & Zevon, M. A. (1998). The structure of work-related stress and coping among oncology nurses in high-stress medical settings: A transactional analysis. Journal of Occupational Health Psychology, **3**: 227–242.

Ghavami, N., Katsiaficas, D. & Rogers, L. O. (2016). Toward an intersectional approach in developmental science: The role of race, gender, sexual orientation, and immigrant status. Advances in Child Development and Behavior, **50**: 31–73.

Gonzalez-Guarda, R. M., Florom-Smith, A. L. & Thomas, T. (2011). A syndemic model of substance abuse, intimate partner violence, HIV infection, and mental health among Hispanics. Public Health Nursing, **28**: 366–378.

Gray, A. M. (1982). Inequalities in health. The Black Report: A summary and comment. International Journal of Health Services: Planning, Administration, Evaluation, **12**: 349–380.

Health Survey for England (2014). Health, social care and lifestyles. See https://digital.nhs.uk/data-and-information/areas-of-interest/public-health/health-survey-for-england-health-social-care-and-lifestyles.

Hudson, C. G. (2005). Socioeconomic status and mental illness: Tests of the social causation and selection hypotheses. The American Journal of Orthopsychiatry, **75**: 3–18.

Jadad, A. R. & O'Grady,L. (2008). How should health be defined? British Medical Journal, **337**: a2900.

Jenkins, R., Bhugra, D. & Bebbington, P. (2008). Debt, income and mental disorder in the general population. Psychological Medicine, **38**: 1485–1493.

Jiang, W., Krishnan, R. R. & O'Connor, C. M. (2002). Depression and heart disease: Evidence of a link, and its therapeutic implications. CNS Drugs, **16**: 111–127.

Jones, M. E., Campbell, G., Patel, D. et al. (2013). Risk of mortality (including sudden cardiac death) and major cardiovascular events in users of olanzapine and other antipsychotics: A study with the General Practice Research Database. Cardiovascular Psychiatry and Neurology, **2013**: 647476.

Karasek, R. & Theorell, T. (1990). Healthy Work-Stress, Productivity and the Reconstruction of Working Life. New York, NY: Basic Books.

Kessler, R. (2003). Epidemiology of women and depression. Journal of Affective Disorders, **74**: 5–13.

Keyes, C. (2002). The mental health continuum: From languishing to flourishing in life. Journal of Health and Social Behaviour, **43**: 207–22.

Khan, M. S., Osei-Kofi, A., Omar, A. et al. (2016). Pathogens, prejudice, and politics: The role of the global health community in the European refugee crisis. The Lancet Infectious Diseases, **16**: e173–177.

Limb, M. (2014). Government is accused of back-pedalling on its commitment to "parity of esteem" between mental and physical healthcare. British Medical Journal, **348**: g3053.

Lindert, J. & Levav, I., editors (2015). Violence and Mental Health: Its Manifold Faces. Berlin: Springer.

Marine, A., Ruotsalainen, J., Serra, C. & Verbeek, J. (2006). Preventing occupational stress in healthcare workers. The Cochrane Database of Systematic Reviews, **2006**: CD002892.

Marmot, M. (2005). Social determinants of health inequalities. The Lancet, **365**: 1099–1104.

Marmot, M. (2006). Health in an unequal world. The Lancet, **368**: 2081–2094.

Marmot, M. & Bell, R. (2016). Social inequalities in health: A proper concern of epidemiology. Annals of Epidemiology, **26**: 238–240.

Marmot, M. A., Goldblatt, J., Boyce, P. et al. (2010). Strategic review of health inequlalities in England post-2010. See http://discovery.ucl.ac.uk/111743/.

McKenzie,K., Bhui,K., Nanchahal, K. & Blizard, B. (2008). Suicide rates in people of South Asian origin in England and Wales: 1993–2003. The British Journal of Psychiatry, **193**: 406–409.

Millard, C. & Wessely, S. (2014). Parity of esteem between mental and physical health. British Medical Journal, **349**: g6821.

Myers, D. G., Neuberger, J. S. & He, J. (2009). Cardiovascular effect of bans on smoking in public places. Journal of the American College of Cardiology, **54**: 1249–1255.

Nieuwenhuijsen, K., Bruinvels, D. & Frings-Dresen, M. (2010). Psychosocial work environment and stress-related disorders: A systematic review. Occupational Medicine (London), **60**: 277–286.

Petticrew, M., Tugwell, P., Welch, V. et al. (2009). Better evidence about wicked issues in tackling health inequities. Journal of Public Health, **31**: 453–456.

Pickett, K. & Wilkinson, R. G. (2015). Income inequality and health: A causal review. Social Science and Medicine, **128**: 316–326.

Sim, F. & Mackie, P. (2006). Health inequalities: The Black Report after 25 years. Public Health, **120**: 185–186.

Singer, M. (2010). Pathogen–pathogen interaction: A syndemic model of complex biosocial processes in disease. Virulence, **1**: 10–8.

Smith, G. D., Bartley, M. & Blane, D. (1990). The Black report on socioeconomic inequalities in health 10 years on. British Medical Journal, **301**: 373–377.

Smith, R. (2008). The end of disease and the beginning of health. See http://blogs.bmj.com/bmj/2008/07/08/richard-smith-the-end-of-disease-and-the-beginning-of-health/.

Social Finance (2009). Social impact bonds: Rethinking finance for social outcomes. See www.socialfinance.org.uk/sites/default/files/publications/sib_report_web.pdf.

Social Finance (2014). Social finance launches 3 social impact bonds to tackle youth homelessness. See www.socialfinance.org.uk/sites/default/files/news/social-finance-fair-chance-fund.pdf.

The King's Fund (2015). Mental health: Our work on mental health and mental health services. See www.kingsfund.org.uk/topics/mental-health.

Thornicroft, G. (2011). Physical health disparities and mental illness: The scandal of premature mortality. The British Journal of Psychiatry, **199**: 441–442.

Vineis, P. (2003). Causality in epidemiology. Sozial und Praventivmedizin, **48**: 80–87.

Vinnerljung, B., Hjern, A. & Lindblad, F. (2006). Suicide attempts and severe psychiatric morbidity among former child welfare clients: A national cohort study. Journal of Child Psychology and Psychiatry, **47**: 723–733.

Whiteford, H. A., Degenhardt, L., Rehm, J. et al. (2010). Global Burden of Disease attributable to mental and substance use disorders: Findings from the Global Burden of Disease Study. The Lancet, **382**: 1575–1586.

WHO (2001). The World Health Report 2001– Mental Health: New Understanding, New Hope. Geneva: World Health Organization.

WHO (2014a). Health impact assessment. See https://www.who.int/hia/about/glos/en/.

WHO (2014b). Global Burden of Disease. See www.who.int/topics/global_burden_of_disease /en/.

WHO (2014c). Social Determinants of Mental Health. Geneva: World Health Organization.

Wilkinson, R. & Pickett, K. (2007). The problems of relative deprivation: Why some societies do better than others. Social Science and Medicine, **65**: 13.

Chapter 7

Laidback Science: Messages from Horizontal Epidemiology

Alarcos Cieza and Jerome E. Bickenbach

Introduction

In the last two decades or so, mental health epidemiology has taught us two important messages. The first is that the personal and social burden of mental health conditions, long underestimated, is significantly higher than prevalent physical health conditions such as cancer or diabetes (Olesen and Leonardi, 2003; Andlin-Sobocki & Rehm, 2005).

Second, the cause of this burden is not mortality, or even morbidity, but disability, and, in particular, a wide range of psychosocial difficulties that shape the lived experience of persons who have these disorders and which profoundly affect their quality of life (WHO, 2006; Murray, et al., 2012). Psychosocial difficulties range from problems with attention and memory, emotional lability and listlessness, to disrupted sleep patterns, problems in managing daily routines and interacting with significant others and difficulties at work. They are best conceptualised as impairments and problems in activities and participation, in the light of the WHO's International Classification of Functioning, Disability and Health (ICF) (WHO, 2001). As such, these difficulties can be understood as outcomes of the interaction between the intrinsic features of a person's health state and both environmental and personal factors. In the ICF, the 'environment' constitutes all features of the external world, from climate, to products and the human-built environment, attitudes and all aspects of the social, economic and political world. It encompasses the entire class of 'social determinants of health' as typically defined (see Marmot & Wilkinson, 1999; WHO–CSDH, 2008). Among other things, psychosocial difficulties explore the boundaries, and impacts, of social connectedness as a primary determinant of mental health and quality of life. These epidemiological insights are entirely empirically grounded and tell us about what it means to live with mental ill health.

Over this same period of time, there has been a dramatic upsurge in interest in mental health diagnostics, with an increased reliance on neuroscience, neurotechnology and genomics, which is represented, for example, in the multi-billion dollar Brain Research through Advancing Innovative Neurotechnologies (BRAIN) Initiative that was launched by the US National Institute for Mental Health (NIMH) in 2013 (NIMH, 2013 and see NIMH, 2008) and other examples of what is called 'precision medicine'. The objective of this research agenda is to fundamentally recast mental health diagnostics in the biological language of the brain sciences to more completely understand the biological determinants of mental illness and enhance our prevention capacities and intervention strategies.

Conceptually, these two approaches represent fundamentally different intellectual strategies for understanding complex phenomena such as human behaviour. The neuroscientist is reductive, seeking more and more singular and linear aetiologies and predictable trajectories of disease processes. The epidemiologist, by contrast, seeks associative patterns in the given complexity, without striving for singular explanations. Recovery and improved quality of life are common objectives of both approaches. But neuroscientists focus the conversation on internal complexities, while epidemiologists seek understanding from external, and primarily social, determinants. Arguably, the future of public mental health depends on recognising this difference with a view to the approaches becoming synergetic rather than antagonistic.

Nonetheless, practically speaking, there is an undeniable tension, which, when it comes to research funding, becomes a direct conflict between the epidemiological exploration of the impact of social determinants and neurobiological research to expose salient biological antecedents of disease for diagnostics. One of the important objectives of the Royal College of Psychiatrists' sponsored seminars, which form the basis of this book, was to lay a foundation for better integrating these streams of research, and to explore health and social care strategies that could implement this coordination (see Chapter 26).

But these are long-term objectives that depend on both approaches being clear about their aims, strengths and weaknesses. Here biological scientists are on firmer ground, not only because the biological sciences are mature and relatively stable, but also because their focus is much more narrow. Social scientists confront a bewildering complexity of highly dynamic social environmental factors involving social identity, relationships of belonging and other experiences that are described in detail in other chapters, for which there are varying degrees of association with people's lived experience of mental health problems. New and radical strategies for making sense of this complexity and identifying social resources and ways of using them effectively need to be explored if our understanding of social determinants is to be transformed into practical actions and interventions in public mental health. The innovation of 'horizontal epidemiology' is one such innovative strategy.

PARADISE

The Conceptual Basis for Horizontal Epidemiology

Horizontal epidemiology was the product of a European Commission-funded, FP7 grant titled 'Psychosocial fActors Relevant to brAin DISorders in Europe' (PARADISE; Cieza et al., 2015b; http://paradiseproject.eu/). PARADISE was conducted with 10 partners from eight European countries and its objective was to develop and test an innovative epidemiological strategy for collecting data about the psychosocial difficulties or disabilities that people who have a variety of psychological and neurological conditions may experience. Instead of using the standard approach of inferring from diagnosis (that is, signs and symptoms) the kinds of problems people are likely to experience, a kind of vertical or 'silo'-like approach, the researchers hypothesised that people with vastly different mental health problems would be likely to experience similar if not identical psychosocial difficulties. In other words, in order to get the data needed to characterise the actual lived experience of people experiencing mental health problems, it makes more sense to go beyond diagnostic differences and collect information 'horizontally' across these conditions. In order to put the 'horizontal epidemiology' hypothesis to the test, the research was conducted with people who had a very diverse group of disorders including dementia, depression, epilepsy, migraine, multiple sclerosis, Parkinson's disease, schizophrenia, stroke and substance dependency.

The intuitions behind the hypothesis of horizontal epidemiology arose primarily from the theoretical model of disability found in the ICF, a model about which there is near complete consensus across the health professions. The ICF characterises disabilities as a complex interaction between underlying health conditions, such as diseases, disorders, injuries and the ageing process, the direct, bodily functional consequences of these interactions, which are called impairments, and the complex range of environmental factors which, once again, include but extend far beyond the standard set of social determinants. The model also assumes that certain personal factors such as coping style, experiences and memories, together with demographic factors, also play a role in the process of creating disabilities. Disabilities are defined as impairments at the level of body function, including mental functions, which, in interaction with environmental and personal factors, creates problems in performing all of the basic and complex actions, behaviours and roles that constitute the experience of human life. They run, for example, from the action of reading a newspaper, to basic and instrumental activities of daily living, to increasingly complex, and socially constructed, actions involved in having a social identity and belonging to various social roles, such as being a student, an employee, a parent or a member of a social, cultural or political organisation.

Disabilities, in short, are any level of decrement in functioning at the body, person or societal levels, which is an outcome of interactions between the intrinsic health state of a person and the complete context in which that person lives and acts, including both environmental and personal factors.

Given this model of what it means to have a disability that is associated with a mental health or neurological condition, it is plausible to assume that features of the lived experience of the mental health problem are likely to be similar, and similarly shaped by those environmental factors that are experienced in common by everyone. For example, the fact that everyone during an economic crisis will be subject to similar stresses and strains means that people, even with very different underlying health conditions, will end up experiencing similar psychosocial problems. Yet, the actual lived experience will be psychologically mediated and filtered through beliefs, values and experiences that transform external events into different, internal meanings. People with profoundly held religious beliefs are likely to experience financial hardship as a challenge or test, rather than the unalloyed adverse event that is experienced by the merchant banker.

Sometimes these similarities can be fully explained by common biological experiences: people with depression, anxiety disorder, schizophrenia, stroke, Parkinson's disease and substance abuse all experience sleep problems, since all of these conditions have impact on daily life patterns. Other commonalities seem explicable in terms of commonly experienced social determinants: stigmatising attitudes impact on the lives of anyone with a visible, socially disvalued condition, be it depression, stroke or substance abuse. Clinicians who work with patients who have neurological and psychiatric disorders are very familiar with the fact that there are common difficulties that their patients experience. There is also some research that supports this clinical experience (Leonardi et al., 2009; and Cieza et al., 2010; Iosifescu, 2012; Nandi, 2012; Finsterer & Mahjoub, 2013).

The conceptual basis of the horizontal epidemiology hypothesis, in short, was the theoretical understanding in the ICF of the nature of disability and the social processes that create, worsen or lessen the experience of disability. It is reasonable to suggest that we should find more commonalities in psychosocial problems that impact on the lived experience of people, because of the similarity of people's experiences of the physical and social determinants of these difficulties, than differences that are linked to purely diagnostic criteria for identifying the underlying mental health condition.

The Evidence in Support of the Hypothesis of Horizontal Epidemiology

Grounded in the ICF understanding of disability, and the resulting intuitions about commonalities in lived experience, the PARADISE project attempted to scientifically verify these intuitions. As with any other radical departure from standard practice, the primary challenge which the researchers faced was that, although there is a wealth of evidence about the psychosocial difficulties that people with mental health problems face in their day-to-day lives, there was no consistency in the literature about how these difficulties were characterised. Similarly, there was no consistency in the methods of assessment, if any, that were used, or the modes of data collection and strategies of data documentation that were reported. Moreover, clinical investigators themselves relied on the silo-like approach, by beginning with specific diagnostic criteria for each condition and restricting their interviews to the difficulties that would seem to flow, a priori, from these criteria. And it was rare for researchers to move beyond a specific health problem to seek to make comparisons across health conditions.

The researchers used a multi-method approach to systematic literature reviews to overcome these substantial obstacles by conducting content analysis of outcomes that were reported by patients, input of clinical expertise and a qualitative study to gather information about the psychosocial difficulties and their determinants, experienced by patients with these mental health problems. The results of the literature review and qualitative study have been published (Cabello et al., 2012; Cerniauskaite et al., 2012; Hartley et al., 2014; Levola et al., 2014; Quintas et al., 2012; Raggi et al. 2012; Switaj et al., 2012). Data about psychosocial difficulties and determinants were harmonised and linked to the ICF. An expert consensus selected 64 psychosocial difficulties and 20 environmental determinants for a data collection protocol questionnaire that was piloted on a convenience sample of 80 people with each mental health problem. The results confirmed the commonality of psychosocial difficulties (56 of the 64) and determinants (16 of the 20) across the nine neurological and mental health conditions (Cieza et al., 2015b).

The environmental determinants disclosed by the PARADISE research included some that could easily be predicted (attitudes of, and level of assistance from, family members and friends, general social attitudes and ease of access to alcohol and illegal drugs). Others were surprising (cost of medication, public transportation, availability of assistive devices and the climate). The accompanying qualitative study (Hartley et al., 2014) used a combination of focus group and key informant interviewing and was able to take advantage of the more nuanced and intense interrogation of the lived experience of people who had these mental health conditions. This research confirmed the quantitative study results, but also revealed that the most impactful positive features of the social environment were a perception of social inclusion, availability of work opportunities and self-help groups, self-determination, contact with motivated professionals and achieving a balance between protection and overprotection (see Haslam et al., 2016).

The confirmation of the hypothesis of horizontal epidemiology was the primary objective of the PARADISE project. Further validation would require a similar methodology to be applied to other health conditions, both mental and physical. Yet, the PARADISE multi-method study was sufficiently powerful to construct a questionnaire using 64 psychosocial difficulties and a total of 59 environmental and personal psychological determinants of those difficulties. This questionnaire was administered as a cross-sectional study to a total of 722 persons with the nine conditions, interviewed in four European countries: Italy, Poland, Spain and Finland. These data were used for a confirmatory analysis to support the hypothesis of horizontal epidemiology. Given the power of these data sets, however, it was also possible to use Rasch analysis to construct a metric to measure the impact of neurological and mental health conditions on people's lives. This metric, called PARADISE 24, based on the resulting reduced number of items needed for the metric, is a potential tool for carrying out cardinal comparisons over time of the magnitude of psychosocial impact (Cieza et al., 2015b).

Besides this technical application, there are clear messages from the PARADISE research and the theory of horizontal epidemiology for public mental health in general, and the concept of social scaffolding that underlies the project represented by this volume in particular.

What are the Messages from Horizontal Epidemiology?

Horizontal epidemiology has its most direct and obvious impact on data collection practices and analysis, and will lead to a more informative and effective epidemiology of mental health. More powerful and relevant epidemiological information benefits clinical and public health practice, rationalisation of health systems, research and policy development. Better data are always welcome. But here the issue is not merely better basic information about prevalence and incidence of mental health and neurological conditions, but information relevant to the lives of people experiencing these conditions.

It is a common complaint in mental health epidemiology that our understanding is limited to the data we collect, and, if all that we know about mental health comes in the form of information collected, silo-fashion, from diagnostically distinct mental health conditions, then our understanding is limited, and, in many respects, distorted. Lacking cross-condition information has the result that diagnosis, treatment planning, treatment evaluation and outcome assessment will be carried out separately for each condition. Yet it is precisely data fragmentation that has led to ad hoc and incoherent public health responses to mental health in Europe and elsewhere (Olesen et al., 2006). Missing, typically, is the full range of information about the social determinants of mental illness, especially those complex experiences of social connectedness that are explored in this book, and which are part of the common background for all persons experiencing mental health problems.

With better, horizontal information about mental health, the door opens to new and more powerful epidemiological tools. As mentioned, given data about common psychosocial determinants, it is possible to develop a true metric of the psychosocial impact of mental health conditions, based on information collected directly from people who have these disorders, rather than, as is done with the disability-adjusted life year measure in the Global Burden of Disease studies, relying on 'disability weights', derived from evaluations by health professionals (Mathers et al., 2003; Salomon et al., 2012). Comparable summary measures of psychometric impact is an extremely valuable epidemiological tool since it makes it possible not only to compare the burden of different mental health conditions, individually and at the population level, but also to determine the effect of clinical and public health interventions on people's actual lived experiences. Given information about the cost of interventions, it would then be possible to make precise cost–benefit evaluations for public mental health policy decisions (Cieza et al., 2015a).

Understanding patterns of determinants of the lived experience of mental health and neurological conditions, and knowing that these determinants are cross-cutting, means what we learn from the effectiveness of interventions to improve the lives of patients with one condition, which can be applied to patients of other conditions. Although dementia and substance abuse are very different problems, people with these conditions commonly experience family breakdown, job loss, isolation, depression, sleep problems and so on. Effective community programming for people suffering from dementia may well be applicable with equal effectiveness to people suffering from substance abuse. Although we cannot assume that interventions are always transferable in this way, our repertoire of potentially valuable public health or clinical interventions will expand, the more we understand patterns of determinants. These patterns further invite longitudinal studies that focus on the psychosocial impact of mental health problems along the continuum of care, in the community and across the lifespan.

The potential beneficiaries of research conducted in terms of horizontal epidemiology are, in the first instance, those people whose lives are disrupted by psychosocial difficulties that are created, not merely by the diagnostic symptoms of their mental health or neurological conditions, but also by the physical, social and attitudinal environment in which they live. Clinicians and researchers who work in public mental health with people who have brain disorders will also benefit, since data comparability, not to mention increased data coverage, is hugely important for successful intervention planning, management and research. Horizontal epidemiology, moreover, is potentially de-stigmatising, since it allows clinicians and researchers to focus on common experiences and detach interventions from particular mental health labels. Finally, those persons who are responsible for social agencies and political and economic infrastructures of mental healthcare are likely to benefit from the production of data that validly describe the lived experience of persons who have mental health conditions. These data are not always directly linked to diagnostic criteria but are features of the experience that people share across diagnoses. This approach will greatly improve policy planning and the cost effectiveness of policy initiatives.

Horizontal Epidemiology, Social Determinants and Public Mental Health

Horizontal epidemiology underscores the epidemiological, clincial and policy importance of understanding patterns in the determinants, not merely of the onset of mental health problems, but of the psychosocial difficulties that people with these chronic conditions experience in their lives. Our knowledge of determinants, risk factors and the aetiology of mental health and neurological conditions has been continuously increasing from evidence of, for example, life-course, risk-modelling exercises (Papachristou et al., 2013) or by focusing on the interactions among determinants during life stages (Colman and Ataullahjan, 2010; Ramagopalan et al., 2010). These efforts are undeniably valuable for primary prevention strategies; yet, given the fact that these conditions tend to be chronic and have a huge impact on daily life, it is essential that we do more about the social and other determinants of the experienced burden of the population who are currently affected by brain disorders. At the end of the day, what matters to people are the lives they live.

It remains a major challenge to resolve the theoretical and practical tension between research that focuses on an epidemiological understanding of the impact of social determinants on the lived experience of persons who have mental health problems and basic neurobiological scientific research that aims to expose biological explanations for mental health diseases and disorders. The aim of this contribution, however, was to suggest one of what are potentially several epidemiological innovations that more crisply highlights the benefits of a better understanding of the determinants of the psychosocial difficulties that can so profoundly impact the lives of persons who are diagnosed with these conditions. With this more robust understanding, it may be possible to supplement our neurological knowledge about aetiology for primary prevention with new ways of acknowledging and understanding the role of social identity and connectedness in their experience of mental health. We may also be able to develop and put into practice new tools for identifying personal and social resources that can be made available. Together, these advancements can be translated into practical actions and interventions that can demonstrably improve the lives of people with mental health conditions.

References

Andlin-Sobocki, P. & Rehm, J. (2005). Cost of addiction in Europe. European Journal of Neurology, **12** (Suppl. 1): 28–33.

Cabello, M., Mellor-Marsa, B., Sabariego, C., et al. (2012). Psychosocial features of depression: A systematic literature review. Journal of Affective Disorders, **141**: 22–33.

Cerniauskaite, M., Ajovalasit, D., Quintas, R. et al. (2012). Functioning and disability in persons with epilepsy. American Journal of Physical Medicine and Rehabilitation, **91**: S22–30.

Cieza, A., Anczewska, M., Ayuso-Mateos, J. L. et al. (2015a). Understanding the impact of brain disorders: Towards a 'horizontal epidemiology' of psychosocial difficulties and their determinants. PLoS One, **10**: e0136271.

Cieza, A., Bostan, C., Oberhauser, C. & Bickenbach, J. (2010). Explaining functioning outcomes across musculoskeletal conditions: A multilevel modelling approach. Disability and Rehabilitation, 32 (Suppl 1): S85–93.

Cieza, A., Sabariego, C., Anczewska, M. et al. (2015b). PARADISE 24: A measure to assess the impact of brain disorders on people's lives. PLoS One, **10**: e0132410.

Colman, I. & Ataullahjan, A. (2010). Life course perspectives on the epidemiology of depression. Canadian Journal of Psychiatry/Revue canadienne de psychiatrie. **55**: 622–632.

Finsterer, J. & Sinda Zarrouk, M. (2013). Fatigue in healthy and diseased individuals. American Journal of Hospice and Palliative Medicine, July 26; doi: 10.1177/1049909113494748.

Hartley, S., McArthur, M., Coenen, M. et al. (2014). Narratives reflecting the lived experiences of people with brain disorders: Common psychosocial difficulties and determinants. PLoS One, **9**: e96890.

Haslam, C., Cruwys, T., Haslam, S. A., Dingle, G. A. & Chang, M.X-L. (2016). GROUPS 4 HEALTH: Evidence that a social-identity intervention that builds and strengthens social group membership improves health. Journal of Affective Disorders, **194**: 188–195.

Iosifescu, D. V. (2012). The relation between mood, cognition and psychosocial functioning in psychiatric disorders. European Neuropsychopharmacology, **22** (Suppl. 3): S499–504.

Leonardi, M., Meucci, P., Ajovalasit, D. et al. (2009). ICF in neurology: Functioning and disability in patients with migraine, myasthenia gravis and Parkinson's disease. Disability and Rehabilitation, **31** (Suppl. 1): S88–99.

Levola, J., Kaskela, T., Holopainen, A. et al. (2014). Psychosocial difficulties in alcohol dependence: A systematic review of activity limitations and participation restrictions. Disability and Rehabilitation, **36**: 1227–1239.

Marmot, M. & Wilkinson R., editors (1999). Social Determinants of Health. Oxford: Oxford University Press.

Mathers, C. D., Murray, C. J., Ezzati, M. et al. (2003). Population health metrics: Crucial inputs to the development of evidence for health policy. Population Health Metrics, **1**: 6.

Murray, C. J., Vos, T., Lozano, R. et al. (2012). Disability-adjusted life years (DALYs) for 291 diseases and injuries in 21 regions, 1990–2010: A systematic analysis for the Global Burden of Disease Study 2010. The Lancet, **380**: 2197–2223.

Nandi, P. R. (2012). Pain in neurological conditions. Current Opinion in Supportive and Palliative Care, **6**: 194–200.

NIHM (2008). Strategic plan for research. See www.nimh.nih.gov/about/strategic-planning-reports/index.shtml.

NIMH (2013). Brain Research through Advancing Innovative Neurotechnologies (BRAIN) Initiative. See www.nih.gov/science/brain/.

Olesen, J. & Leonardi, M. (2003). The burden of brain diseases in Europe. European Journal of Neurology, **10**: 471–477.

Olesen, J., Baker, M. G., Freund, T. et al. (2006). Consensus document on European brain research. Journal of Neurology, Neurosurgery and Psychiatry, 77 (Suppl. 1): 1–149.

Papachristou, E., Frangou, S. & Reichenberg A. (2013). Expanding conceptual frameworks: Life course risk modelling for mental disorders. Psychiatry Research, **206**: 140–145.

Quintas, R., Raggi, A, Giovannetti, A. M. et al. (2012). Psychosocial difficulties in people with epilepsy: A systematic review of literature from 2005 until 2010. Epilepsy and Behavior, **25**: 60–67.

Raggi, A., Giovannetti, A. M., Quintas, R. et al. (2012). A systematic review of the psychosocial difficulties relevant to patients with migraine. Journal of Headache and Pain Management, **13**: 595–606.

Ramagopalan, S. V., Dobson, R., Meier, U. C. & Giovannoni, G. (2010). Multiple sclerosis: Risk factors, prodromes, and potential causal pathways. Lancet Neurology, **9**: 727–739.

Salomon, J. A., Vos, T., Hogan, D. R. et al. (2012). Common values in assessing health outcomes from disease and injury: Disability weights measurement study for the Global Burden of Disease Study 2010. The Lancet, **380**: 2129–2143.

Switaj, P., Anczewska, M., Chrostek, A. et al. (2012). Disability and schizophrenia: A systematic review of experienced psychosocial difficulties. BMC Psychiatry, **12**: 193.

WHO (2001). International Classification of Functioning, Disability and Health: ICF. Geneva: World Health Organization.

WHO (2006). Neurological Disorders: Public Health Challenges. Geneva: World Health Organization.

WHO-CSDH (2008). Closing the gap in a generation: Health equity through action on the social determinants of health. Final Report of the Commission on Social Determinants of Health. Geneva: World Health Organization.

Chapter 8

Parity of Esteem for Mental Health

Sue Bailey

A man's body and his mind, with the utmost reverence to both I speak it, are exactly like a jerkin and a jerkin's lining, rumple one, you rumple the other.

Laurence Sterne from *The Life and Opinions of Tristram Shandy, Gentleman.* 1761

Introduction

This book has considered the nature of health and mental health using the definition of the World Health Organization (WHO) and other definitions in Chapter 6. We now move to considering what the term 'parity of esteem' means. This chapter brings together thoughts about parity of esteem for mental health and mental healthcare with physical health and physical healthcare, and the way in which that reflects the contents and values in this book. I have spoken at international events about this topic on many occasions. My wish is to create a powerful statement that mirrors the contents of this book and exemplifies its value by bringing these ideas together in a single chapter,

There is no doubt that the global burden of disease due to mental ill health exceeds that of physical ill health and yet the resources dedicated to physical ill health far exceed those for mental ill health, worldwide. The reasons for this vary through stigma, discrimination and the emphasis of mind–body dualism. Clinicians have often shied away from advocacy roles, but this is an important responsibility that they should build as health professionals as well as members of society.

Essential reading on this topic is the Royal College of Psychiatrists' Occasional Paper OP88, on whole-person care (Royal College of Psychiatrists, 2013). It sets out definitions of parity of esteem, a vision and what was understood at the time of publication about the stigma and discrimination that people who have mental health problems experience, particularly in relation to their treatment for mental ill health.

In the next section, I define parity and parity of esteem and then move on to explore how human rights underpin mental health policy. I argue that if the concept of parity of esteem were fully embraced, not only would that improve the health of individual people, but also the health and economies of nations.

Defining Parity of Esteem for Mental Health

There are varying definitions of the concept of parity of esteem and many barriers to its application. Millard and Wessely (2014) point to the definitional and practical problems of using the term outside the UK. In Chapters 1 and 6, we distinguish the terms equity and equality, and present those definitions later in this one. Thus, other people have proposed that the issue is not about trying to achieve equality between mental and physical health services but more about creating equity of effective services for those people who use mental health services (Timimi, 2014). However, this will only be achieved if mental health services do not work in isolation but are enabled to bring resources together from a range of linked services, including the public health and criminal justice services.

As used here, the term has its roots in political discourse, linked to the civil rights movement in the USA. Parity of esteem was also enshrined in law in the USA in 2006. It was co-opted into the field of mental health by means of the US Mental Health Parity and Addiction Act of 2008. The following definition of parity has been used in the US literature (Royal College of Psychiatrists, 2013, p. 16):

> The overarching principle of the parity movement is equality – in access to care, in improving the quality of care, and in the way resources are allocated . . . If we stay true to the principle of treating each person with dignity and respect in our health care system, then we should make no distinction between illnesses of the brain and illnesses of other body systems.

In the UK, the principle of parity of esteem is enshrined in legislation by the Health & Social Care Act, 2012. This was the government's response to an initiative led by the Royal College of Psychiatrists, the mental health charity, MIND, and the All Party Parliamentary Group on Mental Health. Mental health has often been seen as not receiving the same level of investment as physical health and that affects quality and access to services. There is now a commitment in the UK to achieve parity of esteem by 2020. The definition of parity of esteem given by the Royal College means: equal access to effective care and treatment; equal efforts to improve the quality of care; equal status within healthcare education and practice; equally high aspirations for service users; and equal status in the measurement of health outcomes (Royal College of Psychiatrists, 2013).

In summary, the essence of parity of esteem is best described as: valuing mental health equally with physical health. This approach recognises the strong relationship between mental health and physical health. It is founded in the UK on an understanding that there is lack of parity in three main areas. The report of the All Party Parliamentary Group on Mental Health's inquiry into parity of esteem for mental health (All Party Parliamentary Group on Mental Health, 2015) records those areas as

- The unacceptably large 'premature mortality gap' for people with serious mental illness;
- An acute shortage of high-quality mental health crisis care; and
- Failure to prioritise mental health promotion and prevention in public health strategies.

Valuing Mental Health Equally with Physical Health

Key features of a parity approach mean applying the principles to: people of all ages, including care prior to conception; and all groups of the population, including those who are most at risk of mental health problems. It also means equality of access to health and social care, including provision of equivalent levels of choice and quality, regardless of condition. Parity is, for these reasons, important not only to people with mental health problems but also for all those people who have learning disabilities and are at even greater risk and have high rates of comorbid mental disorders.

The right to health incorporates civil, social and health dimensions. At its heart is the Universal Declaration of Human Rights (United Nations, 1948) and its 30 articles. In the United

Nations Principles for the Protection of Persons with Mental Illness, adopted in 1991 (United Nations, 1991), there are explicit statements that

- All persons have the right to the best available mental healthcare, which shall be part of the health and social care system. [Principle 1]
- All persons with a mental illness, or who are being treated as such persons, shall be treated with humanity and respect for the inherent dignity of the human person. [Principle 3]
- Every person with a mental illness shall have the right to exercise all civil, political, economic, social and cultural rights as recognised in the UN Universal Declaration of Human Rights, the International Covenant on Civil and Political Rights, and the International Covenant on Economic, Social and Cultural Rights, and in other relevant instruments . . . all persons have the right to the best available mental healthcare. [Principle 5].

The WHO has shown that, even in countries where mental health policies exist (WHO, 2011), there is often a focus on detaining people who have a mental disorder, despite this only being required for a very small proportion of people who have mental disorders, and there can be no parity of esteem in these circumstances. Yamin and Rosenthal (2005) propose that a human rights framework is critical to service planning and delivery, and quality of care must form part of this framework. Bhugra et al. (2015, p. 4) argue that, to avoid discrimination in mental health, service planning and delivery is at the heart of human rights-based parity in psychiatry. They say 'Transparency and accountability within the legal framework and clear indicators and outcomes are essential if parity is to be achieved'.

An example of a values-based approach to mental healthcare is embodied by The Values-Based Child and Adolescent Mental Health System Commission (2016). It acknowledges the concerns about the mental health and wellbeing of children and young people. It proposes a whole schools approach within a system that includes families, communities and healthcare services, which is values-based, thereby resisting the isolation of mental health provision from other elements of health and social care. Public Health England (2015), in 'Promoting Children And Young People's Emotional Health And Wellbeing', describes how a whole schools approach might be implemented. This approach is augmented in *Key Principles for Improving Children and Young People's Mental Health in Schools and Colleges* (Children & Young People's Mental Health Coalition, 2017). It proposes that to create resilient people within resilient organisations, the following key principles need to be adopted by schools and colleges:

- Better balance between wellbeing and attainment;
- Better training and support for school staff on mental health; and
- Better support for children and young people when needed.

Mental health has a significant impact on many areas across physical medicine. In the UK, mental healthcare is a poor relation to physical healthcare and this is demonstrated most starkly by the gaps that exist. The gaps we look at here are mortality, funding and stigma, and they are based on experience in England. Here are some features of the recent circumstances.

The Mortality Gap

The mortality gap, that is, the life expectations for those people who have severe mental illness, is on average 20 years less for men and 15 years less for women than for the population as a whole (Wahlbeck et al., 2011). Common mental disorders such as anxiety and depression also bring with them significant premature mortality (Russ et al., 2012). The experience in England is that, across the lifespan and range of mental disorders, only a minority of people with mental health problems receive any intervention for their problems (McManus et al., 2009).

Funding Gaps

Funding gaps in mental health in 2010 accounted for 22 per cent of life years lost to disability (Murray et al., 2013). Mental health services received approximately 11.1 per cent of the National Health Services (NHS) budget in 2010–2011. Also, as cited at the beginning of this chapter, recent policy in England has agreed a national strategy for mental health services that is set out in 'The Five Year Forward View for Mental Health' (NHS England, 2016), and is supported by implementation and review documents. However, concerns remain about the reality of this funding. Analysis by The King's Fund (2015) suggests that many NHS Trusts had seen real-term decreases in income. The NHS Long Term Plan (2019) for England has been published subsequently and builds on this approach. In response to that publication, the Centre for Mental Health (2019) said 'A truly comprehensive set of access standards, similar to those for physical health services, could help to bring parity a step closer if it is backed up with enough funding and long-term investment in the workforce' (Centre for Mental Health, 2019; NHS England, 2019).

The Stigma Gap

Goffman (1963) has written extensively about stigma in his book of that title. Readers are likely to note that Goffman views stigma as an attribute that is deeply discrediting and which reduces the bearer, as a whole and usual person, to being a tainted, discounted one. Stigma and discrimination contribute significantly to the treatment gap. So, the overarching principles of any parity movement are achieving equity and equality of services in response to people's needs. As we saw in Chapter 1, **equity** means that health systems adequately meet the needs of people in the populations that those systems serve, and **equality** means that health systems treat people with similar needs in similar ways, within and across communities. Yet, it is clear that inequity and inequality continue to strongly influence our societies. If we stay true to the principle of treating each person with dignity and respect in healthcare systems, then we would make no distinction between illnesses of our brains and illnesses of our other body systems (Kennedy, 2010).

This brings us back to the core matter in defining parity of esteem, which is valuing people's mental health equally with their physical health, and mental healthcare equally with physical healthcare.

A Human Rights Approach

At the start of this chapter, I referred to the powerful impact of key stakeholders coming together to work together on the issues of parity and their achievement in enshrining this principle into legislation in the UK. There are two questions that arise when extending the uptake of parity of esteem to a global level. First, what would it take to make it possible to have parity become part of the day-to-day experience for those people who experience an episode of mental illness? Second, how would we know that the outcome of such an approach had been successful? I suggest a successful outcome would be characterised by the capability of people who use mental health services to

- Live without shame;
- Participate in the activities of the community in which they live;
- Enjoy self-respect;
- Live free of the associated risks of mental illness (i.e. relative poverty); and
- Have freedom to live their lives in ways that have real meaning and real value for them.

I propose that we take a human rights approach as a driver for change to transform mental health services. The British Institute of Human Rights (2016) exemplifies this approach in 'Mental Health Advocacy and Human Rights'. It works across health and social care, helping staff to understand rather than fear the application of a human rights approach. This enables everyone who is involved in services to apply human rights in day-to-day care, and to ensure that people in power respect and develop the human rights of people who have mental illness and learning disabilities.

Conclusion

I suggest that achieving parity of esteem requires an approach that is focused on whole persons and whole systems, which should bring with it a values and social identity approach to policy, service design and practice. This should be embedded in a rights parity framework and would give us the best measure of success.

The journey towards parity of esteem means that mental health matters not only to every person but also to the health and economy of any nation. Mental health practitioners and users of services have been pioneers of the approaches such as the recovery movement, coproduction of services and shared decision-making. The thinking that underpins mental health practice can lead the rest of health services as a social movement, moving from vertical systems and care to horizontal systems, moving from asking 'What health services do you want?' to 'What would help you enjoy your life more?' across the now four generational families that occupy Smithtown, which is described in Chapter 30.

This book argues that holistic care, that is, an open-minded approach to whole person care, is essential. Parity is ultimately, as much as anything, a mindset, which involves governments, policymakers, commissioners and providers of services, professional practitioners, researchers and the public taking a values-based approach to applying a 'parity test' both to all their activities and, above all, their attitudes.

References

All Party Parliamentary Group on Mental Health (2015). Parity in Progress. The Report of the Inquiry of the All Party Parliamentary Group on Mental Health's into Parity of Esteem for Mental Health. London: All Party Parliamentary Group on Mental Health.

Bhugra, D., Campion, J., Ventriglio, A. & Bailey, S. (2015). The right to mental health and parity. Indian Journal of Psychiatry, 57: 117–121.

British Institute of Human Rights (2016). A human rights approach to advocacy. See www.bihr.org.uk/a-human-rights-approach-to-advocacy-resources.

Children & Young People's Mental Health Coalition (2017). Key Principles for Improving Children and Young People's Mental Health in Schools. London: Children & Young People's Mental Health Coalition.

Goffman, E. (1963). Stigma: Notes on the Management of Spoiled Identity. Englewood Cliffs, NJ: Prentice-Hall.

Kennedy, I. (2010). Getting It Right for Children and Young People. London: Department of Health.

McManus, S., Meltzer, H., Brugha, T., Bebbington, P. & Jenkins, R. (2009). Adult psychiatric morbidity in England, 2007. Results of a household survey. NHS Information Centre for Health and Social Care and the Department of Health Sciences, University of Leicester. See https://digital.nhs.uk/data-and-information/publications/statistical/adult-psychiatric-morbidity-survey/adult-psychiatric-morbidity-in-england-2007-results-of-a-household-survey.

Millard, C. & Wessely, S. (2014). Parity of esteem between mental and physical health. British Medical Journal, **349**: g6821.

Murray, C. J., Richards, M. A.,Newton, J. N. et al. (2013). UK health performance: Findings of the Global Burden of Disease. The Lancet, **381**: 997–1020.

NHS England (2016). The five year forward view for mental health. A Report for the Independent Mental Health Taskforce to the NHS in England. See www.england.nhs.uk/wp-content/uploads/2016/02/Mental-Health-Taskforce-FYFV-final.pdf.

NHS England (2019). The NHS Long Term Plan 2019. https://www.longtermplan.nhs.uk/wp-content/uploads/2019/01/nhs-long-term-plan.pdf.

Public Health England (2015). Promoting Children and Young People's Emotional Health and Wellbeing: A Whole School and College Approach. London: Public Health England.

Royal College of Psychiatrists (2013). OP88. Whole-Person Care: From Rhetoric to Reality (Achieving Parity Between Mental and Physical Health). London: Royal College of Psychiatrists.

Russ, T. C., Stamatakis, E., Hamer, M. et al. (2012). Association between psychological distress and mortality: Individual participant pooled analysis of 10 prospective cohort studies. British Medical Journal, **345**: e4933.

The Centre for Mental Health. Response to NHS Long Term Plan 2019 (2019). https://www.centreformentalhealth.org.uk/news/nhs-long-term-plan. London: The Centre for Mental Health.

The King's Fund (2015). NHS five year forward view: Our work looking at the vision for the future of the NHS, health and care. See www.kingsfund.org.uk/topics/nhs-five-year-forward-view.

Timimi, S. (2014). Parity of esteem for mental and physical health is a red herring. British Medical Journal, **349**: g6821.

United Nations (1948). The universal declaration of human rights. See www.un.org/en/universal-declaration-human-rights/.

United Nations (1991). The United Nations Principles for the Protection of Persons with Mental Illness. New York, NY: United Nations.

Values-Based Child and Adolescent Mental Health System Commission (2016). What Really Matters in Children and Young People's Mental Health. London: Royal College of Psychiatrists.

Wahlbeck, K., Westman, J., Nordentoft, M., Gissler, M. & Laursen, T. M. (2011). Outcomes of Nordic mental health systems: Life expectancy of patients with mental disorders. The British Journal of Psychiatry, **199**: 453–458.

WHO (2011). WHO Mental Health Atlas 2011. Geneva: World Health Organization.

Yamin, A. E. & Rosenthal, E. (2005). Out of the shadows: Using human rights approaches to secure dignity and well-being for people with mental disabilities. PLoS Medicine, **2**: e71.

Chapter 9

Belonging

Peter Hindley

Attachment Theory, Social Connectedness and Belonging

Attachment theory has become a central concept in our understanding of resilience in children and young people (Fonagy et al., 1994). However, attachment theory is a relatively narrow concept, focused on the relationship between a child and his or her principal caregivers and the child's need to seek comfort when distressed (Waters et al., 2005). Furthermore, attachment theory concerns itself with individual person's relationships, while recognising that children can have multiple attachment relationships. However, we know that children grow up in complex systems (Bronfenbrenner, 1979) and there is a growing recognition that children and young people's sense of belonging (to individuals, groups and organisations) is a key component of resilience (Hart et al., 2008). Thus, the concept of belonging encapsulates children's relationships with their immediate families or carers, their friends and their friends' families, their schools, social activities (Scouts, football clubs, youth clubs) and wider social experiences, such as religious organisations or cultural groups. Thus, it provides a richer field than attachment theory within which to understand children's social existence.

Belonging can be defined as frequent personal contacts or interactions with another person, ideally positive but mainly free from conflict and negative effects; an interpersonal bond or relationship, marked by stability, affective concern and continuation into the foreseeable future; ideally mutual (Baumeister & Leary, 1995). In contrast, Tajfel and Turner (1979) posited belonging firmly within social groups. Baumeister and Leary have suggested that, 'the decisive impact may be the perception that one is the recipient of the other's lasting concern'. Belonging, as an aspect of resilience, has been explored in models of resilience such as a *Circle of Courage* (Brendtro et al., 1990) and *Resilient Therapy* (Hart et al., 2008).

In Chapter 3, Haslam and Haslam highlight the importance of social connectedness as a component of resilience and a protective factor in both mental and physical health. They see social connectedness as: '. . . often reflected in a community's sense of social cohesion, which can be observed and measured in different ways, through trust, cooperation, norms of reciprocity, civic engagement and openness to giving and receiving support'. Belonging can be understood as a component of social cohesion and it particularly encapsulates the importance of mutual concern. This reflects an internalised sense of shared social identity (see Chapter 4) and the role of wider social systems in resilience.

Empirically, a sense of belonging has been found to be an important component of resilience in looked-after children (Schoofeld & Beek, 2005) and in children who are refugees from war-torn areas (Birman et al., 2008). However, as with all aspects of resilience, a sense of belonging can be a double-edged sword. Girls who are gang members, who have often experienced multiple rejections, the opposite of belonging, identify a sense of belonging as the main reason that they belong to gangs. This is despite the fact that they frequently experience sexual exploitation within the gangs (Khan et al., 2013). In a similar vein, the desire for a sense of belonging has been identified as one of the factors that leads to young men becoming involved in religious extremism (Pratt, 2010).

This chapter explores the relevance of a sense of belonging to resilience, both clinically and theoretically, and the risks that a need for belonging can bring to vulnerable individuals and groups.

Belonging and Resilience: Theoretical Aspects

Our understanding of resilience has changed substantially over the past 30 years. Resilience, as originally posited by Rutter (1987), was conceptualised as a function of individual children. Progressively, resilience has been seen as a function of the interaction between children and the environments in which they develop. In recent years, this dynamic view of resilience has come to be seen as an interaction between individual children, their families, wider social settings and cultures. Ungar (2008, p. 225) offers the following definition: 'In the context of exposure to significant adversity, whether psychological, environmental, or both, resilience is both the capacity of individuals to navigate their way to health-sustaining resources, including opportunities to experience feelings of well-being, and a condition of the individual family, community and culture to provide these health resources and experiences in culturally meaningful ways'.

Belonging, as a theoretical construct, fits well in a dynamic understanding of resilience. Early definitions of belonging emphasise its interactional quality, 'sense of being accepted, valued, included, and encouraged by others . . . and of feeling oneself to be an important part of . . . life and activity . . . ' (Goodenow, 1993, p. 25).

More recently, McManus et al. (2012) have argued that belonging should be understood as being intra- and interpersonal, and intra- and intercultural. Thus, belonging may be understood in the following terms: (1) social relationships within dualisms such as man/woman or white/black; (2) an emotional and personalised experience, 'deeply bound up with individual and group identities' (Gorman-Murray et al., 2008, p. 174); and (3) the way social relations, identities and attachments are judged. Therefore, a sense of belonging is created through cultural and social constructions along with local interactions, personal experiences and individual actions and beliefs. In this way, a sense of belonging is significant in linking various scales of behaviour (such as individual and community) and in linking perceptions with actions and impacts.

This suggests that a sense of belonging functions as a component of resilience only when you have somewhere where you can belong and when that place offers you access to health resources and experiences, in culturally meaningful ways. As McManus et al. say (2012, p. 27): 'Clearly, community spirit stems from the interaction of perceptions of community spirit in the past along with perceptions of the physical environment, employment opportunities and sense of belonging. This suggests that resilience and a strong sense of community are influenced by a combination of perceptions about the environment, economy and social belonging.'

Belonging and Resilience: Empirical Findings

Belonging has been found to play an important part in people's sense of resilience in a wide range of studies, from the psychosocial progress of looked-after children (Schofeeld & Beek, 2005) to vulnerable rural Australian communities (McManus et al., 2012).

In adult mental health, a number of studies have shown a correlation between a lack of sense of belonging and depression (Choenarom et al., 2005; McLaren et al., 2007; and see Chapter 4). Lee and Williams (2013, p. 266) found that a sense of belonging was the most powerful protective factor against depression in grown-up children of alcoholic parents. This is confirmed by other studies that have shown that a sense of belonging is negatively correlated with depression (Choenarom et al., 2005; Sangon, 2004; Turner & McLaren, 2011). This echoes findings in young people who are transitioning into adulthood, among whom a sense of belonging in association with the ability to connect with other people, and access to social support, leads to increased resilience. Within educational settings a number of studies have suggested that students' sense of belonging to their school is positively associated with educational and behavioural outcomes (Lovat et al., 2011).

There have been a number of laboratory studies of the function of belonging in group settings (see Hogg et al., 2010, p. 75 for a summary). In general, as uncertainty rises, group identification rises. As Hogg et al. suggest, 'Identification reduces uncertainty because it furnishes a sense of who we are, how we should behave, and how others will treat us . . . '. However, certain types of groups are more effective at reducing a sense of uncertainty. These groups, with high entitativity (the perception of a group as pure entity, abstracted from its attendant individuals), are characterised by clear boundaries, internal homogeneity, social interaction, clear internal structure, common goals and a sense of common fate (Hogg et al., 2010, p. 75). These are common features of fundamentalist religious groups and echo at least one common definition of radicalisation (see Chapter 20).

Fundamentalism and Belonging

> In the absence of actual certainty in the midst of a precarious and hazardous world, men cultivate all sorts of things that would give them the feeling of certainty.
>
> Dewey (1929/2005, p. 33).

As Chapters 3 and 4 point out, membership of a group confers a sense of identity and a means of managing a sense of uncertainty. Religious groups share many common features with non-religious groups: beliefs; attitudes; values; and behaviours that relate to all aspects of life, which are integrated and imbued with meaning by an ideological framework and world view (Hogg et al., 2010). A unique feature of religious groups is the way in which they call upon the sacred and the divine '. . . to provide prescriptive moral guidance for behavioural choices, sacred rituals and quests, and daily life' (Hogg et al., 2010, p. 73). These may be some of the reasons why membership of a religious group confers a wide range of protective factors to its members (e.g. Bullock et al., 2012, and see Chapter 4). However, membership of a fundamentalist religious group is a potential path into religious radicalisation, although as Bhui and Jenkins point out in Chapter 20, it is only one potential path out of many. What part does belonging play in this journey and how can we use the prism of belonging to understand this process?

Pratt (2010) has argued that religious extremism, or fundamentalism, does not represent a move away from the central tenets of a religion but rather an intensification of self-understanding and self-proclamation in relation to these tenets. He goes on to suggest that fundamentalists 'freeze' a moment in time or specific text to define a 'golden' era against which current existence and religious practice should be measured. Impositional fundamentalists then seek to, either overtly or covertly, force everybody to adhere to these beliefs and practices and so belong to a particular group. Thus, the identity of an individual member of a fundamentalist group is inextricably bound up with the identity of the fundamentalist group. Pratt (2010, p. 447) argues that the more assertive the fundamentalism is, the tighter is this bond. Pratt goes on to suggest that, by definition, this stance is completely at odds with a 'liberal' perspective, which allows for uncertainty and multiple possibilities. The impositional religious fundamentalist view sees any alternative view or other identity as anathema, per se.

Belonging and Girls' Membership of Gangs

Impositional fundamentalism seeks to force everybody to belong to the fundamentalist group, overtly or covertly (Pratt, 2010, p. 443). Similarly, with gang membership, there is a sense of total relinquishing of personal identity, at any cost, for the sake of belonging. This can be understood in the context of poor family relationships, particularly experience of sexual abuse, and a lack of a sense of attachment to other people. In this sense, gang membership provides an alternative family. Social inequality and deprivation also are seen as key drivers for gang membership. This is often accompanied by female gang members having difficult family relationships and experiences of sexual abuse. These early adversities are often compounded by school problems, early behavioural difficulties, mental health problems, self-harm, risky sexual behaviour and substance misuse. Paradoxically, gang membership is often seen as offering an alternative to family structures for female gang members and as offering protection in a hostile environment. These negative drivers are compounded by peer pressure and overt physical and sexual intimidation from male and female gang members. However, a sense of belonging is cited as the second commonest reason for people to join gangs (Esbenson & Deschanes, 1998; Wang, 2000).

Khan et al. (2013) recommend the following, 'Programmes for females should foster respectful and positive relationships as an important lever for promoting change when working with young women. Relationships are particularly influential for young women both as a way in to risky activity and as a way out'.

Conclusions

McManus (2012) et al. suggest that a sense of belonging functions as a component of resilience only when you have somewhere where you can belong, and when that place offers you access to health resources and experiences in culturally meaningful ways. A sense of belonging appears to be an important component of resilience for people who belong to intact families and communities. However, when access to the source of resilience is restricted, the need for a sense of belonging can lead to children, young people and adults satisfying that need by joining groups that are not necessarily beneficial to them as individual persons. Members of religious fundamentalist groups relinquish their personal needs in order to achieve a higher purpose by, if necessary, sacrificing their own lives. In Chapter 20, Bhui and Jenkins argue that the process of radicalisation can be compared with the process of grooming young people to enter sexually abusive relationships. Female members of gangs may be subjected to a wide range of abusive experiences in order to be part of a gang. Being part of a gang provides both material protection and a sense of being part of a social group, which was not provided by their families for many young female members.

Ironically, this suggests that for belonging to function effectively as a component of resilience, we should ensure that the other half of belonging, the social organisation to which one wants to belong, is available. In Chapter 20, Bhui and Jenkins suggest that this might be one component of an effective strategy to prevent radicalisation of young people, and they cite how positive affiliation to local cultural practices has been used to encourage young people to leave gangs in the Rio Favelas. Similarly, Khan et al. (2013) cite Girls Circle as an example of a promising intervention for working with female gang members: 'The approach relies on growth-fostering relationships . . . as a primary lever for supporting change'. Finally, in Chapter 4, Haslam et al. clarify how shared group identity enables access to material and emotional support and conveys meaning to group members' actions.

Thus, efforts to promote belonging might be best directed at supporting family and social cohesion in order to ensure that our needs to belong are met by objects that will genuinely treat us as people and valued members of our social groups.

References

Baumeister, R. F. & Leary, M. (1995) The need to belong: Desire for interpersonal attachments as a fundamental human motivation. Psychological Bulletin, **117**: 497–529.

Birman, D., Beehler, S., Harris, E. M. et al. (2008). International Family, Adult, and Child Enhancement Services (FACES): A community-based comprehensive services model for refugee children in resettlement. American Journal of Orthopsychiatry, **78**: 121–132.

Brendtro, L., Brokenleg, M. & Van Bockern, M. (1990). Reclaiming Youth at Risk: Our Hope for the Future. Bloomington, IN: National Education Service.

Bronfenbrenner, U. (1979). The Ecology of Human Development. Cambridge, MA: Harvard University Press.

Bullock, M., Nadeau, L. & Reneaud, J. (2012). Spirituality and religion in youth suicide attempters' trajectories of mental health service utilization: The year before a suicide attempt. Journal of the American Academy of Child and Adolescent Psychiatry, **21**: 186–193.

Choenarom, C, Williams, R. A. & Hagerty, B. M. (2005). The role of sense of belonging and social support on stress and depression in individuals with depression. Archives of Psychiatric Nursing, **19**, 18–29.

Dewey, J. (1929/2005). The Quest for Certainty: A Study of the Relation of Knowledge and Action. Whitefish, MT: Kessinger Publishing.

Esbenson, F. & Deschanes, E. P. (1998). A multisite examination of youth gang membership: Does gender matter? Criminology, **36**: 729–828.

Fonagy, P., Steele, P., Steele, H., Higgitt, A. & Target, M. (1994) The theory and practice of resilience. Journal of Child Psychology and Psychiatry, **35**: 231–257.

Goodenow, C. (1993). The psychological sense of school membership among adolescents: Scale development and educational correlates. Psychology in the Schools, **30**: 79–90.

Gorman-Murray, A., Waitt, G. & Gibson, C. (2008). A Queer Country? A case study of the politics of gay/lesbian belonging in an Australian country town. Australian Geographer, **39**: 171–191; https://doi.org/10.1080/00049180802056849.

Hart, A., Blincow, D. & Thomas, H. (2007). Resilient Therapy with Children and Families. London: Brunner Routledge.

Hogg, M. A., Adelman,J. R. & Blagg, R. D. (2010). Religion in the face of uncertainty: An uncertainty-identity theory account of religiousness. Personality and Social Psychology Review, **14**: 72–83.

Khan, L., Brice, H., Saunders, A. & Plumtree, A. (2013). A Need to Belong: What Leads Girls to Belong to Gangs. London: Centre for Mental Health.

Lee, H. & Williams, R. A (2013). Effects of parental alcoholism, sense of belonging, and resilience on depressive symptoms: A path model. Substance Use and Misuse, **48**: 265–273.

Lovat, T., Dally, K., Clement, N. & Toomey, R. (2011). Values pedagogy and teacher education: Re-conceiving the foundations. Australian Journal of Teacher Education, **36**: 59–72.

McLaren, S., Gomez, R., Bailey, M. & Van Der Horst, R. K. (2007). The association of depression and sense of belonging with suicidal ideation among older adults: applicability of resiliency models. Suicide and Life-Threatening Behavior, **37**: 89–102.

McManus, P., Walmsley, J., Argent, N. et al. (2012). Rural community and rural resilience: What is important to farmers in keeping their country towns alive. Journal of Rural Studies, **28**, 20–29.

Pratt, D. (2010). Religion and terrorism: Christian fundamentalism and extremism. Terrorism and Political Violence, **22**: 438–456.

Rutter, M. (1987). Psychosocial resilience and protective factors. American Journal of Orthopsychiatry, **57**: 316–331.

Sangon, S. (2004). Predictors of depression in Thai women. Research and Theory for Nursing Practice, **18**: 243–260.

Schofield, G. & Beek, M. (2005). Risk and resilience in long-term foster-care. British Journal of Social Work, **35**: 1283–1301.

Tajfel, H. & Turner, J. C. (1979). An integrative theory of intergroup conflict. In Austin, W. G. & Worchel, S., editors, The Social Psychology of Intergroup Relations. Monterey, CA: Brooks/ Cole, pp. 33–47.

Turner, L. & McLaren, S. (2011). Social support and sense of belonging as protective factors in the rumination: Depressive symptoms relation among Australian women. Women and Health, **51**: 151–167.

Ungar, M. (2008). Resilience across cultures. The British Journal of Social Work, **38**: 218–235.

Wang, J. (2000) Female gang affiliation: Knowledge and perceptions of at-risk girls. International Journal of Offender Therapy and Comparative Criminology, **44**: 618–632.

Waters, E., Corcoran, D. & Anafarta, M. (2005). Attachment, other relationships, and the theory that all good things go together.Human Development, **48**: 80–84.

Chapter 10

Families and Communities: Their Meanings and Roles Across Ethnic Cultures

Hinemoa Elder

Ko Parengarenga te moana.
Parengareanga is the ocean.
Ko Tawhitirahi te maunga.
Tawhitirahi is the mountain.
Ko Awapoka te awa.
Awapoka is the river.
Ko Waimirirangi te tupuna.
Waimirirangi is the ancestor.
Ko Potahi te marae.
Potahi is the meeting place.
Ko Te Aupouri, ko Ngātī Kurī, ko Te Rarawa, ko Ngāpuhi nui tonu ōku iwi.
Te Aupouri, Ngāti Kurī, Te Rarawa and Ngāpuhi are my tribal affiliations.
Ko Hinemoa Elder tōku ingoa.
Hinemoa Elder is my name. [1]

He tātai whetū ki te rangi, ko te ira tangata ki te whenua.
Like the ancestry of stars in the heavens so is the essence of humanity in the land.

Introduction

The tradition of taking family and social histories and integrating these aspects into formulations and recommendations is a time-honoured health practice. The role of ethnic cultural understandings of family and community pertinent to this process is less clear. Alongside this, the extent to which contemporary practice keeps up with culturally responsive research, investigating concepts of family and community, is variable. This chapter covers how relevant research and practice-based evidence might inform health practitioners to better engage with concepts of family and community through an ethnic cultural lens. The topic is vast and this chapter presents a pragmatic review of the salient literature together with a tailored critique of key issues that impact on practitioners and policymakers alike.

Why is this an important area to explore? I argue that the ways in which practitioners, and those people who influence the nature of health practice, define and work with ethnic-specific meanings of family and community provide a potent source of potential health gain as well as a means of marginalisation. The fluidity, context specificity and nuances around

[1] This is the pepeha of the author, a formal Māori-specific way of introduction, locating the person according to the landmarks and genealogical origins.

these meanings of family and community across cultures, and their continuing evolution, demands that we maintain competency if we are to develop robust therapeutic relationships and effect change on a wider scale.

Ultimately, families' and communities' self-definitions must be heard and acted on by health practitioners and policymakers. In this way, possibilities for self-determination can be better understood and supported, leading, thereby, to better health outcomes. Indeed, heeding the call from Chapter 6, the very definition of health and wellbeing could be improved and made more meaningful by including group self-determination as a key indicator. In other words, the ability to identify and prioritise options, based on access to the resources of groups through cultural identity.

One of the significant biases of this chapter is that it is written in English and draws on the related literature in the English language. Unfortunately, this approach excludes the richness of other cultural discourses. Another bias is towards using examples from Aotearoa New Zealand, from Māori experience. This relates to my origins, practice and research. I hope that these exemplars will promote broader consideration of ethnic cultural groups with which readers have contact. Alongside that consideration it is the well-recognised issue that cultural competency begins with self-reflective critique of the culture of practice rather than a competency focused on 'other' (D'Souza, 2003; Elder & Tapsell, 2013).

This chapter asks two practical questions. First, what are the influences that might improve how we co-discover a 'family history' with families we work with? Even when we are seemingly working with one person, there are family relationships and histories to carefully consider, including with family members who are no longer alive. What is an expansive and inclusive approach to this aspect of rapport building, assessment and therapy that encompasses the meanings across the dimensions of family and community within a particular ethnic culture? When we consider the aspects included in a family history, what guides the material included? How does this reflect the culture of practice, the structures that we practitioners and researchers represent in our interactions with these communities and our beliefs and values about family and community structures, recognising that almost all health indices are about structural disadvantage, a point that is strongly made in Chapter 6?

Second, what would a culture-specific 'community history' look like? How would a health practitioner, or researcher, go about considering and documenting the necessary elements? I make the case for adding this to the existing suite of historical aspects of assessments. I illustrate with a specific community example. What this shows is that health practitioners and policymakers alike should have some historical knowledge in order to best understand intergenerational influences, particularly of trauma and colonisation, stigma and discrimination, as well as potential that is located within communities.

Family History

Health practitioners are schooled in the practice of taking a family history. This usually involves considering the family history of mental and physical illnesses, substance abuse and suicide. Without doubt, there is real value in understanding these historical aspects, which enable, among other things, discussion and answering family questions about the risk of other family members developing serious mental illnesses. Interestingly, a population study in Denmark, which reviewed 1.74 million people, found that a general psychiatric family history was a confounder between diagnosis of schizophrenia and urbanisation of place of birth (Mortensen et al., 2010). The authors also found that, while schizophrenia was associated with increased rates of schizophrenia in first-degree relatives, almost any other psychiatric disorder among first-degree relatives increased the personal risk of schizophrenia. This highlights the importance of ensuring that quality information is shared about what the family may consider to be subtle changes or culturally bound psychological distress. The importance of community factors, such as urbanisation at birth, is also a feature that practitioners may not be familiar with.

Practice-based evidence tells us that taking a family history commonly means reviewing the pathological aspects, with, perhaps, occasional discretionary references to culturally based strengths. Other items on the history-taking schedule, such as developmental and social histories, capture aspects that might also be understood as lending a deeper shared understanding of each particular family's distinctive experiences. Again, our training emphasises the importance of identifying pathology but with less focus on strengths, let alone cultural strengths. This focus can become the source of dislocation from family and community, both as a contributor to mental illness and as a result of it. Specific family factors, such as intra-familial violence and substance abuse, can be formulated as vulnerability or predisposing factors. The importance of exploration and formulation of family and community dislocation from war, natural and man-made disasters as well as the ongoing effects of colonisation, such as forced closure of communities (McInerney, 2015), is without question. However, this is a necessary but not sufficient approach. Identifying strengths and resilience factors as well as markers of belonging, as highlighted in Chapter 9, is also essential in establishing family identity that is not defined by pathological factors, and provides an opportunity for healing. Unfortunately, I found no papers investigating this issue in family history-taking.

The importance of using culturally relevant approaches in ensuring that a robust family history is obtained has been elegantly articulated (Sheldon, 2001). Sheldon's paper gives a vivid and useful account of the effective means of connecting with aboriginal peoples, living in remote areas. He makes the important point that for them, and I would argue for other cultural groups, 'asking about the presenting illness first baffles most Aboriginal people who feel their problems cannot be properly appreciated unless their relationships in their community and their spiritual beliefs are understood' (p. 440).

Attending to relationships within communities and families, and with health practitioners, is crucial. Health practitioners who assess peoples of different ethnic cultures may find it challenging to understand the meanings associated with their patients' concepts of family and community. There are a number of possible reasons for this. Health practitioners may feel this material is outside their remit. Even if they did begin to understand each family's and community's experiences, they may feel this is an area over which they have little influence. The use of cultural protocols that enhance rapport is one helpful approach. Indeed, some cultural groups do not fully engage until cultural protocols have been completed. In Māori culture, the use of whakawhanaungatanga (establishing connections in relationships) is recognised as a required practice. Some practitioners may find this a challenge as the practice invites the clinician and whānau alike to talk about their origins and identity.

Te Reo Māori, the Māori language, illustrates the sophistication in thinking about connecting with groups of different sizes, as evidenced by the number of pronouns in our language. Te Reo Māori differentiates between pronouns for one, two and three or more people. In addition, pronouns are exact about whether the person being talked to is included or not. These nuances of shared group membership in the language exemplify the importance that is placed on precision when it comes to the shared cultural markers of group identity, aligning with the discussion in Chapter 4. This practice of using whakawhanaungatanga is a valuable way to signal cultural responsivity to the whānau, which is likely to lead to better-quality interactions for whānau and clinicians alike (Elder, 2008). As one of the participants in this study stated, following whakawhanaungatanga, 'and the people would say, "now we can place you, now we know who you are, now we can get on with the clinical bit", but if you didn't do the other bit properly first you never really got to the clinical bit' (Elder, 2008, p. 201).

Researchers are clear that obtaining a thorough family history is important for both genetic and public health screening reasons. However, what constitutes a family history mirrors a focus on disorder rather than strengths (Milne et al., 2008). Ensuring that a holistic and rich understanding, very much in line with the discussion about the horizontal epidemiology approach in Chapter 7, which includes mitigating factors such as resilience within families and community resources, must be taken into account.

Other barriers to well-rounded exploration of family history for health professionals have been identified in the context of Māori with depressive illness (Thomas et al., 2010). These practitioners identified that they face having limited time for assessment and treatment. They are mindful of limited resources and they may feel pressured to deal with physical symptoms first. The importance of improving overall communication with patients to overcome these barriers, in order to ensure Māori with depressive illness are afforded the same options as non-Māori, has been underlined (Thomas et al., 2010).

The issue of racism and discrimination is also relevant here. Racism is well established as a determinant of health for indigenous communities and other cultural groups (Harris et al., 2006; King et al., 2009; Priest et al., 2011; Williams & Mohamed, 2009). Racial disparities in health are well documented and researchers are now calling for a more sophisticated way of measuring and assessing the collective effects of racism with other stressors. It is noted that few measures ask questions about the family experiences of stigmatised social identity, discrimination and racism. Rather the research has been individual-focused, which does not help to illuminate these experiences in collective cultures. Residential segregation of families and communities as an example of how racism can impact on health has been reviewed. However, the links between this and other factors such as internalised racism and their associations with risks to health require further research (Williams & Mohamed, 2009).

In Aotearoa New Zealand, there has been significant exploration of the range of experiences of different cultural groups and their dimensions of the concepts of family and community, and appropriate methods for researching whānau (extended family) experiences (Adair & Dixon, 1998; Cram, 2011; Cram & Kennedy, 2010; Pihama et al., 2002). A special focus on Māori has been important for a number of reasons. These include holding the status of indigenous first nations peoples, as peoples who have a unique relationship with the Crown because of Te Tiriti O Waitangi (The Treaty of Waitangi) and because Māori are vastly overrepresented across all fields of illness, including mental illness. These features drive imperatives for cultural competency in understanding and responsivity of health practitioners and policymakers in order to improve outcomes. As with other ethnic cultural groups, there is variability of expression of cultural values and ways of living across generations of Māori. Despite this, three surveys have found that the majority of Māori are interested in, see value in, and participate in Māori cultural activities and visit their own marae (traditional meeting house on ancestral lands) (Statistics

New Zealand, 2013b; Statistics New Zealand & Ministry of Culture and Heritage, 2003; Te Puni Kokiri, 2010). These findings suggest that, for the majority of Māori, there are shared cultural understandings such that Māori-focused policies and competencies are important (Minister of Health, 2006).

Language use in understanding the nuances of concepts that are associated with the English concept of family warrants attention here. The Māori word 'whānau' expresses the concept of wider extended family. There is no Māori word for 'nuclear family'. Despite colonisation and its ongoing impact on contemporary Māori society, the concept of whānau ora (wellbeing of whānau) is something many Māori relate to, albeit in a range of ways (Boulton & Gifford, 2014). Translating the word whānau to the English word 'family" is common practice in Aotearoa New Zealand, and yet inaccurate. In this way, the English language and culture continues to marginalise Māori cultural meanings of the concept of family. By reducing the concept of whānau to that of family means that health potential and health needs can remain invisible and unmet. In my research, exploring traumatic brain injury for Māori, I found that it was important that whānau were recognised as the unit of healing, rather than the individual or index patient (Elder, 2013a, 2013b). This is in contrast to the existing rehabilitation paradigm, which emphasises the importance of people regaining independence (Stucki, 2005).

There is the lack of recognition by many people, including practitioners, that families have knowledge and skills that are specific to the area of health concern at hand. In the context of traumatic brain injury, whānau have access to considerable cultural knowledge resources, specific to the culturally determined aspects of the injury (Elder, 2013a, 2013b). One such culturally determined aspect of Māori health is called wairua, which is defined here as the uniquely Māori connection with all aspects of the universe. The culturally defined aspects of injury to wairua indicate a cultural response that must be given the same credence as clinical knowledge (Elder, 2013b). Some whānau may not initially realise that they have access to this cultural knowledge. Practice-based evidence shows us that this can be related to their experiences of some health services in which both explicitly and covertly Māori people are encouraged to leave culturally informed understandings at the door. Indeed, international research and local practice-based evidence suggests this kind of cultural imposition has links to indigenous youth suicide.

Other ethnic cultural groups may face similar marginalisation when their concepts of family are constructed only from the perspective of the English word. Bringing this awareness into policy and practice can help to enrich a more authentic and accurate understanding of the impact of the family as understood by that cultural group. This approach also unlocks resources that may otherwise remain unrealised, thereby compromising outcomes such as self-determination.

Family and Community

The critical relationship between family and community and the importance of ethnic culture is highlighted by Sparrow (2011). Sparrow makes the point that research to address behavioural, mood and anxiety difficulties within families and communities has tended to focus on parenting and parenting advice, rather than exploring issues of ethnic culture. This approach to research has led to programmes that are assumed to be generalisable, whereas, in practice, this is not the case: 'often, parenting experts appear to assume a homogenous audience that matches their own culture and circumstances' (p. 138). Sparrow also makes links between community sources that promote vital parental emotional availability, and provides specific examples of working with different cultures in their communities (Sparrow, 2011). The ecological developmental paradigm espoused by Bronfenbrenner (1979) is also consistent with these layers of influence occurring within families and communities although the issue of ethnic culture is not an area specifically developed in that paradigm.

Historically, researchers who are interested in a deeper understanding of community aspects of health have focused on aspects at the child and family level in order to understand risk factors for both illness and resilience. Neighbourhood-focused research, examining collective efficacy, has emerged as a promising area (Odgers et al., 2009; Sparrow, 2011, 2014). Articulating the neighbourhood-level social processes that may contribute to both illness and wellbeing strongly resonates with social identity theory, which is more broadly described in Chapter 4. Rather than being a conglomeration of individual characteristics, the group-directed response is where social capital is mobilised and the community demonstrates openness to a shared experience of checking in and looking after each other for the greater good. In other words, the concept expresses the idea of, 'more than the sum of its parts'. This concept aligns with Māori concepts of manaaki (hospitality, sharing) and kaitiakitanga (guardianship, caring) that are, by their very nature, collectivist and reciprocal (Moko-Mead, 2003).

The histories of communities are powerful sources of understanding in terms of formulating intergenerational aspects of community and family life. Indeed, they are integral to culturally informed formulations and recommendations. I now present the example of an area called Manurewa.

Manurewa is a suburb of Auckland, the largest city in Aotearoa New Zealand. There are two stories about its name from pre-colonial times. One is that it is named after a kite that came loose from its ties and drifted away. Another is that it is named for the soaring of birds in the area. In 1863, when the Waikato wars began, most Māori left the area as they were given an ultimatum by the government; either swear an oath to Queen Victoria or go south of the Maungatawhiri River. In 1874, Manurewa had 11 houses and four mud huts. A school was relocated there in 1906, and roads were gradually improved. There were few jobs there until the 1950s as the area functioned as a dormitory suburb, because most residents worked in other parts of Auckland (Wichman, 2001). According to the census, the population in 2013 was 82,000 people, and 20 per cent of them were Māori. Manurewa is now the most ethnically diverse part of Aotearoa New Zealand. The diversity mix is changing, however; from 2006 to 2013, the Māori population was declining, while Pacific island, Asian, Middle Eastern, Latin American and African communities have been increasing (Statistics New Zealand, 2013a).

Using this community history in working with a Māori whānau is likely to inform possible issues of dislocation from ancestral land or a range of experiences of belonging if they do not originate from the area. Equally, exploration may uncover layers of identity that link to distinctive neighbourhoods as they existed at different times. Investigation of the nuances of neighbourhood in the general South Auckland area found that young Māori identified with specific localities, shops and streets as defining their identity (Borrell, 2005). As other cultures moved into the area, intermarriage with people of other cultures across generations in the community is opening up the possibility of additional group cultural resources, which are not otherwise identified, if a thorough history of the community is not investigated.

This type of community history is a necessary addition to the current history schedules of health assessments in order to gain a broader, culturally nuanced understanding in working with families within their complex community influences. This reflects the state of research in the area of social identity and the social determinants of health.

Discussion

It is notable that I have been able to identify so little research that specifically addresses issues of ethnicity and culture within family and community aspects of health and wellbeing. This is especially interesting because of the ethnic cultural disparities that are faced by indigenous and other ethnic cultural groups and the well-documented effects of racism and structural discrimination (Harris et al., 2006; King et al., 2009). In addition, practice-based evidence shows that these are the issues at the hard end of developing rapport and a shared understanding of circumstances which, when maximised, limit misdiagnosis and promote robust formulation, with likely better outcomes.

How, then, do we infuse healthcare training with cultural competency skills, knowledge and attitudes as well as encouraging culturally rigorous research approaches that continue to build our awareness of the importance of working better with different cultures in different communities and family groups? Various legal requirements are one mechanism, such as those afforded by the New Zealand Health Practitioners Competency Assurance Act 2003, and the cultural competency requirements of medical colleges. They provide a minimum standard, however. Champions who 'walk the talk' and provide teaching and supervision at all levels are critical to meeting the needs of these families and communities. The risk-averse, health-provider organisational structures that have arisen in the last 20 years must also change their focus to one that is open, inclusive and truly family- and community-centred as defined by the families and communities themselves. This would mean giving some of their power back to communities and that is a mechanism that is currently being trialled as a consequence of the Whānau Ora policy and praxis in Aotearoa New Zealand (Turia, 2011). Mainstream healthcare organisations need to take account of and act on their perpetuating of barriers to families and communities taking back their self-determination, particularly where their communities are ethnically determined and therefore face specific stereotypes and stigma.

Conclusions

Practitioners and policymakers must keep up to date with research that illuminates aspects of family and community, and particularly with work that views these matters through an ethnic cultural lens. This is because the communities we work in, advocate for, and influence are increasingly ethnically diverse and include some distinctive ethnic groups, such as indigenous peoples.

Reflective practice that promotes and maintains cultural competence begins with critical analysis of our own cultural backgrounds and the culture of our practice. This is the foundation from which we can begin to thoughtfully explore family and community histories in order to better formulate our patients' circumstances, to support self-determination and to achieve better health outcomes.

I have argued for an in-depth approach to family history-taking, mindful of the nuances within ethnic cultural groups and across generations. A collection of aspects of pathology is insufficient and risks families feeling defined solely by what is challenging. This further limits progress in identifying potential for change and healing. I have argued for the specific exploration of culturally defined strengths and resilience. I have presented evidence that families may have specific cultural understandings, pertinent to particular health conditions, and that wider family knowledge can be usefully regarded as having weight that is equal to clinical knowledge. The importance of using cultural protocols cannot be over-emphasised in order to set the scene for a holistic assessment and therapeutic journey. Use of cultural advisers and cultural workers can assist with ensuring these protocols are handled correctly.

English language translations are problematic and care needs to be taken that English language concepts do not override and marginalise the cultural meanings of family and community. These matters are highlighted by the contrasting cultural values of individuality and collectivism.

Finally, I have put forward the concept of the collaborative discovery of a community history in order that patients, families and health practitioners more fully understand and utilise not only the challenges within their communities but also the potential resources. In this way, the practitioners' gaze is drawn to the wider community issues that invite a broader scope of advocacy and practice. At the same time, each family is more likely to feel that their lives have been more fully understood.

References

Adair, V. & Dixon, R., editors (1998). The Family in Aotearoa New Zealand. Auckland: Longman.

Borrell, B. (2005). Living in the city ain't so bad: Cultural identity for young Māori in South Auckland. In Liu, J. McCreanor, T. McIntosh,T. & Teaiwa, T., editors, New Zealand Identities: Departures and Destinations. Wellington: Victoria University Press, pp. 191–206.

Boulton, A. F. & Gifford, H. H. (2014). Whānau ora; he whakaaro ā whānau: Māori family views of family wellbeing. International Indigenous Policy Journal, **5**: 1–16.

Bronfenbrenner, U. (1979). The Ecology of Human Development: Experiments by Nature and Design. Cambridge, MA: Harvard University Press.

Cram, F. (2011). Whānau Ora and Action Research. Wellington: Te Puni Kokiri.

Cram, F. & Kennedy, V. (2010). Researching with whānau collectives. MAI Review, **3**: 1–12.

D'Souza, R. (2003). Incorporating a spiritual history into a psychiatric assessment. Australaisian Psychiatry, **11**: 12–15.

Elder, H. (2008). Ko wai ahau? (Who am I?). How cultural identity issues are experienced by Māori psychiatrists and registrars working with children and adolescents. Australasian Psychiatry, **16**: 200–203.

Elder, H. (2013a). Indigenous theory building for Māori children and adolescents with traumatic brain injury and their extended family. Brain Impairment, **14**: 406–414.

Elder, H. (2013b). Te Waka Oranga. An indigenous intervention for working with Māori children and adolescents with traumatic brain injury. Brain Impairment, **14**: 415–424.

Elder, H. & Tapsell, R. (2013). Māori and the Mental Health Act. In Dawson, J. & Gledhil, K., editors, New Zealand's Mental Health Act in Practice. Wellington: Victoria University Press, pp. 249–267.

Harris, R., Tobias, M., Jeffreys, M. et al. (2006). Effects of self-reported racial discrimination and deprivation on Māori health and inequalities in New Zealand: Cross-sectional study. The Lancet, **367**: 2005–2007.

King, M., Smith, A. & Gracey, M. (2009). Indigenous health part 2: The underlying causes of the health gap. The Lancet, **374**: 76–85.

McInerney, M. (2015). Australia's remote indigenous communities fear closure. See www.bbc.com/news/world-australia-31846031.

Milne, B. J., Moffitt, T. E., Crump, R. et al. (2008). How should we construct psychiatric family history scores? A comparison of alternative approaches from the Dunedin Family Health History Study. Psychological Medicine, **38**: 1793–1802.

Minister of Health. (2006). Te Kōkiri: The Mental Health and Addiction Plan 2005–2015. Wellington: Ministry of Health.

Moko-Mead, H. (2003). Tikanga Māori, Living by Māori Values. Wellington: Huia.

Mortensen, P. B., Peterson, M. G. & Petersen, C. B. (2010). Psychiatric family history of schizophrenia risk in Denmark, which mental disorders are relevant? Psychological Medicine, **40**: 201–210.

Odgers, C. L., Moffitt, T. E., Tach, L. M. et al. (2009). The protective effects of neighbourhood collective efficacy on British children growing up in deprivation: A developmental analysis. Developmental Psychology, **45**: 942–957.

Pihama, L., Cram, F. & Walker, S. (2002). Creating methodological space: A literature review of Kaupapa Mâori research. Canadian Journal of Native Education, **60**: 30–43.

Priest, N. C., Paradies, Y. C., Gunthorpe, W., Cairney, S. J. & Sayers, S. M. (2011). Racism as a determinant of social and emotional wellbeing for Aborignianl Australian youth. Medical Journal of Australia, **194**: 546–550.

Sheldon, M. (2001). Psychiatric assessment in remote Aboriginal communities. Australian and New Zealand Journal of Psychiatry, 35: 435–442.

Sparrow, J. (2011). Child justice, caregiver empowerment and community self-determination. In Fennimore, B. S. & Goodwin, A. L., editors, Promoting Social Justice for Young Children. New York, NY: Springer, pp. 35–46.

Sparrow, J. (2014). Touchpoints: Linking families, professionals, institutions and communities for children's health, education and wellbeing. In Baylis, N. & Keverne, B., editors, Towards a Science of Happiness. Lisbon: Calouste Gulbenkian Foundation, pp. 137–156.

Statistics New Zealand (2013a). Census profile Manurewa. Retrieved 19 March 2015, from http://www.stats.govt.nz/Census/2013-census/profile-and-summary-reports/quickstats-about-a-place.aspx?request_value=13627&tabname=

Statistics New Zealand (2013b). Te Kupenga. Wellington: Statistics New Zealand.

Statistics New Zealand & Ministry of Culture and Heritage. (2003). A Measure of Culture: Cultural Experiences and Cultural Spending in New Zealand. Wellington: Statistics New Zealand, Ministry of Culture and Heritage.

Stucki, G. (2005). International classification of functioning, disability and health (ICF): A promising framework and classification for rehabilitation medicine. American Journal of Physical Medicine and Rehabilitation, **84**: 733–740.

Te Puni Kokiri. (2010). 2009 rangahau i ngā waiaro, ngā uara me ngā whakapono mō Te Reo Māori. 2009 Survey of attitudes, values and beliefs towards the Māori language. Wellington, New Zealand.

Thomas, D. R., Arlidge, B., Arroll, B. & Elder, H. (2010). General practitioner views about diagnosing and treating depression in Māori and non-Māori patients. Journal of Primary Health Care, **2**: 208–216.

Turia, T. (2011). Whānau ora: The theory and the practice. Best Practice Journal, **3**: 11–17.

Wichman, G. (2001). "Soaring Bird": A history of Manurea to 1965. Auckland. Manurea Historical Society,

Williams, D. R. & Mohamed, S. A. (2009). Discrimination and racial disparities in health: Evidence and needed research. Journal of Behavioural Medicine, **32**: 20–47.

Chapter 11

The Nature of Resilience: Coping with Adversity

Richard Williams and Verity Kemp

Introducing Resilience

This book illustrates the burgeoning literature focusing on the ill effects of many forms of adversity, misfortune and disaster, whether deliberate and human-inspired or of, so-called, natural origins. There appear to be many possible ways in which humans can fare badly in response to endogenous and exogenous stress, inequity and inequality. But, by contrast with the risks and the all-too-real suffering of so many survivors, we are struck by the positive ways in which so many people appear to cope with the stress, strain and potentially deleterious impacts. Indeed, post-traumatic growth and mental health problems that are consequent on disasters do not appear to lie at the opposite extremes of a spectrum of outcome, but may co-occur.

We are moved to ask how so many people do well or reasonably well and in what ways that learning might be applied to preventing people from developing problems in the future. We do not diminish the very real risks to people's physical and mental health and to community infrastructure and services that are posed by adversity and disaster. The North Atlantic Treaty Organization (NATO) Guidance issues a warning when it says, 'Substantial resilience of persons and communities is the expected response to a disaster, but is not inevitable' (Department of Health, 2009; NATO/EAPC, 2009). And we are aware that more serious untoward events and circumstances, which produce distress for most people, also precipitate new episodes of pre-existing mental ill health or cause new disorder. These disorders may be long-term for a minority of persons affected.

Our work on psychosocial care in response to adversity and disasters has a two-pronged approach. One is about what families, friends, the helping agencies, employers, societies and states could and should do to prevent people from experiencing problematic responses to short-term and sustained adversity and stress. The second concerns the best ways to produce timely assessments and interventions, including treatments, for people who are at higher risk of becoming mentally unwell as a consequence of those stressors. Thus, we work with governmental bodies to set out evidence- and values-based strategic approaches to assisting people in need after their exposure to disasters of all kinds (e.g. Department of Health, 2009; Ministry of Health, New Zealand, 2016; NATO/EAPC, 2009).

This chapter focuses on the preventative avenue by exploring the nature and meaning of resilience. We survey definitions that are used to identify many different, but overlapping ways in which the term is used. Then, we focus on the social interactions and processes that assist people, families, people at work and existing and emergent communities to show resilience in adversity and crises. Thus, we focus most on the intrapersonal and interpersonal, or collective, processes whereby people express personal and community psychosocial resilience.

Defining Resilience

The Challenge

An immediate challenge is the ubiquitous use of the term resilience: it has given rise to misunderstanding and criticism. Robinson's words (2015, p. 13) resonate, 'There is wide variation in what is taken to represent resilience'. Grünewald and Warner (2012) ask if resilience is a buzz word or useful concept and fear that, if the term were to mean all things to all people, it could become an empty shell. We agree that greater clarity of definition and awareness of its nature and origins is required if we are to use the term advisedly and reap the benefits.

We summarise research on six ways in which the concept of resilience is used to identify the problems with using the term in undefined ways.

(1) Defining resilience is complicated by the levels at which the term is used. Commonly, resilience is used in relation to: society; culture; policy; strategic planning, management and integration of regions; communities; families; and people and their emergent relationships when they face challenge. The literature also shows that the term is used to describe very many features of countries' infrastructure, resources, plans and approaches to disaster risk reduction and intervening, after untoward events and in adversity.

(2) We have observed that resilience is often used to reassure people that ill effects of untoward events are not inevitable and that government departments anticipate that people will be able to protect themselves. While this may be a laudable objective, it is insufficient without empirical evidence.

(3) Our experience is that resilience is often used to describe desired endstates after untoward events in which people remain well despite facing great adversity and/or stress. The research by Patel et al. (2017) and Ntontis et al. (2018) supports our experience. We witness the term resilience being used as a social construction that argues backwards from desired outcomes to presume people's capabilities or traits that have, arguably, contributed to good outcomes. We see many people in the policy, clinical and research fields falling prey to the temptation to define resilience as being evident when people do NOT develop problems, symptoms or disorders or when they cope without seeking professional help after their exposure to adversity, traumatic or other stressful events. We agree with Almedom and Glandon (2007) that it is unhelpful to use resilience as a synonym for good outcomes or apply it to describe what is, too often, an undefined force for good.

(4) In respect of community resilience, Ntontis et al. (2018) have analysed governmental and other guidance on community resilience. Their analyses show that 'treating resilience as the opposite of vulnerability and vulnerability as the opposite of resilience can lead to circular reasoning . . . in which the concept of resilience is employed by certain institutions as an explanatory concept to account for individuals' and communities' resilience'.

(5) Ntontis et al.'s other main finding is that 'the reification of resilience can be problematic since it occludes the processes that lead a community to being resilient in the first place'. They argue that, 'This reification can become even more problematic when such representations are placed descriptively together with other reified concepts, like that of vulnerability, especially when social processes and dynamics are not considered'.

(6) In our opinion, the concept of resilience has become a strong example of concepts that are 'deeply rooted in metaphorical ways of thinking' (Haslam et al., 2017). In this case, the metaphors include those drawn from metallurgy and horticulture. While initially helpful, these metaphors have tended to simplify and, arguably, oversimplify, the concept, allowing it to become reified and for circularity of statements made about it to appear even in governments' guidance. Norris et al. (2008) summarise an array of theoretical models. They, too, identify the diversity of understandings of the nature of resilience in their analysis. They identify the metallurgical metaphor in which resilience concerns how groups of people, communities and public systems cope with, and spring back from, major problems, adversity and untoward events to regain effective functioning. Arguably, that metaphor is now outdated by research from both the social sciences and neurobiology.

Pragmatically, we are sympathetic to the view of Warner and Grünewald (2012) that, 'A facilitating approach to "resilience" helping people to help themselves might . . . [point to] the role that public- and private-sector actors can play in supporting . . . local capabilities'. This is closer to using resilience as a term that summarises the relational processes that take place when people pursue social causation.

These findings shape this chapter. We endeavour to look beneath the surface to better understand psychosocial resilience as a way of describing how people and groups of people cope, recover and develop when they face adversity and challenge.

Resilience as an Ecological Concept

The United Nations Office for Disaster Risk Reduction (UNISDR) defines resilience as 'The ability of a system, community or society exposed to hazards to resist, absorb, accommodate to and recover from the effects of a hazard in a timely and efficient manner, including through the preservation and restoration of its essential basic structures and functions' (UNISDR, 2009). This, and a number of other definitions, is based on ecological concepts that appear to focus on resilience as describing how systems and communities resist and are restored to the status quo ante, after the effects of hazards.

Resilience in Disasters, Emergencies and Adversity

The Department for International Development (DFID, 2011, p. 6) defines resilience as 'The ability of countries, communities and households to manage change, by maintaining or transforming living standards in the face of shocks or stresses – such as earthquakes, drought or violent conflict – without compromising their long-term prospects'. The Organisation for Economic Co-operation and Development (OECD, 2013, p. 1) definition is 'The ability of individuals, communities and states and their institutions to absorb and recover from shocks, whilst positively adapting and transforming the structures and means for living in the face of long-term changes and uncertainty'. These definitions agree about absorbing stress, maintaining standards and recovering, but the OECD goes further than do UNISDR and DFID by adding the processes of adapting and transforming.

Combaz (2014) asks, 'What is disaster resilience?', and provides a useful orientation to the way in which the word is used in disasters. The definition which that report adopts is, 'Disaster resilience is the ability of individuals, communities, organisations and states to adapt to and recover from hazards, shocks or stresses without compromising long-term prospects for development'. Thus, the notions of long-termism and preserving capacities for development are added by Combaz and DFID to the processes taken as defining resilience.

Others (e.g. Howell & Voronka, 2012) criticise the ways in which the construct of resilience is often misunderstood. Some critics say that policymakers may place too much responsibility on individual persons and wider society rather than on responsible authorities that have the potential power to address the underlying causes of risk.

Psychosocial Resilience

We use the term 'psychosocial resilience' to separate uses of the construct that relate to human systems from the broad, general and, very often, undefined uses of the term. In this context, the adjective 'psychosocial' refers to:

> ... the cognitive, emotional, social and physical experiences of particular people and of collectives of people ... in the context of particular social and physical environments. It ... is used to describe the psychological and social processes that occur within and between people and across groups of people ... [and] these processes as they occur before, during and after events that may be variously described as emergencies, disasters and major incidents. (Department of Health, 2009)

Layers of Psychosocial Resilience

Psychosocial resilience embraces the notions of coping, adapting in response to challenge in order to recover well, and transforming in order to mitigate the effects of future challenges. But, even at this personal level, Southwick et al. (2011) report Layne et al. (2007) as finding at least eight distinct meanings.

Helpfully, Dückers (2017) describes a multilayered psychosocial resilience framework that conceptualises and connects capacities at individual, community and society levels. The first layer concerns each person's reactions to adversity and potentially or actually traumatic events. He sees community resilience as centring on the neighbourhoods and cities in which people live. We extend the notion of communities to include workplaces, schools, clubs and other groups in which people associate. As we shall see, some communities arise in emergent circumstances. Dückers points out that the capacity of societies to return to a stable order depends on the presence of socio-economic, political and institutional conditions together with operational structures and resources (p. 183).

Here, we focus on the personal, group and community levels at which resilience is used. We adopt the term 'psychosocial resilience' when we use the construct in this way and we note that it takes in a number of Smith's dimensions of the human condition that he covers in Chapter 2.

We perceive two main streams of theory and research regarding resilience at personal, family and community levels that, despite opposing assertions, we see are not conceptually or practically discrete. We see them as being concerned with similar aspects of people's lives and experiences when faced with events of sudden onset or longer-term adverse circumstances. They are:

- How people develop through childhood into adulthood and learn to construct positive relationships, acquire the capacity to create new ones and mourn the loss of others, while they adapt and transform as life events impact; and

- How people process the most challenging, traumatic and tragic crises in their lives and present their experiences in their emotional, cognitive, social and behavioural responses.

In Chapter 9, Hindley quotes Ungar's definition of resilience (Ungar, 2008, p. 225): 'In the context of exposure to significant adversity, whether psychological, environmental, or both, resilience is both the capacity of individuals to navigate their way to health-sustaining resources, including opportunities to experience feelings of well-being, and a condition of the individual family, community and culture to provide these health resources and experiences in culturally meaningful ways.' This approach brings in the notions of help-seeking and the importance of culture, and it identifies the reciprocal relationships on which resilience turns. Similarly, our use of the concept is entirely compatible with people experiencing rather than resisting short-term distress if it is not associated with prolonged or sustained dysfunction. Importantly, Elder explores the importance of families and culture in more detail in Chapter 10.

Recovery is a word that is often used in relationship to both traumatic events and mental ill health. Each use describes active, positive approaches that are taken by particular people to manage their environments in the context of supportive groups of other people and the resources that they have available. Deegan (1988) describes:

> . . . recovery as a process, a way of life, an attitude and a way of approaching the day's challenges. It is not a perfectly linear process. At times our course is erratic and we falter, slide back, regroup, and start again . . . The need is to re-establish a new and valued sense of integrity and purpose within and beyond the limits of the disability . . .

People who are resilient in the face of adversity and crisis have similar experiences. Studies of how humans behave during and after complex situations that demand change show that tipping the definition of resilience towards adaptability, transformation and sustainability rather than solely resistance to change and absorbing stress provide a substantial model for understanding how people achieve these things and a more adequate picture of their needs. We see the twin tracks of coping in the face of adversity, on one hand, and adaptability and transformation, on the other, as the key features of human resilience.

Many authors point out that people who face stressful challenges may show uneven functioning, which reflects their having capabilities in some domains, but not in others (e.g. Southwick et al., 2011, p. xi, p. 6). This observation, together with current dynamic, interactive models of resilience (Masten et al., 2011), explain why these characteristics may vary with time and may be specific to particular circumstances, social networks and events so that psychosocial resilience varies with social settings rather than it being a constant personal characteristic or trait.

Three Generations of Resilience

Bonanno (2004), quoted by Dückers (2017), sees resilience as differing from recovery, which he describes as 'a trajectory in which normal functioning temporarily gives way to . . . psychopathology . . . usually for a period of at least several months and then gradually returns to pre-event levels . . . By contrast, resilience reflects the ability to maintain a stable equilibrium' (p. 20). We prefer an approach that adopts the notion of trajectories, but which turns less on psychopathology and which borrows from the recovery approach that we touched on earlier. We think that the features that we have identified so far in this account are summarised by the three 'generations' of resilience that are informed by the opinions of Omand (2010). We identify:

- First-generation resilience: the ability to cope reasonably well with events and their immediate aftermath. This use embraces the ecological approach, but goes beyond resistance to stress.
- Second-generation resilience: the ability to adapt and recover from events.
- Third-generation resilience: the ability of people to transform themselves, their relationships and the organisations that impact on them in the light of lessons learned from events. This use of the term takes into account the potential for challenging circumstances and events to evoke growth in certain people in certain circumstances despite the unwelcome nature of the events through which they go and the possibility that they may develop mental health problems.

First-generation psychosocial resilience describes robustness and coping, and that resonates with the horticultural metaphorical construct of hardiness. A difficulty emerges if we try to align the notions of how humans adapt and recover from challenges with their resisting change as the concept of hardiness might imply. Indeed, adaptation implies that the object of recovery after an adverse event is not to resist changes but to embrace them in order to return to coping well. The second generation focuses on recovering with fortitude and without giving up cherished values, which we see as core to psychosocial resilience. The third generation concerns how people cope better in the future and it includes transformability and sustainability among its components.

Community Psychosocial Resilience

Patel et. al. (2017) have published a systematic review of the literature on community resilience, based on a qualitative review of 80 papers and grey literature to May 2015, concerning disasters that met the UNISDR definition including 'acts of violence such as war and terrorism as well as natural disasters' (Patel et. al., 2017, p. 4).

That review corroborates our view of the diversity of, and difficulty with, definitions. The authors found more than 50 different definitions and came to the view that it is 'an amorphous concept that was understood and applied differently by different research groups' (p. 8). They concluded that 'community resilience can … be seen as an ongoing process of adaptation, the simple absence of negative effects, the presence of a range of positive attributes, or a mix of all three' (p. 8).

Consequently, Patel et al. (2017) commend focusing on the elements that have been identified as contributing to resilience. Their literature review identified nine main elements and 19 sub-elements, through inductive thematic analysis of the sources, and they are illustrated in Table 11.1. Their opinion is that 'use of the phrase community resilience, and attempts to define the concept, may be unhelpful if it obscures the importance of these … elements' (p. 14).

Dückers draws attention to Adger's (2000) definition of community resilience. It is 'the ability of human communities to withstand external shocks or perturbations to their infrastructure, such as environmental variability or social, economic or political upheaval, and to recover from such perturbations'.

Norris et al. (2008) assert that community resilience 'emerges from four primary sets of adaptive capacities – economic development, social capital, information and communication, and community competence – that together provide a strategy for disaster

Table 11.1 Elements of community resilience (from Patel et al., 2017)

Main elements	Sub-elements
Local knowledge	Factual knowledge base
	Training and education
	Collective efficacy and empowerment
Community network and relationships	Members of communities are well connected
	Members of communities form a cohesive whole
Communication	Effective communication
	Strong communication networks
	Risk communication
	Crisis communication
Health	Health services can be disrupted so build hospitals to higher structural standards
	Sustain delivery and quality of care for people who have physical and mental health problems
Governance and leadership	Infrastructure and services
	Public involvement and support
Resources	Natural, physical, human and social resources
Economic investment	Economic programming
	Economic development of post-disaster infrastructure
Preparedness	
Mental outlook	Hope
	Adaptability
	Acceptance of uncertainty and change

preparedness'. We quote their definition of resilience later, but believe that their approach should be adapted to take in developments in social science of the last decade.

The significance of Dückers' (2017) multilayered framework is that he shows that an important component of community resilience is that it should link the capacities and processes that support resilience, at society and individual levels. He says that the time stages before, during and after a crisis are relevant for coping and adaptive capacities with respect to the levels of his framework. He observes that, when a crisis occurs, it is tackled by networks of organisations (p. 184) and the linkages between them are vital to resilience. Thus, coordination and alignment are important matters in promoting resilience and recovery. This emphasises the importance of connectedness and agency.

The Origins of Psychosocial Resilience

Sapienza and Masten (2011) observe that models of what we call psychosocial resilience have become more dynamic and systemic with time. They describe four waves of research that have ensued since the importance of resilience was recognised and show a progressive shift from: work to identify the nature and properties of what constitutes resilience; how it operates through interactive, multilevel and multidisciplinary processes; through to the current concern with 'the dominant models of resilience [which are] . . . dynamic, focused on processes linking neurobiology to behavior [and] to environmental conditions'.

We summarise a range of theoretical approaches to the origins of resilience in this section. They contribute to the research findings which show that the potentially adverse effects on persons, families and communities of adversity, emergencies and disasters can be mitigated by dynamic human social systems (Williams & Hazell, 2011).

Genetics and Neuroscience

Genetics are highly relevant to understanding resilience (Levin, 2009). But, because this book focuses on social influences on health, we do not pursue genetics though we recognise their relevance.

We take a similar position concerning neurobiology. Fortunately, a contemporary, authoritative review of the neurobiology of resilience is available (Osório et al, 2016). Its authors identify in the research literature to 2014, ' . . . some of the neural, neurochemical, genetic and epigenetic components that may characterize vulnerability, and conversely resilience . . . '. That review allows us to focus here on a selection of the many social and developmental influences that fall into Smith's dimensions of sociability, cognition and agency (see Chapter 2).

Child Development

Hindley introduces us to attachment theory, belonging and resilience as linked constructs that affect children and young people in Chapter 9. He covers a number of aspects of children's and young people's resilience. Therefore, we cover other aspects of resilience as it applies to children and young people in this chapter.

One of those matters concerns whether or not younger children can be resilient given their psychosocial and physical immaturity and the process of rapid development on which they are bound. Southwick et al. say, 'Children, in general, are remarkably resilient' (Southwick et al., 2011, p. xiv) and, 'What information that does exist suggests that children cope as well as, if not better than adults' (p. xii). But, a journal editorial on the effects of early trauma and deprivation on human development says that the papers in that journal provide ' . . . compelling cross-sectional and longitudinal evidence that early experiences of inadequate input (neglect/deprivation) and unwanted input (threat/trauma) – remembered or not – led to long-term developmental and clinical abnormalities' (Zeanah & Sonuga-Barke, 2016, p. 1101). Importantly, they draw attention to papers that '. . . demonstrate that the presence and behavior of caretakers moderate the effects of early adversity and response to interventions' (Zeanah & Sonuga-Barke, 2016, p. 1101). Once again, the transactional nature of resilience arises.

That same editorial also draws attention to the cumulative risk model, showing that 'long-term adverse outcomes are better predicted by the total number, rather than the specific nature of environment risk exposures'. It has become the dominant thesis on how 'environmental exposures to different adverse experiences and events early in life produce negative outcomes many years later' (Zeanah & Sonuga-Barke, 2016, p. 1099).

Another research review focuses on resilience in child development and the variety of circumstances in which neurobiology, social ecology, nutrition and adjustment impact on the children's resilience. As one of the papers states, '. . . this body of knowledge supports a perspective of resilience as a complex dynamic process driven by time- and context-dependent variables, rather than [it being] the balance between risk and protective factors with known impacts on mental health' (Panter-Brick & Leckman, 2013).

Belonging, Attachment and Resilience

Pathways that protect children and young people and enable them to develop well and express resilience include '. . . factors such as attachment[s], social support, religion, intelligence and problem-solving ability, and cognitive flexibility . . . ' (Southwick et al., 2011, p. xii).

In Chapter 9, Hindley substantiates the importance of children accumulating experiences of relating to other people, and the power of their sustained sense of belonging, to their social and emotional development, which projects through their lives. We also see psychosocial resilience as resting on attachment and relational skills, social identity, dependable social networks and availability of social support as well as certain personal attributes. Elder makes very important points about families and culture in Chapter 10.

In our opinion, it is likely that the dependency of children and young people on adults around them for food, safety, security, caring, nurturing, warmth and learning is the factor that may render them more vulnerable to the ill effects of adversity and untoward events. These requirements, which are ordinarily intense in children and young people who are developing rapidly, may be threatened by the impacts on adults' abilities to offer parenting and social support during adversity and after major incidents. We think that these social understandings begin to resolve the tension between recognising why children and young people are widely held to be more vulnerable to adversity and major incidents than are adults while some researchers assert that they can cope as well as do adults. Perhaps, children's dependencies on social connectedness are more powerful than are the limitations of all but young children in being able to summon the personal capacity for resilience (Sheikh et al., 2016)?

People's attachment capacities, which are usually developed in early childhood and thereafter, link them with the power of social support. Mawson (2005, p. 95) argues that, 'the typical response to a variety of threats and disasters is not to flee but to seek the proximity of familiar persons and places . . . ' and he proposes a social attachment model that recognises the '. . . gregarious nature of human beings and the primacy of attachments'. This opinion endorses the low frequency of mass panic (see Chapter 16). Nonetheless, the common occurrence of panic remains an opinion that is held strongly by many responsible authorities despite this not being supported by evidence. The myth of panic impacts strongly but erroneously on policy and practice (Carter et al., 2013).

People's attachment capacities and styles may partially explain the origins of psychosocial resilience. These capacities enable them to benefit from enduring social connections, create emergent links with people who find themselves in similar critical situations and benefit from the power of social support (Bryant & Foord, 2016). Bryant's opinion is that, 'There is overwhelming evidence that social attachments play a critical role in how humans manage adversity', and 'Individual differences in how we seek out and benefit from attachments impact on the actual availability of social connections' (Bryant, 2016, p. 5).

Bryant reviews the literature that shows how attachment styles are likely to be associated with benefiting from social support. He says, 'Individual differences in how we seek out and benefit from attachments impact on the actual availability of social connections, which in turn can markedly impact on how we think, feel and behave' and, 'The accumulating evidence suggests that social support will be variably helpful to people after trauma, depending on one's attachment style . . .' (Bryant, 2016, p. 5). But, he also points to literature showing that people who have insecure and avoidant attachment styles may also convey advantages on groups of people when they face challenges.

Personal and Collective Characteristics of Psychosocial Resilience

Previously, Williams and Drury have described two interacting – personal and collective – contributions to psychosocial resilience. But, the evidence of the intersection of personal and collective attributes is such that we think now that the distinction is difficult, given the power of social connectedness, social processes and social support. People who are more poorly connected tend to receive less social support and, consequently, fare less well. Perceived emotional and instrumental support, availability of support from families and network size have been reported as protective factors for common mental disorders, and the particular type of social support may be important (Smyth et al., 2014).

Nonetheless, some people who become isolated may do well. Perhaps they are able to sustain themselves by rehearsing, in their inner worlds, mental images and thoughts of their connectedness? Bryant and Foord (2016) say, 'Attachment theory posits that activation of mental representations of attachment figures can reduce stress and boost coping [and] consolidation of emotional memories can be moderated by activation of attachment representations'.

Robinson says, 'Rutter ... draws on research to propose a series of mechanisms that might mediate the interaction of the risk and protective variables in a positive direction [by]: reducing the risk impact, possibly by altering the risk or by reducing exposure to the risk; reduction of negative chain reactions; promoting self-esteem and self-efficacy; and providing opportunities' (Robinson, 2015; quoting Rutter, 1987).

Our reading of the literature has led us to the opinion that psychosocial resilience is not best understood as a trait within persons but as linked to the inner representation of their interactions, attachments and identifications, between them and other people. However, a number of personal psychological capabilities overlap with, or are included within, the attributes of psychosocial resilience. They include: hardiness, sense of coherence, engagement and cognitive emotional regulation (Kobasa, 1979; Kobasa et al., 1982; Williams & Kemp, 2017). In addition, engagement theory considers that resilience describes processes that people use to regulate their distress and their trajectories of engagement and adaptation. A cognitive emotional regulation framework for coping is based on people using regulation of their emotions to change adaptively their appraisal of the stressors they experience and, thereby, moderate those stressors' impacts on their coping (Troy & Mauss, 2011).

Collective psychosocial resilience illustrates the relationship between social context, culture and how people respond to each other, and how they cope with crises and adversity. It describes how people behave when they are in groups, and how they deal with and recover from adverse events (Department of Health, 2009; Williams & Drury, 2011). Drury and Williams define collective psychosocial resilience as 'the way in which groups of people and crowds of people express and expect solidarity and cohesion, and thereby coordinate and draw upon collective sources of support and other practical resources adaptively to deal with adversity' (Department of Health, 2009; Williams & Drury, 2011). Research indicates the benefits for people of creating shared social identities include making available to them peers' perceptions and appraisals of risk against which they can calibrate their own judgements and perceptions of how the world is, and how it should be. This can be the basis of group consensus (Haslam et al., 1998). Certainly, stress is reduced when collective support is forthcoming.

While attachment capabilities may partially explain the origins of psychosocial resilience, our evaluation of the evidence is that it does not explain sufficient of the facts without combination with findings from social psychology. Drury and colleagues, for example, showed that in the London bombings, in 2005, altruistic behaviour was far more frequent than selfish behaviour and yet most people were not with others they knew beforehand.

Until quite recently, the social supportive actions that people in mass emergencies exhibit was thought to be dependent on pre-existing social relationships (Mawson et al., 2005). A very important development in the research on collective resilience has described a dynamic model, based on a social identity theory (Haslam, 2004; Turner et al., 1987). This approach has developed from studying how crowds respond to crises. We think that this approach makes a huge contribution to understanding resilience and we acknowledge empirical evidence that the social identity model has stronger explanatory value for how social support operates than does the stress buffering hypothesis (Praharso et al., 2016).

Drury et al. (2009a; Chapters 15 and 17) argue that the social identity model suggests that there is a move from focusing on 'me' to focusing on 'we' and, thereby, a shared social identity, when people suffer extreme events together. He describes the experience of shared fate in particularly troubling emergency situations as providing the means by which people rapidly form and share social identities with strangers. Thus, shared fate enables groups of people to offer each other social support as a result of their shared experience (Cocking et al., 2009; Drury et al., 2009b). People involved in the London bombings shared possessions and offered social support to people to whom they might, otherwise, not have talked, to the point of putting themselves at risk (Williams & Drury, 2010, 2011). This research illustrates that resilient, adaptive behaviours do develop without social relationships that have been established before events occur.

This approach identifies gaps in understanding, to date, the mechanisms whereby shared fate occurs. Perhaps, exposure to substantial stress evokes inner attachment primes, which propel people to seek social connectedness. If so, coming into contact with people in similar situations brings the sense of a shared fate. This cues rapid, if temporary, attachments to people who are also seeking proximity, and processes that generate shared identities, which might be described as collective resilience, are evoked.

An Integrated Approach

Six Dimensions of the Human Condition

We see psychosocial resilience as a set of systemic, dynamic processes in which people's social connectedness, social identities and attachment capacities play strong parts. It describes social processes by which people act singly or together to mitigate, moderate or adapt to the effects of events. It is a dynamic construct that describes how people cope with, adapt to and transform their lives over time in response to acute and/or chronic challenges rather than indicating a set of personal traits or attributes.

In Chapter 2, Smith asks that we consider the social determinants of mental health fully; we must not only uncover the social processes of social causation concerning the epidemiology of mental illness and mental health, but also those processes of social construction that affect how notions of illness, health and wellbeing are defined, given meaning or responded to within social contexts. In all probability, psychosocial resilience sits across the processes of social causation and social construction. It is clear that many of the definitions turn less on scientific examination of how human systems behave when challenged and more on construction of ways of thinking. 'How we function in our social world after trauma is a highly complex issue' (Bryant, 2016, p. 5). We think that the origins and impacts of psychosocial resilience can be found in each of Smith's six dimensions of the human condition and particularly in our experiences of sociability, cognition, evaluation and agency.

Adaptive Capacities

Norris et al. define resilience as a process linking a set of adaptive capacities to a positive trajectory of functioning and adaptation, after a disturbance (Kaniasty & Norris, 2004; Norris et al., 2008, 2009). This is our preferred definition.

We concur with Robinson, who points out that Rutter argued 30 years ago that vulnerability and protection are two ends of the same concept and that, 'The vulnerability or protective effect is evident only in combination with the risk variable . . . the terms "process" and "mechanism" are preferable to "variable" or "factor" because any one variable may act as a risk factor in one situation but as a vulnerability factor in another' (Rutter, 1987; Robinson, 2015).

We have already drawn attention to research indicating that resilience may be context- and role-specific (Panter-Brick & Leckman, 2013). So, it is inappropriate to describe people as inherently resilient or vulnerable without referring to their particular circumstances and the risks that they face. The contemporary circumstances in which people find themselves, the people with whom they relate at the time, their present needs and the resources available also have enormous impacts on how well they cope and flexibly use a variety of coping strategies that are associated with resilience (Southwick et al., 2014). These horizontal epidemiological factors (Chapters 7 and 13 in this book) resonate with what we know of the power of peer groups. Certainly, this approach is not intended to diminish the '. . . profound influence of early life experiences (biological embedding) as another predisposing factor for life stressors and the cumulative burden . . . ' or awareness '. . . of the capacity of the brain to store memories of a lifetime, as well as the capacity of the brain for plasticity . . .' (Sapienza & Masten, 2011). But it does argue for a broad approach in which resilience is considered among a range of factors that influence people's needs and responses to events.

The literature (Williams et al., 2014) suggests that the core features of people who show good psychosocial resilience, as defined by Norris et al. (2008, 2009), are:

- They perceive that they have, and actually receive, social support. We think that the abilities of people to accept and use social support and the availability of it are two of the core features of resilience.
- They tend to show acceptance of reality.
- They have belief in themselves that is supported by strongly held values.
- They have abilities to improvise.

People respond to stressors by mobilising their inner, personal resources and, in parallel, the support provided by their families, colleagues, friends and the people with whom they are in contact, when untoward events occur, is critically important. Together, these resources enable people, families and communities to generate adaptive capacities that assist them to cope reasonably well, recover from events and learn lessons for the future.

Thus, personal and collective processes come together to underpin individual psychosocial resilience. Community psychosocial resilience may emerge when people interact as members of groups. Sometimes, interactions occur between recognised or established groups of people and, as Drury et al. show in Section 3, these relationships may also arise emergently in crises when groups of people who are thrown together by events share a fate that promotes social identity, however transiently.

Distress, Disorders and Psychosocial Resilience

People facing adverse circumstances are likely to experience stress because these situations may undermine their positive perceptions of the environment and themselves, their senses of control and feelings of worth. They may have insufficient emotional, cognitive, social or physical resources to cope with events. Typically, these experiences are described as distress, which describes 'the experiences and feelings of people after external events that challenge their tolerance and adaptation . . . Distress is an anticipated human emotion, not a disorder, when it and any associated psychosocial dysfunction emerges and persists in proportion to external stressful situations' (NATO/EAPC, 2009).

It is important to distinguish people's distress, consequent on their involvement in a crisis or longer-standing adversity, from mental disorder. This might be challenging because their experiences or symptoms may be similar. The distinction turns on the pathways or trajectories of people's responses over time and the severity and duration of any associated dysfunction. Furthermore, distress may lead to people's dysfunction, which may be temporary, or more sustained, and can, in some circumstances, lead to or be a component of mental disorders. Masten et al. (2011) offer examples of resilience pathways in the context of acute trauma and chronic adversity and Norris et al. (2009) describe people's stress trajectories. Hobfoll et al. (2011) offer principles that show how engagement and distress interact.

Bryant et. al. (2016), 'provide the first evidence of disorder-specific patterns in relation to [their] social connections after disasters. Depression appears to co-occur in linked [people] whereas PTSD [post-traumatic stress disorder] risk is increased with social fragmentation'. We agree with Bryant et al., that, 'These patterns underscore the need to adopt a sociocentric perspective of postdisaster mental health in order to better understand the potential for societal interventions in the wake of disaster'.

An Alternative Model for Psychosocial Resilience

This chapter summarises a number of concepts, constructs, theories and processes taken from the work of a variety of scientific disciplines that all contribute to the overarching concept of psychosocial resilience. We illustrate how the term, resilience, is frequently used as a shorthand to describe: complicated functions of organisations when they face challenging events; or people's behaviour and their responses to adversity and challenge. This wide use of the term is unsatisfactory.

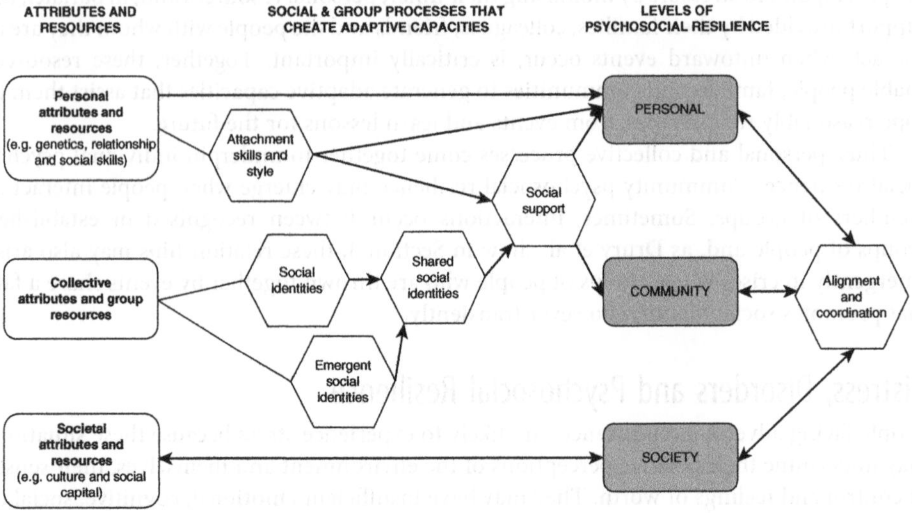

Figure 11.1 Attributes, social processes and levels of psychosocial resilience

Instead, we propose a transactional and contextual model for psychosocial resilience. We see personal factors, which include people's experience of events and a range of social contextual factors, as interacting over time with factors that emerge from participants' membership of groups, relationships and their attachment styles. The model brings together processes from:

(1) Social–ecological models of recovery (Maercker & Hecker, 2016; Maercker & Horn, 2013);
(2) Social identity approaches (Drury et al., 2009b; Williams & Kemp, 2016, 2017); and
(3) Attachment theory (Fonagy et al., 2014; Nolte et al., 2011; Sharp et al., 2012).

Figure 11.1 summarises diagrammatically some of the topics, social processes and layers of psychosocial resilience that this chapter covers. It is superimposed on Dückers' description of levels of resilience (2017).

Panter-Brick (2015) provides a forward-orientated exploration of the relationships between culture and resilience. In the context of culture, it is clear to us that, while resilience may appear at first sight as a straightforward way in which to express how so many people recover after serious events and cope in adversity, it is also a challenging topic. We would not wish to lose it. Therefore, continuing research and refinement of the construct is necessary. Importantly, we have covered a rich variety of observational and theoretical perspectives. Panter-Brick and Leckman (2013) point out that, 'A lens on resilience shifts the focus of attention from efforts to appraise risk or vulnerability, towards concerted efforts to enhance strength or capability. It also shifts the focus of analysis … to asking more complex questions regarding wellbeing, such as when, how, why and for whom do resources truly matter'.

The extent to which people are able to display psychosocially resilient social processes is influenced by many factors including: their social connectedness (emergent connections, relationships and attachments); their capacities to adapt, transform their connectedness and use their experiences; the particularities of the events and circumstances; genetics and neuroscience; and, how all these elements interplay. We, too, may have fallen prey to reification and circular arguments. Nonetheless, we hope that the topics covered help readers in taking the journey towards a better understanding of what resilience is.

Practically, we concur with Ntontis et al. (2018) who propose that the following points should be considered by people who use the construct of resilience in their work:

> (i) 'It is better to avoid using simple, reified, and static definitions of . . . resilience . . . since they lack explanatory power, as well as clear directions for future action in preparedness and response'; (ii) 'Circularity (using resilience to explain resilience itself) should be avoided, since it lacks focus on its more specific, core parts and, thereby, risks overemphasising empirical support for actions that are proposed'; and (iii) 'A focus on enhancing some specific core aspects of . . . resilience [is likely to be] more fruitful than attempts to enhance resilience in abstract'.

References

Adger, W. N. (2000). Social and ecological resilience: Are they related? Progress in Human Geography, **24**: 347–364.

Almedom, A. M. & Glandon, D. (2007). Resilience is not the absence of PTSD any more than health is the absence of disease. Journal of Loss and Trauma, **12**: 127–143.

Bonanno, G. A. (2004). Loss, trauma, and human resilience. Have we underestimated the human capacity to thrive after extremely aversive events? American Psychologist, **59**: 20–28.

Bryant, R. A. (2016). Social attachments and traumatic stress. European Journal of Psychotraumatology, **7**: article 29065; http://dx.doi.org/10.3402/ejpt.v7.29065.

Bryant, R. A. & Foord, R. (2016). Activating attachments reduces memories of traumatic images. PLoS One, **11**: e0162550. doi: 10. 1371/journal.pone.0162550.

Bryant, R. A., Gallagher, H. C., Gibbs, L. et al. (2016). Mental health and social networks after disasters. American Journal of Psychiatry, November; doi: 10.1176/appi.ajp.2016.15111403.

Carter, H., Drury, J., Rubin, G. J., Williams, R. & Amlôt, R. (2013). Communication during mass casualty decontamination: Highlighting the gaps. International Journal of Emergency Services, **2**: 29–48; doi: 10.1108/IJES-06-2012-0026.

Cocking, C., Drury, J. & Reicher, S. (2009). The psychology of crowd behaviour in emergency evacuations: Results from two interview studies and implications for the fire & rescue services. Irish Journal of Psychology, **30**: 59–73.

Combaz, E. (2014). Disaster Resilience: Topic Guide. Birmingham: GSDRC, University of Birmingham.

Deegan, P. E. (1988). Recovery: The lived experience of rehabilitation. Psychosocial Rehabilitation Journal, **11**: 11–19.

Department of Health (2009). NHS Emergency Planning Guidance: Planning for the Psychosocial and Mental Health Care of People Affected by Major Incidents and Disasters. London: Department of Health.

DFID (2011). Defining Disaster Resilience: A DFID Approach Paper. London: DFID.

Drury, J., Cocking, C. & Reicher, S. (2009a). Everyone for themselves? A comparative study of crowd solidarity among emergency survivors. British Journal of Social Psychology, **48**: 487–506.

Drury, J., Cocking, C. & Reicher, S. (2009b). The nature of collective resilience: Survivor reactions to the 2005 London bombings. International Journal of Mass Emergencies and Disasters, **27**: 66–95.

Dückers, M. L. A. (2017). A multi-layered psychosocial resilience framework and its implications for community-focused crisis management. Journal of Contingencies and Crisis Management, **25**: 182–187.

Fonagy, P., Lorenzini, N., Campbell, C. & Luyten, P. (2014). Why are we interested in attachments? In Holmes, P. & Farnfield, S., editors, The

Routledge Handbook of Attachment: Theory. Hove: Routledge, pp. 31–48.

Grünewald, F. & Warner, J. (2012). Resilience: Buzz word or critical strategic concept? Humanitarian Aid on the Move, **10**: 1–7.

Haslam, S. A. (2004). Psychology in Organizations: The Social Identity Approach. London: Sage.

Haslam, S. A., Cornelissen, J. P. & Werner, M. J. (2017). Metatheories and metaphors of organizational identity: Integrating social constructionist, social identity, and social actor perspectives within a social interactionist model. International Journal of Management Reviews, **19**: 318–336; doi: 10.1111/ijmr.12150.

Haslam, S. A, Turner, J. C., Oakes, P., McGarty, C. & Reynolds, K. (1998). The group as a basis for emergent stereotype consensus. European Review of Social Psychology, **28**: 203–239.

Hobfoll, S. E., Hall, B., Horsey, K. J. & Lamaoureux, B. E. (2011). Resilience in the face of terrorism: Linking resource investment with engagement. In Southwick, S. M., Litz, B. T., Charney, D. & Friedman, M. J., editors, Resilience and Mental Health: Challenges Across the Lifespan. Cambridge: Cambridge University Press, pp. 253–263.

Howell, A. & Voronka, J. (2012). Introduction: The politics of resilience and recovery in mental health care. Studies in Social Justice, **6**: 1–7.

Kaniasty, K. & Norris, F. H. (2004) Social support in the aftermath of disasters, catastrophes, and acts of terrorism: Altruistic, overwhelmed, uncertain, antagonistic, and patriotic communities. In Ursano, R. J., Norwood, A. E. & Fullerton, C. S., editors, Bioterrorism: Psychological and Public Health Interventions. Cambridge: Cambridge University Press, pp. 200–229.

Kobasa, S. C. (1979). Stressful life events, personality, and health: An inquiry into hardiness. Journal of Personal and Social Psychology, **37**: 1–11.

Kobasa, S. C., Maddi, S. R. & Kahn, S. (1982). Hardiness and health: A prospective study. Journal of Personal and Social Psychology, **42**: 168–177.

Layne, C. M., Warren, J. S., Watson, P. J. & Shalev, A. Y. (2007). Risk, vulnerability, resistance, and resilience: Towards an integrative conceptualization of posttraumatic adaptation. In Friedman, T. K. M & Resick, P., editors, Handbook of PTSD: Science and Practice. New York: Guilford Press, pp. 497–520.

Levin, A. (2009). Genes influence vulnerability to posttrauma disorders. Psychiatric News, **44**: 17.

Maercker, A. & Hecker, T. (2016). Broadening perspectives on trauma and recovery: A socio-interpersonal view of PTSD. European Journal of Psychotraumatology, **7**: 29303; doi:10.3402/ejpt.v7.29303.

Maercker, A. & Horn, A. B. (2013). A socio-interpersonal perspective on PTSD: The case for environments and interpersonal processes. Clinical Psychology and Psychotherapy, **20**: 465–481.

Masten, A. S., Monn, A. R. & Supkoff, L. M. (2011). Resilience in children and adolescents. In Southwick, S. M., Litz, B. T., Charney, D. & Friedman, M. J., editors, Resilience and Mental Health: Challenges Across the Lifespan. Cambridge: Cambridge University Press, pp. 103–119.

Mawson, A. R. (2005). Understanding mass panic and other collective responses to threat and disaster. Psychiatry, **68**: 95–113.

Ministry of Health, New Zealand (2016). Framework for Psychosocial Support in Emergencies. Wellington: Ministry of Health.

Nolte, T., Guiney, J., Fonagy, P., Mayes, L. C. & Luyten, P. (2011). Interpersonal stress regulation and the development of anxiety disorders: An attachment-based developmental framework. Frontiers in Behavioral Neuroscience, 21 September; http://doi.org/10.3389/fnbeh.2011.00055.

Norris, F. H., Stevens, S. P., Pfefferbaum, B., Wyche, K. F. & Pfefferbaum, R. (2008). Community resilience as a metaphor, theory, set of capacities, and strategy for disaster readiness. American Journal of Community Psychology, **41**: 127–150; doi: 10.1007/s10464-007-9156-6.

Norris, F. H., Tracy, M. & Galea, S. (2009). Looking for resilience: Understanding the longitudinal trajectories of responses to stress. Social Science and Medicine, **68**: 2190–2198.

NATO/EAPC (2009). Psychosocial Care for People Affected by Disasters and Major Incidents. Brussels: North Atlantic Treaty Organisation–Euro-Atlantic Partnership Council.

Ntontis, E., Drury, J., Amlôt, R., Rubin, G. J. & Williams, R. (2017). Emergent social identities in a flood: Implications for community psychosocial resilience. Journal of Community and Applied Social Psychology, 26 July: 1–12; https://doi.org/10.1002/casp.2329.

Ntontis, E., Drury, J., Amlôt, R., Rubin, G. J. & Williams, R. (2018). Community resilience and flooding in UK guidance: A critical review of concepts, definitions, and their implications. Journal of Contingencies and Crisis Management, 2018: 1–12; doi: 10.1111/1468-5973.12223.

OECD (2013). What does 'resilience' mean for donors? An OECD factsheet. See www.oecd.org/dac/conflict-fragility-resilience/docs/May%2010%202013%20FINAL%20resilience%20PDF.pdf.

Omand, D. (2010). Securing the State. London: C. Hurst & Co (Publishers) Ltd.

Osório, C., Probert, T., Jones, E., Young, A. H. & Robbins, I. (2016). Adapting to stress: Understanding the neurobiology of resilience. Behavioral Medicine, **43**: 307–322; doi: 10.1080/08964289.2016.1170661

Panter-Brick, C. (2015). Culture and resilience: Next steps for theory and practice. In Theron, L. C., Liebenberg, L. & Ungar, M., editors, Youth Resilience and Culture: Commonalities and Complexities. New York, NY: Springer, pp. 233–244.

Panter-Brick, C. & Leckman, J. F. (2013). Editorial commentary: Resilience in child development – interconnected pathways to wellbeing. Journal of Child Psychology and Psychiatry, **54**: 333–336.

Patel, S. S., Rogers, M. B., Amlôt, R. & Rubin, G. J. (2017). What do we mean by 'community resilience'? A systematic literature review of how it is defined in the literature. PLoS Currents Disasters, February 1; 9: ecurrents.dis.db775aff25efc5ac4f 0660ad9c9f7db2.

Praharso, N. F., Tear, M. J. & Cruwys, T. (2016). Stressful life situations and wellbeing: A comparison of the stress buffering hypothesis and the social identity model of identity change. Psychiatry Research, **247**: 265–275; http://dx.doi.org/10.1016/j.psychres.2016.11.039

Robinson, A. (2015). The resilience motif: Implications for youth justice. Youth Justice, 1–16. doi: 10.1177/147322541 5587601.

Rutter, M. (1987). Psychosocial resilience and protective mechanisms. American Journal of Orthopsychiatry, **57**: 316–331.

Sapienza, J. K & Masten, A. S. (2011). Understanding and promoting resilience in children and youth. Current Opinion in Psychiatry, **24**: 267–273.

Sharp, C., Fonagy, P. & Allen, J. (2012). Posttraumatic stress disorder: A social-cognitive perspective. Clinical Psychology: Science and Practice, **19**: 229–240; doi: 10.1111/cpsp.12002.

Sheikh, T. L., Mohammed, A., Eseigbe, E. et al. (2016). Descriptive characterization of psycho-trauma, psychological distress, and post-traumatic stress disorder among children and adolescent internally displaced persons in Kaduna, Nigeria. Frontiers in Psychiatry, 7: 179; doi: 10.3389/fpsyt.2016.00179.

Smyth, N., Siriwardhana, C., Hotopf, M. & Hatch, S. L. (2014). Social networks, social support and psychiatric symptoms: Social determinants and associations within a multicultural community population. Social Psychiatry and Psychiatric Epidemiology, **50**: 1111–1120; doi: 10.1007/s00127-014-0943-8.

Southwick, S. M., Bonanno, G. A., Masten, A. S., Panter-Brick, C. & Yehuda, R. (2014). Resilience definitions, theory, and challenges: Interdisciplinary perspectives. European Journal of Psychotraumatology, 5: 25338; doi:http://dx.doi.org/10.3402/ejpt.v.

Southwick, S. M., Litz, B. T., Charney, D. & Friedman, M. J. (2011). Preface. In Resilience and Mental Health: Challenges Across the Lifespan. Cambridge: Cambridge University Press, pp. xi–xv.

Troy, A. S & Mauss, I. B. (2011). Resilience in the face of stress: Emotion regulation as a protective factor. In Southwick, S. M., Litz, B. T., Charney, D. & Friedman, M. J., editors, Resilience and Mental Health: Challenges Across the Lifespan. Cambridge: Cambridge University Press, pp. 30–44.

Turner, J. C., Hogg, M. A., Oakes, P. J., Reicher, S. D. & Wetherell, M. S. (1987). Rediscovering the Social Group: A Self-Categorization Theory. Oxford: Blackwell.

Ungar, M. (2008). Resilience across cultures. The British Journal of Social Work, **38**: 218–235.

UNISDR (2009). Terminology on Disaster Risk Reduction. Geneva: United Nations Office for Disaster Risk Reduction.

Williams, R. & Drury, J. (2010). The nature of psychosocial resilience and its significance for managing mass emergencies, disasters and terrorism. In Awotona, A., editor, Rebuilding Sustainable Communities for Children and Their Families After Disasters: A Global Survey. Newcastle upon Tyne: Cambridge Scholars Publishing.

Williams, R. & Drury, J. (2011). Personal and collective psychosocial resilience: Implications for children, young people and their families involved in war and disasters. In Cook, D., Wall, J. & Cox, P., editors, Children and Armed Conflict. New York, NY: Palgrave McMillan, pp. 57–75.

Williams, R. & Hazell, P. (2011). Austerity, poverty, resilience, and the future of mental health services for children and adolescents. Current Opinion in Psychiatry, **24**: 263–266.

Williams, R. & Kemp, V. (2016). Psychosocial and mental health care before, during and after emergencies, disasters and major incidents. In Sellwood, C. & Wapling, A, editors, Health Emergency Preparedness and Response. Wallingford: CABI, pp. 83–98.

Williams, R. & Kemp, V. (2017). Psychosocial resilience: Psychosocial care and forensic mental healthcare. In Bailey, S., Tarbuck, P. & Chitsabesan, P., editors, Forensic Child and Adolescent Mental Health: Meeting the Needs of Young Offenders. Cambridge: Cambridge University Press, pp. 24–39.

Williams, R., Kemp. V. & Alexander, D. A. (2014). The psychosocial and mental health of people who are affected by conflict, catastrophes, terrorism, adversity and displacement. In Ryan, J., Hopperus Buma, A., Beadling, C. et al., Conflict and Catastrophe Medicine. Berlin: Springer, pp. 805–849.

Zeanah, C. H. & Sonuga-Barke, J. S. (2016). The effects of early trauma and deprivation on human development: From measuring cumulative risk to characterizing specific mechanisms. Journal of Child Psychology and Psychiatry, **57**: 1099–1102.

Chapter 12

The Value of Tolerance and the Tolerability of Competing Values

Jonathan Montgomery

Introduction

Earlier and later chapters in this book explore the importance of membership of communities of values; whether gangs or sports teams, or in sharing adversity such as natural disasters (see, for example, Chapters 3, 4, 11, 16 and 17). At this point, and before moving into some specific scenarios in Section 3, and a closer examination of practical aspects of social identity theory in Section 4, we see it as important to take stock, on one hand, and set some challenges for social scientists to reflect upon later in this book. Section 1 identified the lens of sociability through which we are examining the human condition together with recent approaches to understanding the power of social connectedness and, within that, social identity, for our health. Chapter 13 brings together many of the concepts covered in Sections 1 and 2.

While we accept that community membership is an important source of social support and psychosocial resilience, we also contend that it cannot be accepted uncritically as an unalloyed good. We must understand the possible costs as well as the benefits of strong communities. This is covered briefly in the book thus far. There are two key questions that we need to consider when assessing the resilience that comes from identification with communities. Furthermore, if we are prepared to benefit from social support delivered by group membership, do we also acquire responsibilities for not only members of the groups of which we are members but, possibly, too, for people who are not assisted in this way?

The first question concerns the value of tolerance, and we highlight that below in the light of heresy and apostasy. Here the issues relate to the protections for individual persons from their communities. A second key question concerns the limits of our respect for the values of others; the tolerability of competing values. Here the issue is understanding whether there are specific values or value communities that should not be tolerated even within a political framework that values tolerance for the resilience and other benefits that it brings. Further, we should also consider how membership of a profession serves to constrain personal values, and generates expectations of actions that sometimes create tensions for those persons who engage in the work with which we are concerned.

Communities of Value and Communities of Resistance

There can be a positive, constructivist, angle to community bonds. They provide a sense of shared purpose and experience that enables people to make sense of uncertainty and vulnerability. This could be described as an inclusive dynamic; psychosocial resilience comes through belonging (Cruwys et al., 2013; Chapters 9 and 11). Here, what is shared is a degree of common values (even if this is no more than a preference for soccer over rugby).

It is important to foster value communities such as these if we are to support people's resilience.

Community membership can also provide a foundation for solidarity in the face of adversity (Williams & Drury, 2009; Chapters 16, 17, 23, 25 and 30). This has a different dynamic that could be characterised as exclusive; resilience through difference. The inclusive dynamic draws resilience from identification with fellow members of the community and contemplation of the shared experiences and values that define it and hold it together. The exclusive dynamic draws resilience from resistance. It does not require there to be shared values, only shared enemies. Thus, Christians, Jews and Muslims might share in a community of resistance to secularism but be engaged in internecine conflict with each other on matters of faith and doctrine (Williams, 2012). Scotland, Ireland and Wales may compete vigorously with each other at sports, but unite in opposition to England. This means that solidarity is highly context-dependent. Adversity in the form of external threats may itself strengthen the affective bonds within a community and thus foster resilience (Taiffel, 1982). This suggests that we should promote tolerance of different value systems, as it promotes the possibility of resilience coming through the sense of common adversity. This would not be available if there were a single monochrome value system.

Thus, community membership can work inclusively, but it may also manifest itself through a sense of identity as differentiation. Courts in the UK and Europe are grappling with this over the acceptability of symbols of religious identity; crosses, hijab, burkas (Hunter-Henin, 2012). These can be seen as 'rituals of resistance', drawing strength not from their theological significance so much as their function as badges of belonging. Thus, community members who might not usually be 'observant' adopt the symbols of their faith communities to demonstrate solidarity (Beetham, 1971; James, 1974; Taiffel, 1982). This may enhance the resilience of some people but at the expense of others; both outside the community of value and also within it. Stronger community identity may go hand in hand with a sense of superiority and with denial of respect for others. The challenge is to promote strong communities without disrespect.

Heresy and Apostasy

If psychosocial resilience can be drawn from belonging to an affective community of shared experience and value, then it is in the 'public interest' to support and tolerate these communities. However, it is not necessarily the case that all members of those communities benefit equally from being permitted to live according to their value systems. Some may wish to escape what they see as limitations on their flourishing. We must consider problems of both heresy and apostasy.

A heretic is someone who is both within and apart from a value system. A Muslim is not a Christian heretic but a member of a different faith. In contrast, a heretic is someone who accepts their identity in the faith, but rejects some of its orthodoxies. There may be issues of personal resilience here. If you believe that floods are divine retribution for recognising gay marriage, what does this tell you about your own wickedness if your house is flooded? If you believe in miraculous healing and the power of prayer, how will you react if your tumour is not cured? There may also be problems of repression.

An apostate is someone who previously adhered to, but has now left, the community – an ex-member. It is typical for strong value communities to regard this as a betrayal and quite different to non-membership.

An uncritical acceptance of value community-based psychosocial resilience might benefit some members at the expense of others, and even increase their vulnerability either as current members who are uncomfortable with the values (heretics) and those who suffer more greatly when they reject their former beliefs and leave than they would had they never been members (apostates). Support for apostates can be provided without interfering with the value communities themselves, because they are likely to have extracted themselves. It is important to recognise the impact on them of the fact that they have detached themselves from a source of support, which may leave them more exposed than they would have been if they had never been associated with it. Support for heretics raises a rather different challenge because it requires interference with the value community itself. This raises our second problem.

Liberalism and Value Communities

The significance of community membership to social support and, thereby, psychosocial resilience presents a challenge to the dominant western political ideology of toleration. Liberal societies pride themselves on toleration and it is sometimes claimed that it is the very essence of liberalism that it is neutral between competing values (Raz, 1986).

J. S. Mill's famous essay, *On Liberty*, first published in 1859 (Mill, 1972), championed men's (sic) rights to develop their own sense of individuality without having conceptions of the 'good' imposed upon them. He argued that two things followed from this. First, that there are areas of our lives that should be regarded as private (self-regarding) and immune from public intervention (both in the form of social disapproval and state regulation). Second, that there are limits to the type of argument that could properly be used to justify state intervention into people's personal choices. Thus, it is not permissible for the state to constrain choices that people make by claiming that it is in their own interests; this is a type of paternalism that substitutes the judgement of the state about what is good for a person for their own assessment.

Mill suggested that it is, however, legitimate for the state to regulate private choices in order to protect others from being harmed. This 'harm criterion' is a type of argument that was thought to be neutral between the personal preferences of individual people, but legitimate in assessing the exercise of public power. This framework has resonated powerfully in UK politics, including in the debate over the legalisation of homosexual activity in the 1950s (Wolfenden, 1957) and, more recently, discussions about using technologies to assist human reproduction (House of Commons Committee on Science and Technology, 2005), and the permissibility of assistance in dying (Montgomery, 2006; R [Nicklinson] v Min Justice [2014], United Kingdom Supreme Court 38). It may provide a solution to the problems of heresy and apostasy.

The idea of 'political liberalism' of John Rawls develops further the idea that there is a distinctive logic to 'public reason' that is independent of particular communities of values to which individual persons belong (Rawls, 1971, 1993, 1999). He is particularly concerned with the problems created for the USA by the formal separation of church and state in a country that remains strongly religious. On his account, the value systems that come with membership of a religion are 'thick' and cover the full breadth of people's lives. However, these 'thick' systems of value are bound to come into conflict with other such systems when deployed in relation to political decisions, and they need to be set aside in favour of 'thin' systems which are more limited in their ambition but can allow public institutions to operate in the face of competing and conflicting 'thick' systems of value. While liberalism has served the interests of toleration, its contribution to creating and supporting people's resilience is weak. Its neutrality between values means that it fails to create affective inclusivity because it does not stand for any particular community.

This is noted by communitarian political theorists, who argue that value-neutral liberalism is too 'thin' and only a satisfactory account of human flourishing when combined with the acceptance of communities of value (Taylor, 1989; Walzer, 1983). These communities can be a significant source of resilience. However, because they may also mask patterns of power and inequalities that may be detrimental to members, it is necessary to establish frameworks from which it is possible to judge when challenge is appropriate.

Illiberal Communities?

The value communities which we have discussed all operate within and across other societal arrangements. Most people belong to more than one value community. To pursue the sporting analogy; two people might share an identity as Londoners but also separate identities through their support of the local rival football teams, Arsenal and Tottenham. They might be both British and Muslim. This may provide resources on which we can draw to help identify the limits of our tolerance.

First, there is the idea of 'common values' among our differences (Haslam, 2004). This works by focussing on the values that are shared rather than those on which we disagree. It is not necessary that we agree on the reasons for thinking these values are important. The fact of our agreement is sufficient to enable them to operate as a basis for a community of communities. John Rawls has described this as an 'overlapping consensus' – the common ground shared by the various value communities. These common values can constitute a 'public morality', on the basis of which it is legitimate to be critical of specific instances where a community fails to respect those values (Rawls, 1971, 1993).

The foundation of such common values can be justified in various ways. First, there might be an empirical approach, seeking those values that seem to be universally adopted. This raises significant challenges, however, as was acknowledged even in ancient western philosophy in relation to the apparent ubiquity of the institution of slavery. Philosophers and theologians were reluctant to accept that the universal practice of slavery in the world known to them meant that it was to be accepted as part of the divine order. This was an illegitimate shift from empirical fact ('is') to value ('ought').

Nevertheless, the empirical turn remains attractive, at least politically, as it enables bridges to be built between communities on the basis of apparently shared commitments. They include obligations of reciprocity and mutual respect under which those who accept the benefits of common life can reasonably be expected to offer others those same benefits. This type of argument justifies limitations on 'hate speech' and racist political protests, on the basis that it is implicit in the choice to exercise rights of free expression and democratic protest that you accept its importance. It is, therefore, inconsistent and self-defeating for people who exercise such rights to deny them to others. Consequently, those who live as members of a common society, especially one in which different value communities co-exist, bind themselves to some common values by their practices. This can be understood as a development of a form of social contract theory based on tacit agreements, implicit in their communal actions (Weale, 2013). It is reasonable to regulate so as to ensure people behave consistently.

However, any such consensus may be superficial. This can be seen in relation to two social institutions that are often seen as fundamental and plausible candidates for universal support. The first is the institution of property, seen by many as being essential to social order. It may be correct to suggest that some form of enduring arrangement around who has legitimate access to land and other means of production is essential to community living. However, it does not follow, as some have argued, that *private* property is natural. There are many other forms of property, including common and communal systems, and even most developed private property systems recognise that some goods (e.g. air) are outside the scope of ownership (Waldron, 1990). In a number of cultural systems, typically those of indigenous communities that have been overtaken by invading forces, land is outside the scope of property systems because it is a common and natural good. Technically, English land law still holds this formal structure, with all ownership being notionally derived from that of the Crown (state) (Cooke, 2012). Thus, the fact that the *concept* of property is widespread and that some property type arrangements are almost universally in place does not legitimate a particular *conception* of property rights.

Nor does it suggest that property is an absolute good that outweighs other values. John Locke's argument for property being derived from the exertion of labour was based on the proviso that this was justified only while 'as much and as good' was available for others to cultivate and so earn their own property (Locke, 1988, originally published in 1689). It was a limited justification. Further, the suggestion that I own something does not permit me to use that property free from social constraints or responsibilities. Thus, ownership of a knife does not legitimate its use for murder. Nor is taxation incompatible with the idea of private property.

These two points – the first about the difference between a universal concept and its particular conception in any given value system and the second about the relative value of such concepts and other important issues – can be seen in relation to the institution of the family. It is probably right that some system of affiliation or belonging is universal and exists in all societies – this is a way of describing the psychosocial connections that make a collection of people a group. It does not follow that such connections need to be based on genetic or marital ties. Yet, it is not uncommon (e.g. in discussions on homosexual marriage) for the variety of familial ties to be ignored in favour of some universalist claim.

Marriage, like other family arrangements, differs across societies, so that the claim that it is a common institution is misleading. It also differs over time in the same societies. In addition, the family can be both a source of strength and of repression. While strong familial structures can enhance psychosocial resilience (Wakefield et al., 2015), they may nevertheless be unjust. The attempts of legal systems to distinguish between arranged and forced marriages can be seen as a context in which the limits of liberalism are being tested. Western cultures find the concept of arranged marriage strange against a background of their modern (and rather recent) myths of individualised romantic love. Consequently, we tend to discuss this as an issue of Asian religious culture. However, the novels of Jane Austen and plot of Downton Abbey are just as concerned with the interplay of societal expectations and personal choice over marriage plans, all made in the shadow of socio-economic property transactions.

Feminist analyses of the consequences of treating family life as a private rather than public matter have shown how this categorisation can be used to mask imbalances of power and as an excuse to resist state intervention to protect those who suffer abuse of various kinds within families (Olsen, 1983). Similar points have been made about the potential for multiculturalism to mask and enhance the structural inequalities faced by women (Okin, 1999; but see Kymlicka, 1999).

An appeal to the idea of common values may be helpful in the politics of intercommunal relationships because it does not require the values of a community to be confronted. However, in order to assure ourselves that it is legitimate to accept values that are widely held, we need to identify a normative not merely descriptive account of the values that are at stake. This is a contemporary debate in relation to the practice of female genital mutilation (FGM). There is an international global consensus that the practice is unacceptable. In the UK, the attempt to stamp out this cultural practice has led to specific criminal sanctions, and mandatory reporting requirements for health professionals in relation to vulnerable children. Yet the practice of male circumcision has been accommodated and is not seen as a harmful in the same way. Both practices are understood by proponents as initiation rites, but irrespective of prevalence, we feel able to draw a line between them because of the level of harm caused by FGM. This holds even in the face of the fact that most practitioners of FGM are female.

The problem, therefore, is to identify minimum standards that are non-negotiable and can be enforced irrespective of their actual acceptance by others. Natural rights theorists, such as John Finnis, contend that this can be achieved by objective rational consideration, and that if we spent time reflecting on the requirements for human flourishing we would all come to realise that there are certain fundamental and irreducible goods that need always to be respected (Finnis, 1980). Social contract theorists suggest that even if we are not logically committed to such a position, something like it can be generated by agreement. John Rawls used a thought experiment to generate the idea that we would sign up to certain societal ground rules, in relation to public institutions at least, if we asked ourselves what sort of society we would choose if we had to design it without knowledge of precisely what characteristics and socio-economic (dis)advantages we would have (Rawls, 1971). These approaches give us reasons to accept values as morally binding upon us. However, they remain the subject of argument and dispute.

A more positivist approach would be to concentrate on the institutionalisation of such common values through instruments such as international conventions on human rights. This enables immediate practical decisions to be based on carrying through such agreements without being paralysed by intellectual doubt. It defers the conceptual problems of the philosophical and political foundations of universal values to the sphere of diplomatic negotiations. This approach can accept the provisionality of human rights norms, but build on their legal validity as a basis for action. Joseph Raz has argued that one of the key functions of human rights is to legitimate criticism of non-compliant states and to justify intrusions into their sovereignty (Raz, 2010). The problem about the limits of tolerance of value communities is closely analogous to that function.

Human rights can, therefore, be a pragmatic basis for defining the 'public' values that can be brought to bear when conflicts need to be resolved. On this basis, we can argue that it is appropriate to support a 'dissident' member of a community in denying the legitimacy of its values when those values compromise the fundamental human rights of the member. Identifying when this is the case is not straightforward, but a methodology for doing so can be found in human rights law. It also provides processes for resolving disputes.

Professional, Personal and Public Values

This analysis has identified the importance of personal membership of value communities in gaining the social support which most of us crave, and establishing psychosocial resilience (e.g. see Chapters 11 and 13). Health and social care professionals, like everyone else, draw their own resilience from such communities. We have also identified the importance of 'public' values for guiding responses to conflicts between individual persons and the value communities with which they are connected. We need to recognise that professionals may also find themselves conflicted. The expectations of public value may not be consistent with their own personal beliefs.

European courts tend to grapple with this as an issue of religious (broadly defined) freedom. The European Court of Human Rights has upheld the analysis that, while people are entitled to believe that homosexuality is contrary to the rule of God, they are not entitled to use that belief to refuse to fulfil their contractual responsibilities to register civil partnerships, and now homosexual marriages. The logic is that they do not need to work as registrars of births, deaths and marriages and, if they choose to do so, they accept some limitations on the values they can express in their work (Eweida & others v UK [2013], 57 European Human Rights Reports 213). The UK Supreme Court has also considered the issue in relation to the scope of the statutory rights of conscientious objection conferred by the Abortion Act 1967, which were narrowly construed (Greater Glasgow Health Board v Doogan [2014], United Kingdom Supreme Court 68).

Among other things, professions are value communities. In some cases, those values are formally expressed within documents such as the General Medical Council's (GMC's) Good Medical Practice. They are also conveyed by employing institutions and expressed through educational practices. Professional values are a form of public values, albeit with less claim to universalism than human rights. They are located within a specific form of social contract that sets out, among other things, the expectations of non-judgemental and non-discriminatory service. In the UK, but not necessarily elsewhere in the world, this expectation played an important part in protecting those contracting HIV/AIDS from discrimination. Professionals play a key role in ensuring 'public values' drive the services that are available to people who are in need of support. However, at times, that may involve suppressing their own personal values.

Statutory rights of conscientious objection in the UK are limited to abortion, embryo research and infertility treatments. However, the guidance from the GMC, the regulator of the medical profession in the UK, goes further and allows for general rights of conscience. This is illustrated by reference to the right to refuse to provide contraception, which is said to extend even to emergency contraception, though, in contrast, statutory rights do not permit doctors to avoid responsibility for abortions in emergencies. This suggests a shift in the balance between personal and professional values that may enable intolerance to spill over into the clinic. This is limited by anti-discrimination requirements. A similar pattern is seen with other professions. This raises the question of whether we are loosening our expectation that professionals should be more tolerant of the values of people who seek their services than we can expect of individual members of society (Montgomery, 2015).

Conclusion

Earlier chapters in this book have explored the significance of social identity and belonging in supporting resilience. This has led us to appreciate the importance of sustaining communities of values and tolerating differences between them. It is the essence of the meaning of toleration that it restrains inclinations to intervene in the lives of others, interventions that could be justified for reasons such as preventing injustice were it not for the value of tolerance (Raz, 1986). The concerns in this chapter are with probing the limits of such toleration and exploring the conceptual resources on which we might draw in addressing the tensions that emerge if we promote value pluralism.

We return in Chapter 24 to consider how values framed in public health ethics may be used to resolve differences of priority, preference and opinions between different groups of people. We see these approaches as important, given the lessons that emerge in this book about the powerful influences of shared social identity that marks group membership.

References

Beetham, D. (1971). Transport and Turbans. Oxford: Oxford University Press.

Cooke, E. (2012). Land Law. Oxford: Oxford University Press.

Cruwys, T., Dingle, G. A., Haslam, C. et al. (2013). Social group memberships protect against future depression, alleviate depression symptoms and prevent depression relapse. Social Science and Medicine, **98**: 179–186.

Finnis, J. (1980). Natural Law and Natural Rights. Oxford: Oxford University Press.

Haslam, S. A. (2004). Psychology in Organizations: The Social Identity Approach. London: Sage.

House of Commons Committee on Science and Technology. (2005). Human Reproductive Technologies and the Law (HC Paper 7 2004–5). London: The Stationery Office.

Hunter-Henin, M. (2012). Why the French don't like the Burqa: Laïcité, national identity and religious freedom. International Comparative and Law Quarterly, **61**: 1–27.

James, A. (1974). Sikh Children in Britain. Oxford: Oxford University Press.

Kymlicka, W. (1999). Liberal complacencies. In Cohen, J., Howard, M. & Nussbaum, M. C., editors, Is Multiculturalism Bad for Women? Princeton, NJ: Princeton Univerisity Press, pp. 31–34.

Locke, J. (1988). In Laslett, P., editor, Two Treatises of Government. Cambridge: Cambridge University Press (originally published in 1689).

Mill, J. S. (1972). On Liberty. London: JM Dent (originally published in 1859).

Montgomery, J. (2006). The legitimacy of medical law. In Maclean, S., editor, First Do No Harm: Law, Ethics and Medicine. Aldershot: Ashgate, pp. 1–16.

Montgomery, J. (2015). Conscientious objection: Personal and professional ethics in the public square. Medical Law Review, 23: 200–220.

Okin, S. M. (1999). Is multiculturalism bad for women? In Cohen, J., Howard, M. & Nussbaum, M. C., editors, Is Multiculturalism Bad for Women? Princeton, NJ: Princeton Univerisity Press, pp. 41–46.

Olsen, F. (1983). The family and the market: A study of ideology and legal reform. Harvard Law Review, **96**: 1497–1578.

Rawls, J. (1971). A Theory of Justice. Cambridge, MA: Harvard University Press.

Rawls, J. (1993). Political Liberalism. New York, NY: Columbia University Press.

Rawls, J. (1999). The Law of Peoples. Cambridge, MA: Harvard University Press.

Raz, J. (1986). The Morality of Freedom. Oxford: Oxford University Press.

Raz, J. (2010). Human rights without foundations. In Besson, S. & Tasioulas, J. editors, The Philosophy of International Law. Oxford: Oxford University Press.

Taiffel, H. (1982). The social psychology of minorities. In Husband, C., editor, Race in Britain. London, Hutchinson.

Taylor, C. (1989). Sources of the Self: The Making of the Modern Identity. Cambridge: Cambridge University Press.

Wakefield, J. R., Sani, F., Herrera, M., Khan, S. S. & Dugard, P. (2015). Greater family identification – but not greater contact with family members – leads to better health: Evidence from a Spanish longitudinal study.

European Journal of Social Psychology, 46: 506–513.

Waldron, J. (1990). The Right to Private Property. Oxford: Oxford University Press.

Walzer, M. (1983). Spheres of Justice. Oxford: Blackwell.

Weale, A. (2013). Democratic Justice and the Social Contract. Oxford: Oxford University Press.

Williams, R. (2012). Faith in the Public Square. London: Bloomsbury.

Williams, R. & Drury, J. (2009). Psychosocial resilience and its influence on managing mass emergencies and disasters. Psychiatry, 8: 293–296.

Wolfenden. (1957). Report of the Committee on Homosexual Offences and Prostitution. London: HMSO.

Chapter 13

Towards Partnerships in Health and Social Care: A Coloquium of Approaches to Connectedness

Richard Williams, Sue Bailey and Verity Kemp

Partnerships in Thinking, Theorising and Approach

While there is great optimism for healthcare to be gained from developments in neuroscience, genetics and epigenetics, the social contexts and social approaches revealed by research, including much that we cover in this book, are also very powerful contributors to our health and recovery from ill health. As Nestler et al. say, 'Psychiatric disorders are complex multifactorial illnesses ... While genetic factors are important in the etiology of most mental disorders, the relatively high rates of discordance among identical twins ... clearly indicate the importance of additional mechanisms' (Nestler et al., 2016, p. 447).

This book focuses on social and environmental mechanisms; this chapter draws together a selection of the topics raised in Sections 1 and 2. We link facets of the social science that have come up thus far with concepts that are implicit in public physical and mental healthcare, and we summarise the concept of mental health recovery. Our overall aim is to show how recent research indicates why healthcare staff should recognise and use lessons from the social sciences more widely to complement the neurosciences and other sciences. We draw together a selection of the constructs and theories to show connections and overlaps between the concepts that appear in this book. This makes us enthusiastic about what further research and developmental thinking in partnership will yield. Later, we devote Section 4 of this book to considering how theoretical approaches to partnerships identified in Sections 1, 2 and 3 might be developed and applied in the real world. Section 3 provides graphic examples of why social connectedness and partnership are important.

In Chapter 7, Cieza and Bickenbach identify powerfully how many very different diseases and disorders have similar impacts on people who suffer them, which they link to impairment of functioning, despite the very different arrays of symptoms and signs of each one. In this book, we consider carefully the observations made by Cieza and Bickenbach about different disorders having similar impacts on the lives of people who are affected. We also recognise that the impacts of those disorders differ and depend on people's social circumstances, employment, relationships and commitments, in addition to the nature of their ill health.

The variations in the ways in which people experience their health and ill health is picked up by Heath's quote from Tolstoy (Heath, 2011), 'No complaint affecting a living being can ever be entirely familiar, for each [person] ... has his own individual peculiarities and whatever his disease it must necessarily be peculiar to himself'. Thus, no two people experience health, illness, disease or disability in the same way. But, these influences go well beyond being mere context. This chapter illustrates how these personal differences arise and how person-, family- and community-centred approaches to caring can be based on broad approaches to the theoretical notions about what ails us. Curiously, this approach is also propelled by the similarities of functional impairment covered in Chapter 7 by the construct of horizontal epidemiology.

The Human Condition

Chapter 2 presents the six dimensions of the human condition and the wider range of our being that impacts on our experiences of embodiment and finiteness. In this context, Heath (2011) has opined that gentleness is the key to the future of medicine and that it is more important to attempt to identify and support people's resources and capacities for creating health than to concentrate on risk, ill health and disease. This fits with our focus on public health and the social determinants of health in Chapters 3, 4, 6, 7, and 9–11.

These considerations underpin our opinion, which is that harnessing the advantages from scientific developments turns not only on adequacy of resources but also on our attending to lessons from diverse fields. They include how populations of people can be assisted to benefit from health promotion, public healthcare and public mental health-care and how people who wish to be more healthy or who need healthcare are included in conversations about their preferences, social circumstances and expectations. The intention is that they should be actively engaged as coproducers through approaches that recognise and tackle the social impacts of their illnesses. We pick up these matters in Chapters 23–26.

Social Connectedness, the Social Determinants of Health and Social Exclusion

Already, this book has illustrated the power of social connectedness in promoting people's health and in harnessing the benefits of the physical sciences in future approaches to designing and delivering health services. Haslam and Haslam, in Chapter 3, point out that 'Social relationships affect health. Of that we are certain. People who are more strongly connected live longer, are in better health and experience better wellbeing. None of us is immune to these effects . . .'. These authors also focus on the social determinants of health and mental health. They summarise how '. . . poverty, inequality and age, among other factors, contribute to, and exacerbate the consequences of social disconnection'. Bhui et al, in Chapter 6, also summarise the literature on the benefits of social equality by looking at its antithesis. Yet it is also important to understand the different meanings of equity and equality when designing and delivering services (see Chapter 1).

The determination to tackle social exclusion has underpinned certain policies of past governments in the UK (Khan et al., 2015). It has been defined as, 'A shorthand label for what can happen when individuals or areas suffer from a combination of linked problems such as unemployment, poor skills, low incomes, poor housing, high crime environments, bad health and family breakdown' (Khan et al., 2015). The term, and its associated cross-departmental policies, clearly imply that the government recognised the untoward impacts of people having restricted access to social relationships, organisations and other resources. Levitas et al. (2007) define social exclusion as, '. . . a complex and multidimensional process [that] . . . involves the lack or denial of resources, rights, goods and services, and the inability to participate in normal relationships and activities, available to the majority of people in a society, whether in economic, social, cultural or political arenas. It affects the quality of life of individuals and the equity and cohesion of sociality as a whole'.

By contrast, Chapters 3 and 4 consider how social connectedness may operate powerfully and positively to support people within families, communities and other groups. Thus, social exclusion denies people access to resources and opportunities that could be greatly beneficial to them rather than solely to the niceties of living.

Horizontal Epidemiology, Syndemics and the Recovery Approach

Horizontal Epidemiology

Cieza and Bickenbach begin Chapter 7 of this book by pointing out that

> In the last two decades or so, mental health epidemiology has taught us two important messages. The first is that the personal and social burden of mental health conditions, long underestimated, is significantly higher than prevalent physical health conditions such as cancer or diabetes.
>
> Second, the cause of this burden is not mortality, or even morbidity, but disability, and, in particular, a wide range of psychosocial difficulties that shape the lived experience of persons who have these disorders and which profoundly affect their quality of life.

Now, we recognise that the burden and costs of mental disorders are high for people who have these problems but also for their relatives and friends. As Cieza and Bickenbach say in Chapter 7 and the contents of Chapter 6 illustrate, there is evidence that the personal, social and economic costs of mental health problems and mental disorders have been underestimated in the past. As Bhui et al. summarise in Chapter 6, valid and reliable information now makes us aware of the full range of psychosocial problems that shape the lived experiences and the quality of life of persons who have these disorders.

However, the construct of horizontal epidemiology goes beyond our recognising the true and broad impacts of mental health problems. Core to the premise of horizontal epidemiology is the observation that the psychosocial difficulties that are faced by people and their relatives, associated with mental disorders, are by no means exclusively determined by diagnosis. Horizontal epidemiology focuses on the experiences of people who have disorders and concentrates on what is relevant to their lives to improve planning of interventions and their quality of life. We assert that similar circumstances apply to physical disorders. Core to our considerations in this book is how people's personal experiences, relationships and their circumstances shape their health and their recovery from ill health.

Cieza and Bickenbach conclude that:

> Horizontal epidemiology underscores the epidemiological, clincial and policy importance of understanding patterns in the determinants, not merely of the onset of mental health problems, but of the psychosocial difficulties that people with these chronic conditions experience in their lives. Our knowledge of determinants, risk factors and the aetiology of mental health and neurological conditions has been continuously increasing from evidence of, for example, life-course, risk-modelling exercises or by focusing on the interactions among determinants during life stages . . .

Syndemics

A concept that, arguably, overlaps with the thinking that lies behind horizontal epidemiology, and with the foci of this book, is that of syndemics. It is raised by Bhui et al. in Chapter 6. The notion was introduced in the 1990s, but developments were summarised in a series of papers in *The Lancet* in 2017. According to an editorial (The Lancet, 2017, p. 881):

> A syndemic, or synergistic epidemic, is more than a convenient portmanteau or a synonym for comorbidity. The hallmark of a syndemic is the presence of two or more disease states that adversely interact with each other, negatively affecting the mutual course of each disease trajectory, enhancing vulnerability, and which are made more deleterious by experienced inequities.

The Lancet's editorial (p. 881) continues:

> Perhaps the most unique feature of the syndemic approach to understanding various disease states and the way in which they cluster is the emphasis on the situation and circumstances in which individuals live. In other words, syndemics fundamentally rely on context.... The observation that these factors did not merely exist in parallel, but were intertwined and cumulative, offered a branch point for clinical medicine and public health interventions.

We think that the common ground between the constructs of horizontal epidemiology, the social determinants of health and syndemics lies in their emphases on contexts, and the intertwining and cumulative interactions of people's social environments and the inequities and inequalities they experience with their health needs. All three approaches serve to remind us to look beyond embodiment and finiteness when we assess people's health and to avoid silo approaches to considering people's comorbidities.

The Recovery Approach

Recovery refers to people living as well as they are able to, after untoward events, during adversity and after ill health. This construct also takes us beyond returning to how we were before we became unwell to our developing new meaning and purposes in our lives as we grow beyond the effects of our health problems. The focus should be on salutogenesis (Antonovsky, 1979) rather than pathogenesis.

Recovery involves creating new layers of positive identity, amplifying use of personal strengths and social resources and discovering that lived experiences can be assets and not just risk factors, and that everyone has something to offer as well as needing support from others (Slade, 2010). Again, these processes are germane to the messages in this book. Horizontal epidemiology, and the research quoted in Chapter 7, provide the scientific underpinning for the recovery approach, and the recovery approach represents a practical form of taking horizontal epidemiology into wider healthcare practice, planning and policy.

Roberts and Boardman published two reviews of mental health recovery (Roberts & Boardman, 2013, 2014). The principles of recovery they summarise are now core to thinking about mental healthcare in the UK and in a number of countries around the world, and they are underpinned by approaches built on connectedness and partnerships.

Arguably, the principles represented by horizontal epidemiology and the recovery approach are applicable to the whole of healthcare: the social determinants of health point strongly in this direction. Certainly, we have seen these principles in action when stroke teams take into account the breadth of people's disabilities and personal experiences in practicing good aftercare; though we suspect that many practitioners might not recognise them as implicit in their good practice.

Healthcare is in major transition in the UK and elsewhere. We think it critical that practitioners and researchers understand what recovery means for our work and our relationships with patients and their families. These implications are also represented in moves towards coproduction. As we have said previously (Bailey & Williams, 2014):

> Recovery adds educational, human rights and social justice orientations to the responsibilities of society. It collapses the traditional separation between health promotion and illness prevention on one hand and treatment and rehabilitation on the other. That dichotomy of approach has contributed, albeit unwittingly, to stigmatising people who have mental disorders and possibly excluded mental health professionals from efforts to increase the well-being of populations.

The concept of *horizontal epidemiology* should be a vital influence on public health and *psychosocial care* for people who are unwell. The former recognises the centrality to the quality of people's lives of the circumstances in which they live, while the latter recognises that people's personal and collective strengths may surface in times of adversity (Williams and Drury, 2011).

Social Connectedness and Social Identity

Each of the concepts we have summarised implies trying to alter the circumstances in which people relate, live and work in order to provide them with opportunities to achieve satisfying social connections and derive support from their shared identities as members of networks and groups. Roberts and Boardman (2013, 2014) teach us just how important patients' shared social identities are to their wellbeing and their ability to live as well as they are able.

In Chapter 4, Haslam et al. present a nuanced analysis, showing that our social connectedness has an especially important, dynamic bearing on our health. The authors' exposition of shared social identity provides insight into certain mechanisms by which social connectedness works as an agent in health and healthcare.

Social identity is based on views we take into ourselves of who we are on the basis of our membership, however loose or tight, of a range of social groups. We define and evaluate our social identities in relation to other groups. Shared social identity is the basis of productive social interactions, including communication, family life, social support, leadership, motivation, cooperation and trust. As Haslam et al. say, '... social identities are beneficial to health because they are the basis for meaningful forms of group life and hence give us access to important social and psychological resources'. We direct attention to Figure 4.1, showing that the resources conferred by our shared social identities include those of people deriving support, meaning and a sense of control from their feeling connected to other people.

Haslam *et al.* also say in Chapter 4:

> ... if our capacity to form meaningful social connections is compromised because, for example, we lose or lack social identities or because our social identities are stigmatised, then this is likely to limit our access to these same social and psychological resources and hence constitutes a significant threat to our psychological and social functioning. This can

> also be true if, as a function of their particular nature, groups exert a negative influence on our lives because the content of a given social identity . . . is harmful in some way.

This points up the possibility of our social connectedness being a force for good or ill. Arguably, the social identities of patients and relatives in Mid Staffordshire (Francis, 2013) and the residents of Winterbourne View and their families (Department of Health, 2012) were deeply affected by their hugely aversive experiences and we guess that there was too little positive sharing of identities between staff and patients or residents.

As we shall see in Section 3, Drury et al. take these initial conceptions much further in Chapters 15 and 17 by exploring the implications of shared social identity for the behaviour of people in crowds, and when they are affected by emergencies and disasters.

Belonging, Attachment and Psychosocial Resilience

Hindley says in Chapter 9 that attachment relationships have

> . . . become a central concept in our understanding of resilience in children and young people. However, attachment theory is a relatively narrow concept, focused on the relationship between a child and his or her principal caregivers . . . [W]e know that children grow up in complex systems and there is a growing recognition that children and young people's sense of belonging (to individuals, groups and organisations) is a key component of resilience.

Chapters 9 and 11 show that, if they have developed reasonably secure attachment styles from earliest childhood and through life, people's capacities for attachment, explain, in part at least, how they form supporting relationships with other people, including strangers, when the challenges they face are substantial. Research has demonstrated the substantial effect sizes of social support on physical and mental health (Jetten et al., 2012).

Hindley defines belonging as 'Frequent personal contacts or interactions with another person, ideally positive but mainly free from conflict and negative effects; an interpersonal bond or relationship, marked by stability, affective concern and continuation into the foreseeable future . . .'.

Psychosocial resilience explores a preventive dimension, concerning the factors and experiences that enable people to cope with and recover from distress in the face of many differing adversities. Chapter 11 provides a substantial account of the nature of this construct. It shows that neurobiological and socio-ecological perspectives are among many disciplinary findings that are contributing to our growing understanding. Thus, resilience is a process of harnessing biological, psychosocial, structural and cultural resources to sustain wellbeing (Panter-Brick & Leckman, 2013). It draws on the personal and collective resources that people and their peers mobilise to avoid becoming more affected by adverse events than they otherwise might be. Tol et al. (2013) raise, albeit without using the terms we explore here, striking resonances between the notions of horizontal epidemiology, recovery and resilience when they conclude that the 'body of knowledge supports a perspective of resilience as a complex dynamic process driven by time- and context-dependent variables, rather than the balance between risk and protective factors with known effects on mental health' (p. 445).

Insecure and Other Attachment Styles

As Hindley shows in Chapter 9, while attachment theory has been a central concept of understanding resilience in children and young people, its very narrowness and focus on individual relationships does not allow for the multiplicity of relationships and connections that people usually have. Rather, Hindley argues, we should focus on the richer field of the concept of belonging and its role as an aspect of resilience. Hindley further suggests that efforts to promote belonging might be best directed at supporting family and social cohesion in order to ensure that our need to belong is met by persons who genuinely treat us as people and valued members of our social groups.

Thus, we see horizontal epidemiology, recovery and psychosocial resilience as related and overlapping constructs, albeit with differing focuses for action. They share strikingly similar principles and the notions of our social connectedness and shared social identities are intricately involved in each one. Furthermore, they relate to the six dimensions of the human condition.

The Psychosocial Approach and Psychosocial Care

Patel (2014) points out that there is a gap between the way in which mental health specialists apply the terms 'mental health' and 'mental disorder' and the broader conceptualisations of psychosocial suffering that affect very many more people than those who may require specialist mental healthcare.

The number of people who require supporting interventions to assist them to cope with distress and disabilities consequent on their experiences of poverty, adversity and ill health is very substantial. Many of them may be psychosocially resilient despite their distress. But, intervening early when people are affected by stressful situations can reduce the risks of their developing disorders later. We term these interventions as 'psychosocial care'. By contrast, mental healthcare refers to delivering biomedical interventions from which people who have disorders may benefit.

The psychosocial approach we commend here espouses current professional opinion (Patel, 2014), which recommends:

- Distinguishing people who are distressed from those who require biomedical interventions;
- Providing assistance for the greater number of distressed people through lower-intensity psychosocial interventions; and
- Basing the distinctions between the two sorts of conditions on patterns and trajectories of people's experiences as observed in general populations.

The implications of drawing together the constructs we summarise in this chapter, which form the substance of Sections 1 and 2 of this book, are that there are two important conclusions for planning and delivering healthcare. First, it is important to recognise and respond to the broad range of people's psychosocial needs without limiting that to mental health problems or their needs for physical healthcare. Second is providing effective, evidence-based interventions that are informed by the relevant scientific evidence. Our experience is that people who have health problems require psychosocial care that focuses on their wider experiences and needs, alongside high-quality mental and physical healthcare. This is another reason why we propose that it is important to found a comprehensive approach to healthcare on solid partnerships that are able to provide a platform of psychosocial care and education in which people's social, educational and communication needs are considered alongside effective interventions to promote their health and/or treatments for their ill health, including mental disorders.

Coproduction and Partnerships

This takes us to coproduction as a way forward. A balanced plan for effective psychosocial and healthcare requires us to learn from a range of perspectives about how best to understand and respond to the needs of populations, and to optimise their care. We should take full account not only of risk and protective factors, but also of time, context, connectedness, collective experiences and relationships, and other horizontal epidemiological factors. Thereby we are enabled to seek new alignments between patients, the people who provide their support and practitioners in services, and to create effective, coproductive relationships, involving the public, practitioners and policymakers.

In its People Powered Health programme, Nesta UK makes the case for changing the ways in which all healthcare is organised, by showing how the very best scientific and clinical knowledge can be better combined with the expertise and commitment of patients (Horne et al., 2013). Nesta advocates:

- Changing consultations to create purposeful, structured conversations that combine clinical expertise with patient-driven goals and build networks of support;
- Commissioning new services that provide more than medicine to complement clinical care, by supporting long-term behaviour change, improving wellbeing and building social support networks; and
- Patients and professionals co-designing pathways that focus on long-term outcomes, recovery and prevention.

Concluding Comments

Horizontal epidemiology, recovery, attachment, social identity, psychosocial resilience and psychosocial care and the proven power of certain types of social connectedness and shared social identity remind us to look beyond illness and on into the hopes and aspirations of patients as multifaceted human beings. People live in society, not in health services.

There are implications for the quality, culture and values of our services and professional behaviour that are reflected in each of the related concepts that we have drawn together. These opportunities are to be embraced rather than feared. We must spread our learning to take into practice developments in the social sciences. We must use understanding of belonging, social identity, resilience and social networks because these are the sources of social support that can have substantial effect sizes (Jetten et al., 2012). Failing to follow this route could threaten the gains for people's health that should come from the rich developments in the physical sciences.

We believe that people who live with any health condition should be central to planning and delivering their care: these partnerships can help to reduce inequalities and promote equity. This virtuous, coordinated delivery system is radical: it requires colleagues to revisit their relationships across health and social care. If we are to promote people's health, including their mental health, while mitigating and moderating the risks of ill health and reducing blockages to recovery, we also require values-based approaches to better recognising and actively harnessing the social determinants of health. These approaches require us to see patients in their whole contexts and this agenda fits well with delivering safe care with compassion and dignity.

In parallel, we must improve the psychosocial safety of working environments for practitioners, especially in a climate that remains risk-averse rather than promoting positive risk-taking. This propels us to improve the psychosocial safety of the environments in which all practitioners work and the leadership and peer support that practitioners require if they are to build on their strengths and sustain their resilience (Edmondson, 1999, 2003). A key challenge is how we embed this approach across our training and in day-to-day practice.

References

Antonovsky, A. (1979). Health, Stress and Coping. London: Jossey-Bass Publishers.

Bailey, S. & Williams, R. (2014). Towards partnerships in mental healthcare. Commentary on: Understanding 'recovery' and becoming a recovery-oriented practitioner. Advances in Psychiatric Treatment, **20**: 48–51; doi: 10.1192/apt.bp.113.011270.

Department of Health. (2012). Department of Health Review: Final Report Transforming Care: A National Response to Winterbourne View Hospital. London: Department of Health.

Edmondson, A. (1999). Psychological safety and learning behaviour in work teams. Administrative Science Quarterly, **44**: 350–383.

Edmondson, A. (2003). Managing the risk of learning: Psychological safety in work teams. In West, M., Tjosvold, D. & Smith, K., editors, International Handbook of Organizational Teamwork and Co-operative Working. Chichester: John Wiley & Sons.

Francis, R. (2013). Report of the Mid Staffordshire NHS Foundation Trust Public Inquiry. London: Controller of Her Majesty's Stationery Office; ISBN: 9780102981476.

Heath, I. (2011). Divided We Fail: The Harveian Oration 2011. London: Royal College of Physicians.

Horne, M., Khan, H. & Corrigan, P. (2013). People Powered Health: Health for People, by People and with People. London: Nesta.

Jetten, J., Haslam, C. & Haslam, S. A., editors (2012). The Social Cure: Identity, Health and Well-Being. Hove: Psychology Press.

Khan, S., Combaz, E. & McAslan Fraser, E. (2015). Social Exclusion: Topic Guide, Revised edition. Birmingham: GSDRC, University of Birmingham.

Levitas, R., Pantazis, C., Fahamy, E. et al. (2007). The Multidimensional Analysis of Social Exclusion. London: Department for Communities and Local Government.

Nestler, E. J., Peña, C. J., Kundakovic, M., Mitchell, A. & Akbarian, S. (2016). Epigenetic basis of mental illness. The Neuroscientist, **22**: 447–463; doi: 00.1177/1071073858415608147.

Panter-Brick, C & Leckman, J. F. (2013). Editorial commentary: Resilience in child development – interconnected pathways to wellbeing. Journal of Child Psychology and Psychiatry, **54**: 333–336.

Patel, V. (2014) Rethinking mental health care: Bridging the credibility gap. Intervention, **12**: 15–20.

Roberts, G. & Boardman, J. (2013). Understanding 'recovery'. Advances in Psychiatric Treatment, **19**: 400–409.

Roberts, G & Boardman, J. (2014). Becoming a recovery-oriented practitioner. Advances in Psychiatric Treatment, **20**: 27–47.

Slade, M. (2010). Mental illness and well-being: The central importance of positive psychology and recovery approaches. BCM Health Services Research, **10**: 26.

The Lancet (2017). Editorial. Syndemics: Health in context. The Lancet, **389**: 881.

Tol, W. A., Song, S. & Jordans, M. J. D. (2013). Annual research review: Resilience and mental health in children and adolescents living in areas of armed conflict – a systematic review of findings in low- and middle-income countries. Journal of Child Psychology and Psychiatry, **54**: 445–460.

Williams, R. & Drury, J. (2011). Personal and collective psychosocial resilience: Implications for children, young people and their families involved in war and disasters. In Cook, D., Wall, J. & Cox, P., editors, Children and Armed Conflict. New York, NY: Palgrave McMillan; doi: 10.1057/9780230307698_5.

Chapter 14

Commentaries on Core Themes in Section 2

Jonathan Montgomery, S. Alexander Haslam, Adrian Neal and Richard Williams

Richard Williams' Introduction

This chapter rounds off Section 2. In it, one of the authors, Jonathan Montgomery, begins by highlighting his view of the recurrent themes that arise from all eight chapters in this section.

Then, one of the editors, Alex Haslam, responds by substantially agreeing with Jonathan Montgomery. However, Haslam takes the opportunity to clarify one of the points that Montgomery makes with the intention of drawing attention to a key issue that runs like an artery through the body of this book. This concerns the nature of personalised healthcare and how this should best be understood and delivered. Haslam cautions that, in the process of developing personalised care, we should avoid the temptation to reduce peoples' maladies to their individual conditions.

Jonathan Montgomery's Commentary on Section 2

There are some important themes that run through the chapters in this section of the book. The first is about the complexity of the social interactions that combine to constitute our mental health and wellbeing. Reductionist neurobiology is no more able to give a full account of mental health than are the materialist and determinist versions of social identity that suggest we are simply what our socio-economic context dictates. We have explored the social nature of identity and the coping mechanisms with which it is connected. Linked to this is a second theme about the need for a broad and interdisciplinary approach to understanding the resources and interventions that are available to people, services and policymakers. A third theme is the significance of appreciating people's lived experiences and the importance of integrating them into planning and personalised care. This generates a related point about the adverse impact of loss of control, otherwise styled as agency in this book, and 'being done to' even when interventions are thought by outsiders to be appropriate responses to the diagnoses that have been applied to categorise people's ailments.

This leads us to seek to revise the scope of our understanding, both more broadly to accommodate significant factors in play that go beyond the silos for which we have been trained and also more precisely in order to personalise that understanding to the circumstances as they are actually experienced. The analysis requires professionals to loosen the grip of their expertise and step outside their comfort zones in order to recognise the power of less-familiar forces. We should be wary, however, of assuming that this improved understanding of the scope of our work determines the values to which it should be directed. Recognising the contingent complexities of our lives does not require us to accept them passively. The practical and moral power of human agency remains a key characteristic of the 'good life'.

One of the insights of the recovery model is that success must be measured from the point of view of people living real lives. However, professionals must still reflect on the risks of simply assuming that what is the case should be the case. We cannot abandon the professional responsibility to make choices about what is the right thing to do. The broader insights into the scope of our work may require us to challenge things that have previously been accepted to empower patients as well as to abandon some paternalistic assumptions about what makes for good mental health.

Alex Haslam's Commentary on Section 2

Jonathan has done a great job in identifying many of the core themes in Section 2 of this book, and I think the core points he makes in relation to them are well taken and would be accepted by most of the authors. Certainly, I agree that a key point is that understandings of health must be grounded in the lived experiences of those people who have or do not have health problems. So too do I agree with the point that solutions must mesh with, and make sense from, the perspective of those lived experiences. Among other things, this means that if intervention is about imposition and authority, rather than coproduction and empowerment, it will fail. I agree wholeheartedly too with the conclusion that developing understanding and the delivery of solutions necessarily requires us all to engage with complexity and to be multidisciplinary.

Nevertheless, there is one point in Jonathan's characterisation of the landscape here with which I want to take issue; although, in so doing, I realise that this may be unfair, because it is a point Jonathan makes only parenthetically. At the same time, though, I note that this is a point that is rarely placed front and centre stage in these debates, but, rather frequently, creeps unchecked into discourse on these issues. This point concerns Jonathan's observation that '[we seek] to revise the scope of our understanding . . . more precisely to personalise that understanding to the circumstances as they are actually experienced.'

Again, I agree completely that understanding and treatment must be personalised. All too often, however, I think that 'personalised' is taken to mean 'individualised'; as if the experiences and problems of those people who come under our explanatory and therapeutic gaze are only ever experienced by individual persons as individuals. As each of the chapters in Section 2 of this book show, and the general thrust of work on social determinants of health attests, they are not.

Instead, a great many health problems arise from, and should tackled through the lens of, people's experiences as group members. As immigrants, as mothers, as homeless persons, as unemployed people, as widowers, as council tenants, as victims of domestic violence, as gay people, as prisoners, as Māori, as health service staff. A large part of the challenge of understanding is, therefore, to appreciate the nature of these collective experiences, and then to do something meaningful to improve them; in other words to develop ways of working with relevant groups rather than just with people on their own.

Caring for Staff of the Health and Social Care Services

A Commentary from Alex Haslam with a Contribution on Schwartz Rounds by Adrian Neal

My preceding point also applies to healthcare staff. Again, as well as being intensely personal, many of the experiences that staff have are shared. The importance of recognising this in the process of caring for them is demonstrated by Melanie George's (George, 2016) excellent work on the efficacy of Schwartz Rounds. This shows how Schwartz Rounds can help health service staff cope more effectively with the stress of their work because their structure recognises that many of the stressors that those staff have to deal with are anything but unique. As she reports (George, 2016, p. 9), the introduction of Schwartz Rounds:

> ... was associated with a reported upsurge in feelings of interconnectivity and compassion towards colleagues. More traditional forms of individualised staff support were in contrast, viewed as unhelpful. In particular, the offer of counselling sessions was resented by many staff because it carried the implicit message that the problem arose from a deficiency or weakness within them. New performance management policies compounded this problem and left many feeling blamed and punished for their stress.

Schwartz Rounds are intended to help foster a culture of compassionate patient care by offering healthcare staff from all occupational disciplines the opportunity to meet once a month and reflect on the stresses, dilemmas and successes that they have faced while caring for patients. In short, they provide staff with the opportunity to deal with the psychological, moral and ethical aspects of work that is not only demanding in itself but also high in emotional labour. Schwartz Rounds were specifically referred to, and recommended in Robert Francis QC's report (Francis, 2013) into the complex systemic failings within Mid-Staffordshire Hospital's National Health Service (NHS) Trust.

The Schwartz Center for Compassionate Healthcare (www.theschwartzcenter.org) was founded in Boston, USA in 1995. The centre was named after Kenneth Schwartz, a healthcare attorney who, when diagnosed with terminal lung cancer, observed the importance of the human connection between caregiver and patient. As he put it, 'the smallest acts of kindness made the unbearable bearable' (Schwartz, 1995). Schwartz Rounds have subsequently been implemented in more than 320 organisations across the USA, and over 70 organisations in the UK.

Schwartz Rounds are highly structured forums, involving providing lunch for staff, followed by an hour-long facilitated discussion. Rounds can vary in size from 10 to 100 people attending, and each is themed (e.g. 'Why I come to work'). Discussion begins with a verbal presentation from two or three panellists, who briefly share a personal story that is related to the chosen theme. The discussion that follows is facilitated so as to promote reflection and sharing experiences between peers, rather than problem-solving. Considerable attention is paid to making the rounds feel as safe and supportive as possible.

Research shows (Goodrich, 2012) that the benefits of Schwartz Rounds are manifest at at least three levels. They impact on:

(1) Practitioners, by providing a focal point and opportunity to talk about individual and collective roles;
(2) Teams and staff relationships, by increasing respect, empathy and understanding between staff, and promoting more collaboration between persons and teams; and
(3) The wider hospital/healthcare culture, and help to embed positive values.

Pepper et al. (2012) reflect on their experience at the Royal Brompton and Harefield NHS Trust when they say Schwartz Rounds 'nurture the relationships between patients and all members of staff, and lead those in positions of power in the hospital to re-think the way we organise ourselves and seek to find better solutions'.

Echoing these observations, one of our problems with many workplace stress programmes, as well as with certain forms of psychotherapy, and the theory that underpins them, is that they seek to individualise what are often shared social problems. In the process, they all too easily, and often implicitly and unwittingly, shift the curative burden onto individual persons. Conveniently too, this takes that burden off the shoulders of those people who might not only be expected to bear at least some of it, but also be in a better place to do so. This is true not only of healthcare employers, but also of local councils, housing agencies, corporations, employers and, of course, governments.

There is also a macro-practical dimension to this. This relates to the fact that if we are to successfully tackle the great health challenges of our time, we are unlikely to do so, one person, or one psychotherapy session, at a time. More controversially, we suggest that, by attempting to do so, we may actually be making things worse.

This point can be made in relation to Mary and Dave, our two case studies in Chapter 6. Their difficulties are intensely personal, and they appear to be entirely alone in their suffering. Yet if our efforts at intervention are focused on 'individualising' their problems, there is a real risk that they may ultimately only compound them; not least by making Mary's and Dave's social isolation more corporeal.

Alongside individualised concern, what we really need, then, are solutions that are altogether more 'socialising'. This is a theme that is explored in nearly all of the chapters in Section 2; in some chapters it is overt, while in others it is latent, e.g., as seen in discussions of social justice and belonging. Critically, too, it is a theme that this book as a whole is motivated both to highlight and flesh out. It is also a conversation that is long overdue.

Richard Williams' Response to Jonathan Montgomery and Alex Haslam

Here I make two points. My first is to say that, surely, the core point that emerges from Section 2 is that of highlighting that there is a difference between the importance of personalising health and social care and reducing peoples' maladies to their being seen as lying either simply or solely at the level of individual persons. I describe the latter approach as 'individualising health and social care'. This point is raised in many forms and guises in this book; it arises powerfully in horizontal epidemiology and when studying psychosocial resilience, for example. So, I take this opportunity to thank Alex Haslam for raising this matter. Furthermore, Elder reminds us in Chapter 10 that 'This [broader] approach … unlocks resources that may otherwise remain unrealised … '.

This was a vital point that lay at the core of the training in family therapy that I undertook in Wales, in 1973. That was among the first courses in this therapeutic modality ever run in the UK. Looking back, the effect on my practice has been profound. It has proved to be much more powerful than I thought it might be when the course concluded in 1974, and the messages have remained with me through the last 45 years. The importance of interpersonal and transpersonal group processes was the focus of my training in large group psychotherapy in 1974–75. Perhaps, then, my experience of group-based interventions and the unconscious biases that may arise from our own upbringings and training, for example, also explains why I still find the word 'individual' so tricky. It appears very frequently in scientific writing. But, whatever my colleagues' intentions in using that word, I continue to read it as a cool and distanced reference to particular people that seems to diminish their interconnectedness and interdependencies and remove their families, friends and colleagues from consideration. Thus, I prefer to write of people and persons because those terms appear to me to be warmer but also hint at the kinds of relationships that most people have, even if they are not the subject of particular research or practice. In line with this sentiment, Jonathan Montgomery and I return to explore a group-orientated approach to public health ethics in Chapter 24, in Section 4.

My second point is to briefly identify a contemporary but vital theme that has sat with us as we have written this book. It concerns how we care for staff of health and social care services and apply our learning to meeting their needs. They give so much of themselves in pursuing their patients' and clients' needs, but reciprocally, they too have and acquire needs. Haslam and Neal's discussion of Schwarz Rounds is a helpful way of bringing this issue into focus, while also pointing to the power of collective self-directed solutions. We return to the impact of Schwarz Rounds and to the importance of working to support staff in Chapters 26–28, in Section 4 of this book.

References

Francis, R. (2013). Report of the Mid Staffordshire NHS Foundation Trust Public Inquiry. London: Controller of Her Majesty's Stationery Office; ISBN: 9780102981476.

George, M. S. (2016). Stress in NHS staff triggers defensive inward-focussing and an associated loss of connection with colleagues: This is reversed by Schwartz Rounds. Journal of Compassionate Health Care, 3: 9–26. doi: 10.1186/s40639-016-0025-8.

Goodrich, J. (2012). Supporting hospital staff to provide compassionate care: Do Schwartz Centre Rounds work in English hospitals? Journal of the Royal Society of Medicine, **105**: 117–122.

Pepper, J, Jagger, S. I., Mason, M. J., Finney, S. J. & Dusmet, M. (2012). Schwartz Rounds: Reviving compassion in modern healthcare. Journal of the Royal Society of Medicine, **105**: 94–95.

Schwartz, K. (1995). A patient's story. The Boston Globe, July 16.

Chapter 15

Crowds and Cooperation

John Drury, Hani Alnabulsi and Holly Carter

Introduction

This chapter does two things. First, it shows how social identity principles can explain the basic psychological and behavioural effects of crowd membership. Second, it describes some recent research and applied work that shows how these basic effects operate to contribute to harmonious outcomes in potentially dangerous crowd events.

We begin by explaining some of the fundamental psychology of crowd membership in the next section.

Crowds and Relatedness

In their study of crowd experiences and behaviour at different types of crowd event, Neville and Reicher (2011) distinguish between two different forms of social identification. On the one hand, there is *social identification with a social category*, and, on the other hand, there is *shared social identification with others in the crowd.* The first refers to an abstract group which may not be physically present, whereas the second refers specifically to the people who are physically present and in proximity to oneself. The distinction is crucial for understanding behaviour within a crowd.

Thus, for example, one's identification as a supporter of Manchester United football team may be important and may be salient, but, if other people present in the crowd are not seen as genuine Manchester United supporters or are supporters of another team, this situation has very different implications for how one feels about and responds to them compared to the circumstances in which they are fellow supporters of the same team. Identification with a social category – the cognitive transformation from 'me' to 'we' – entails a shift in one's values and norms, and in one's definition of 'self-interest', which becomes re-defined at the collective level. But this is not enough, in itself, to produce the motivations for providing social support for other people around the person unless there is *shared* social identity with them. Shared social identification with others in the crowd entails a *relational* transformation – or what Neville and Reicher (2011) term a change towards greater relatedness – which will be evident in the quality of intragroup social interactions. When people identify with others in a crowd, they expect social support around shared aims and values, so there are increases in intragroup trust, expected agreement, intimacy and comfort in close proximity (Novelli et al., 2010). Moreover, as other people are no longer 'other' but, instead, are included in the collective self, there are also increases in helping behaviours and willingness to cooperate.

This relational transformation can in turn lead to an *emotional* transformation (Neville and Reicher, 2011; Reicher, 2011). Expected social support, in particular, enables people in groups to coordinate their activity – that is, *to act as one.* The capacity to act as one empowers members to translate their aims and values into reality. This realisation (or objectification) of the collective self feels good, especially for those groups that are subordinate in everyday life and whose actions serve to reverse relations with otherwise dominant outgroups (Drury & Reicher, 2005).

The ability to act together to realise (or impose) ingroup norms operates at the intragroup as well as the intergroup level. If people feel there is consensus and that they will be supported when enacting ingroup norms, they feel confident enough to collectively self-regulate – by acting against the people within the group who don't conform or whose 'deviant' actions put the group interests or identity at risk (Stott et al., 2007).

While these transformations describe a process *within* crowds and other groups, there is a further dimension to understanding crowds and crowd behaviour. Crowds do not exist in isolation but rather in relationships with other groups (Reicher, 2011). This is true of public events such as ceremonies, situations of crowd conflict, such as protests and riots, and emergencies. The perceptions and actions of professional groups that are managing safety or responding to the event mean that crowd psychology is intergroup as well as intragroup. Professional groups outside the crowd can shape the experience of the people within a crowd (Stott & Reicher, 1998). This may be in ways not intended; or, based on an understanding of crowd psychology, the professionals' interventions may operate to facilitate some of the positive processes (cooperation, coordination) that are described above. Therefore, to enhance both crowd experience and crowd safety, the relevant groups should properly understand crowd behaviour and, as a consequence, be able to reflect upon how their actions may be perceived by a crowd (Stott et al., 2007; Stott & Reicher, 1998). Are their actions threatening or supportive, appropriate or inappropriate, inclusive or differentiating? More specifically, the actions of professional groups outside the crowd can, whether deliberately or inadvertently, undermine or enhance the level of shared social identity in the crowd and, in this way, affect levels of coordination and cooperation. Part of the job of successfully managing crowd safety is, therefore, to harness the power of the crowd in question by creating a shared social identity, involving the safety managers and the crowd.

In the remainder of this chapter, we describe some of the empirical support for these ideas, with the emphasis on how the intra- and intergroup processes that we have described contribute to disaster prevention. We will show, first, how social support, which is both expected and provided within the crowd, and collective self-regulation operated to maintain safety in a crowd event that was widely seen as a near disaster. Second, we show how similar crowd processes, based on shared social identification and social support, contributed to safety at the largest crowd event in the world, even at objectively dangerous levels of crowd density. Third, we show the practical application of social identity principles through recent work on the management of chemical, biological, radiological, nuclear and explosive (CBRNe) incidents.

A Near Disaster

In 2002, Big Beach Boutique II, a free music event, attended by around 250,000 people, took place on Brighton beach. The event was described afterwards as a near disaster (Drury et al., 2015). The organisers had planned for a crowd of around 65,000, and so facilities, stewarding organisations and emergency services were overwhelmed by the numbers. As well as filling the beach, the crowd spilled onto the road on the upper promenade, limiting access for vehicles and blocking emergency exit routes. There were also specific incidents that came close to disaster. First, some people climbed up the lighting rigs, putting themselves and others in danger. Second, part of the crowd was close to the waterline; as the tide came in and reduced space, there was a crowd surge as people tried to evacuate the beach; there was a risk of crushing, and some participants became distressed. Yet the event was not, in the end, the disaster that some had feared. The reported number of minor injuries and hospital admissions for this event were not out of line with the expected patient presentation rate for a mass gathering of this size and audience profile. Organisers agreed that it was a near miss rather than a catastrophe.

We surveyed a sample of participants at this event, most of whom described themselves as regular party-goers. We also carried out interviews and analysed all the comments on social media that were posted immediately afterwards (Drury et al., 2015; Novelli et al., 2013). We found that, despite the conditions, many party-goers indicated that they enjoyed the event – some even described it as the best night of their lives. Moreover, many also indicated that they felt safe during the event, and indeed the average rating for 'feeling safe' in the survey was significantly greater than the scale midpoint, despite participants also stating that they felt the stewarding organisations and safety professionals had lost control of the event.

The survey allowed us to examine some of the processes underlying this sense of safety. One factor we investigated was party-goers' identification with the rest of the crowd. The crowd was mixed in that, along with people who regularly attended dance parties, there were also more casual party-goers. The people who identified strongly with the crowd, who saw the crowd as 'us', were much more comfortable with the levels of density than were those who identified with the crowd only weakly. Identification with the crowd also predicted feeling safe. It seemed that the reasons for this were trust and expected support, two of the relational consequences of shared social identity that we described earlier. Shared identification increased the expectation that other people in the crowd, including strangers, would help, if needed, and that they could be trusted to act appropriately in an emergency. We found that both expectations of help and trusting others mediated the relationship between social identification with the crowd and feeling safe.

This study included interviews and other accounts, such as debriefing minutes from the people who managed crowd safety during the event, that is, police officers, ambulance officers, stewards and council officials. Analysis of these accounts revealed a number of contrasts. Thus, some of the people in authority emphasised danger and risk in the crowd; police in particular highlighted what they saw as hostility and antisocial disinhibition across the crowd as a whole. By contrast, crowd participants minimised the issue of disorder, stating that only 'a minority' misbehaved and that there was 'generally good behaviour'. In those instances in which disorder was seen as a problem, party-goers who witnessed it said that it was successfully managed from within the crowd, with little fuss.

While some of the professional groups that attempted to manage safety referred to their own organisation's heroism, resilience or even use of force, when explaining how disaster had been averted, the stewards referred to the capacity of the crowd to self-organise and gave examples in which their own actions built upon this capacity. They said that mutual aid within the crowd helped to prevent disaster:

> . . . the key to the event, the key to the fact that it didn't go wrong is only really because the crowd allowed it not to go wrong – they were happy, they were content, they were informed, and the mood was great.
>
> (Safety advisory group member, Big Beach Boutique, 2002)

This extract indicates the importance of communication with the crowd. Other examples included crowd members giving others privacy to urinate, coordinating their evacuation in an orderly way up the narrow steps and encouraging others not to climb the lighting rigs. The enforcement of norms like these was only possible where there was a strong sense of 'we-ness' or shared social identity.

How Social Identification Moderates the Effect of Crowd Density on Safety at the Annual Hajj

The annual Hajj, or Muslim pilgrimage to Makkah in Saudi Arabia, is one of the world's largest mass gatherings. The Hajj involves rituals at specified spiritual locations during a certain five-day period each year. Therefore, given the number of people seeking to be in the same locations at the same time, one possible threat to crowd safety is the level of crowd density. At densities of over five people per square metre (5 ppm^2), crowds are vulnerable to shock waves, which can easily injure or kill through compressive asphyxiation (Still, 2014).

There have been a number of tragic accidents at the Hajj in the past, including in 2006, when 346 pilgrims died as they attempted to 'stone the devil' at Jamarat Bridge, Mina, and, in 2015, when more than 2,000 people died outside the holy city of Mina in crossflow. And yet, given that crowd densities routinely reach dangerous levels, at Al-Masjid Al Haram, the Grand Mosque, in Makkah, levels of 6–8 ppm^2 are regularly observed during the opening and closing Hajj rituals. It is, perhaps, remarkable that there are so few fatalities as a consequence of crowd crushes. The development of a more scientific approach to risk assessment is part of the explanation for this, alongside the large numbers of Saudi staff who are present at the event. But the sheer number of pilgrims, all in one place at one time, means that these factors cannot be the complete explanation, and, therefore, we must look more closely at the conduct of the crowd itself to see how safety is managed informally from within.

We surveyed over 1,000 pilgrims during the Hajj in 2012, at which the numbers of people attending were officially estimated to be over three million, on their experiences of crowd density and their subjective relations with the people around them (Alnabulsi & Drury, 2014). We trained a small team of research assistants to approach the crowd in and around the Grand Mosque and to estimate the density of the crowd before administering the questions.

A first finding, and perhaps not a surprising one, was that, as crowd density increased, so pilgrims' feelings of safety decreased. The results became more interesting as we began to look at the predictors of this feeling of safety and, in particular, at the relationship between these predictors. Each of the following factors was associated with high levels of feeling safe: the perceived competence of the authorities; social identification; and expected social support from others in the crowd. Based on the distinction made by Neville and Reicher (2011), we measured social identification both in terms of identification with a relevant social category (identification as a Muslim) and in terms of shared social identification with other people in the crowd. We also took a further measure of shared social identification in the crowd by asking pilgrims about the extent to which they felt that others in the crowd identified as a Muslim. While, of course, everyone at the Hajj would identify as a Muslim, feelings about and perceptions of the rest of the crowd could be expected to vary, as some might regard others as not sufficiently spiritual, or too dogmatic, for example.

We expected, and found, social identification as a Muslim to be less important than shared social identification with the crowd in explaining feelings of safety and relations with others in the crowd. Strikingly, we found that social identification moderated the effect of crowd density on the crowd – but only in the case of identification with the crowd and other people's identification as a Muslim. Only people who were low in identification with the crowd felt less safe as crowd density increased. Even more strikingly, for those high in identification with the crowd, as density increased, so feelings of safety actually increased.

The social identity principles outlined in this chapter suggest that the closer one feels psychologically to those around one, the more support one should expect. In a dense crowd, there is a need to know that others will not let me stumble, would not tread on me if I fell and would protect me from pressure if they could. Hence, as expected, we found that expectations of social support mediated the relationships between shared social identification – for both identification with the crowd and the perception that others identify as Muslim – and safety. In other words, it was because shared social identification with others enhanced expectations of support that it moderated the effect of crowd density on safety.

As in the case of the Big Beach Boutique II, participants' statements that they feel safe are of course not the same as objective measures of safety. In fact, feeling safe in the crowd might lead people to gravitate to the most dense areas of the crowd (Novelli et al., 2013), thereby increasing risk. Moreover, the finding that feelings of safety increased in denser crowds for high-identification pilgrims should not be taken as indicating a simple linear function; at a certain level (> 7–8 ppm^2), people lose the ability to move independently (Fruin, 1993) let alone to be considerate or give support to others. Nevertheless, the Hajj study offers a suggestion on how it is that an event that routinely reaches levels of density that most experts would regard as dangerous has involved relatively few fatalities over the years. As with Big Beach Boutique II, the answer has to do with the capacity for cooperation and order of the psychological crowd that is based on a shared social identity.

Facilitating Crowd Cooperation in CBRNe Mass Decontamination

Incidents classified as CBRNe are very different from most other kinds of emergencies in that they require the people who are affected to remain at the scene, even if they are showing no symptoms of injury or illness, and to be decontaminated. In most other emergencies, for example, bombings, fires, earthquakes, those unharmed and the walking wounded make their way away from the source of danger and, indeed, are moved and kept away from the scene by the emergency services' cordons. In the case of CBRNe incidents, however, if people leave the scene of the incident and return to their homes and communities when they are still contaminated, they risk spreading the harmful substance and so causing illness and even mass fatalities. The role of the professional emergency responders in communicating the need for, and purpose of, decontamination to the people affected is vital. This should help people to understand the importance of remaining at the scene, and promote public compliance with the decontamination process. If the incident is large, the ratio of responders to members of the public is likely to be such that, even if they wanted to, emergency responders would be unable to coerce the crowd to take part in decontamination. There is, therefore, a fundamental need for affected members of the public to internalise and to take ownership of the operation, that is, to become active agents, not passive recipients, in their own healthcare.

However, when we surveyed the existing literature and guidance on mass decontamination and reviewed reports of previous small-scale incidents, we found almost no mention of communication and the social aspects of mass decontamination (Carter et al., 2013b). Overwhelmingly, the guidance focused on the technical side of decontamination, such as setting up and operating the decontamination equipment. Where psychology and the crowd were referred to it was simply in terms of mass panic or disorder (see Chapters 16 and 17). There was also an absence of recognition that any crowd disorder and anxiety might be a response to the professional responders' own, insensitive, actions. Instead, the behaviour of affected people was treated as an inherent feature of the psychology of the crowd that was involved.

Our analysis of volunteers' experiences during mass decontamination exercises found that participants were much more willing to undergo the process when responders communicated and showed respect for participants' dignity (Carter et al., 2012, 2013c). We used a large-scale multi-agency decontamination exercise in a major UK city to examine the extent to which social identity processes in the crowd, and between the crowd and the responders, explained this pattern, with a view to eventually making recommendations to improve decontamination procedures (Carter et al., 2013a). Based on social identity research on dynamics between police and football crowds (Stott et al., 2007), we hypothesised, and found, that if the responders' communication was perceived as being honest and practically useful, and if people's privacy was respected, the perceived legitimacy of responders' actions was enhanced. Enhanced responder legitimacy was associated with two important effects. First, it directly predicted increased willingness of the affected people to undergo decontamination. Second, in line with the idea that the public needs to internalise the aims of decontamination, it predicted increased identification with responders.

As stated earlier, a key aim of professional responders and managers who are responsible for the safety of crowds should be to facilitate the crowd's shared social identification, which is the basis of cooperative and coordinated behaviour, both between members of crowds and with the relevant professionals. Importantly, identification with responders was, indeed, associated with enhanced identification among crowd members. This identification with the crowd appeared to have two consequences. First, it was associated with enhanced cooperative behaviour within the crowd. People need to cooperate with each other by, for example, helping with undressing, preserving dignity and washing, and to queue in an orderly manner, if mass decontamination is to be efficient and effective. Shared social identity is an important basis of this cooperation and order. Second, in our research, enhanced identification with the crowd was also associated with members' increased willingness to undertake decontamination. Again, this suggests that the internalisation process that was required had occurred.

These important results were not a one-off. They have been replicated in a laboratory-based visualisation experiment (Carter et al., 2014a) and then extended to a large-scale field experiment in which we not only measured but also manipulated the quality of communication (Carter et al., 2014b). The results of this field study suggested that the mechanism through which shared social identity in the crowd enhanced both cooperation and willingness to undertake decontamination was the increase in peoples' beliefs in efficacy regarding their own ability.

Conclusion

In each of the research examples described in this chapter, participants' identification with the crowd enhanced social-relational factors such as trust and expected social support. This evidence has been used to support the argument that identification with a crowd enables the cooperation, coordination and shared perspective required to prevent disaster in large crowd events and hazardous incidents.

The practical significance of this argument is that, in many large crowd events and incidents, there simply will not be enough responders or crowd safety professionals available to secure safety. Crowd participants must act themselves, either taking the initiative, in which case the professionals' role is to build upon the adaptive capacity and norms of the crowd, or actively giving consent to the actions of responders and safety professionals. The professionals' manner and social skills, including showing respect for crowd members' norms and dignity and explaining how their actions meet the needs of the public, can enhance legitimacy and, therefore, increase cooperation, not only within the crowd but also between the crowd and the professionals. In summary, the concepts of social identity and relatedness in crowds, and the supportive evidence presented here, offer a new way of thinking about the role of crowds in both emergency preparedness and crowd safety management.

Acknowledgements

The research described in this chapter was collaborative and involved the following colleagues: David Novelli (University of Hertfordshire); Clifford Stott (Keele University); Richard Williams (University of South Wales); Richard Amlôt (Public Health England); and G. James Rubin (King's College London). We acknowledge financial support from the following funders: the Leverhulme Trust (Ref. F/00 230/AO), the Ministry of the Interior (Kingdom of Saudi Arabia) and the Health Protection Agency (UK). We also thank the following institutions for their practical support for some of the research described here: the Custodian of the Two Holy Mosques Institute of Hajj Research; and the Centre of Research Excellence in Hajj and Omrah.

References

Alnabulsi, H. & Drury, J. (2014). Social identification moderates the effect of crowd density on safety at the Hajj. Proceedings of the National Academy of Sciences of the United States of America, **111**: 9091–9096.

Carter, H., Drury, J., Rubin, G. J., Williams, R. & Amlôt, R. (2012). Public experiences of mass casualty decontamination. Biosecurity and Bioterrorism, **10**: 280–289.

Carter, H, Drury, J., Amlôt, R., Rubin, G. J. & Williams, R. (2013a). Perceived responder legitimacy and group identification predict cooperation and compliance in a mass decontamination field exercise. Basic and Applied Social Psychology, **35**: 575–585.

Carter, H., Drury, J., Rubin, G. J., Williams, R. & Amlôt, R. (2013b). Communication during mass casualty decontamination: Highlighting the gaps. International Journal of Emergency Services, **2**: 29–48.

Carter, H., Drury, J., Rubin, G. J., Williams, R. & Amlôt, R. (2013c). The effect of communication during mass decontamination. Disaster Prevention and Management, **22**: 132–147.

Carter, H., Drury, J., Amlôt, R., Rubin, G. J. & Williams, R. (2014a). Effective responder communication, perceived responder legitimacy and group identification predict public cooperation and compliance in a mass decontamination visualisation experiment. Journal of Applied Social Psychology, doi: 10.1111/jasp.12286.

Carter, H., Drury, J., Amlôt, R., Rubin, G. J. & Williams, R. (2014b). Effective responder communication improves efficiency and psychological outcomes in a mass decontamination field experiment: Implications for public behaviour in the event of a chemical incident. PLoS One, **9**: e89846.

Drury, J. & Reicher, S. (2005). Explaining enduring empowerment: A comparative study of collective action and psychological outcomes. European Journal of Social Psychology, **35**: 35–58.

Drury, J., Novelli, D. & Stott, C. (2015). Managing to avert disaster: Explaining collective resilience at an outdoor music event. European Journal of Social Psychology, **45**: 533–547.

Fruin, J. J. (1993). The causes and prevention of crowd disasters. Originally presented at the First International Conference on Engineering for Crowd Safety, London, March. (Revised exclusively for crowdsafe.com, January 2002.)

Neville, F. & Reicher, S. (2011). The experience of collective participation: Shared identity, relatedness, and emotionality. Contemporary Social Science, **6**: 377–396.

Novelli, D., Drury, J. & Reicher, S. (2010). Come together: Two studies concerning the impact of group relations on 'personal space'. British Journal of Social Psychology, **49**: 223–236.

Novelli, D., Drury, J., Reicher, S. & Stott, C. (2013). Crowdedness mediates the effect of social identification on positive emotion in a crowd: A survey of two crowd events. PLoS One, **8**: e78983.

Reicher, S. (2011). Mass action and mundane reality: An argument for putting crowd analysis at the centre of the social sciences. Contemporary Social Science, **6**: 433–449.

Still, G. K. (2014). Introduction to Crowd Science. Boca Raton, FL: CRC Press.

Stott, C. & Reicher, S. (1998). Crowd action as inter-group process: Introducing the police perspective. European Journal of Social Psychology, **28**: 509–529.

Stott, C., Adang, O., Livingstone, A. & Schreiber, M. (2007). Variability in the collective behaviour of England fans at Euro2004: 'Hooliganism', public order policing and social change. European Journal of Social Psychology, **38**: 75–100.

Chapter 16

Emergencies, Disasters and Risk Reduction: A Microcosm of Social Relationships in Communities

Tim Healing, Anthony D. Redmond, Verity Kemp and Richard Williams

Disasters as a Microcosm of Societies' Problems

Disasters and major incidents, while uncommon in each country, occur sufficiently frequently worldwide and have such societal impacts that they make headlines on most days. Perhaps, paradoxically, emergencies are so common as to be almost ordinary, if only in purely statistical terms, if it were not for the human impact, worry and suffering that is involved. This chapter shows how disasters are integral to and, thus, present a microcosm of our worlds. Our intention is to use them, in common with each of the topics in Section 3 of this book, to explore social influences on how people, communities and societies respond to and cope with the physical and psychosocial impacts of major events. This chapter links John Drury et al.'s exploration of the contribution of social psychology to crowd science in Chapter 15 with Drury and Alfadhli's Chapter 17, on disasters. We intend that Chapters 15, 16 and 17 provide another window on the human condition, the importance of social relationships and the powerful influences of social identity.

Initially, this chapter clarifies what we mean by disasters and disaster risk reduction. Then, we examine the ways in which nations endeavour to reduce risk, highlighting the importance of including people's psychosocial experiences in this process. Next, we examine the impact of various types of disasters, including complex emergencies, on the survivors and responders who are involved, using examples drawn from the developed world and third worlds. Finally, we look briefly at post-disaster recovery and the intersection of disasters with the six features of the human condition that are covered in Chapter 2.

What is a Disaster?

The definition of a disaster given on the United Nations Office for Disaster Risk Reduction (UNISDR) website is: 'A serious disruption of the functioning of a community or a society at any scale due to hazardous events interacting with conditions of exposure, vulnerability and capacity, leading to one or more of the following: human, material, economic and environmental losses and impacts' (www.unisdr.org, accessed June 2017).

An annotation to the definition notes that 'the effect of the disaster can be immediate and localized, but is often widespread and could last for a long period of time. The effect may test or exceed the capacity of a community or society to cope using its own resources, and therefore may require assistance from external sources, which could include neighbouring jurisdictions, or those at the national or international levels'.

This definition implies a human element regardless of its cause and while some events, such as tsunamis, may do vast damage to the environment, they do not fall within this definition unless they impact upon human populations.

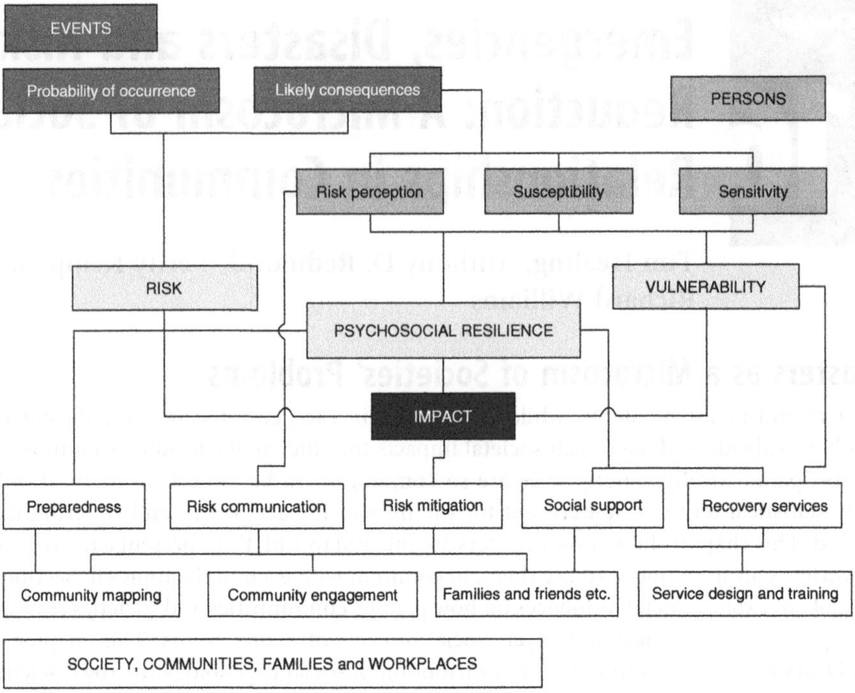

Figure 16.1 The psychosocial components of disasters (copyright R. Williams, 2010. All rights reserved and reproduced with permission.)

Disasters are often broadly divided into 'human-made' and 'natural' and may be subdivided into sudden-onset or 'big bang' disasters (such as earthquakes, tsunamis, terrorist attacks, etc.) and slow-onset or 'rising tide' events (e.g. droughts, famines). Increasingly, the concept of a wholly 'natural' disaster is being challenged as it implies an air of inevitability. There are natural phenomena; but the disaster when it follows is too often the result of a failure to mitigate known risks and vulnerabilities. Human-made disasters include items such as industrial accidents, transport accidents and terrorism. The most extreme types are 'complex emergencies', wars and civil wars with the concomitant problems of violence, injury, loss of life, damage to societies and economies, human rights abuse, population displacement, food shortages, the need for extensive aid and significant risks for aid workers. Figure 16.1 provides an overview of the many psychosocial aspects of disasters.We focus on just a small selection of these topics.

Risk and Risk Reduction

Risk is a function of two variables: *likelihood* (the probability of an event occurring); and *impact* (the likely effects of that event). The likelihood that a disaster will occur is determined by factors such as the type of hazard, the type and location of the community, the geology of the area, weather conditions etc. The impact depends on the nature of the community affected and the degree to which disaster mitigation or prevention activities have or have not been undertaken.

Disaster risk reduction is defined on the UNISDR website as 'processes designed to reduce the damage caused by natural hazards like earthquakes, floods, droughts and cyclones, through an ethic of prevention'. Interestingly, the United Nations incorporates a human element because its approach is based on the premise that there is no such thing as a 'natural' disaster, only natural hazards.

According to the UNISDR, reducing risk depends on reducing either, or both, of the variables, likelihood and impact, by:

- Reducing people's exposure to hazards;
- Reducing the impact on the people affected and their property;
- Proper land and environment management;
- Improved preparedness; and
- Early warning of adverse events.

Commonly, a number of social factors are in play. It is highly unlikely that the responsible authorities can change the location of a community in a situation in which the community faces a hazard such as flooding, for example. But providing better flood defences (e.g. raised banks, berms etc.), modifying structures, such as raising stores and dwellings above ground level, and developing appropriate skills and responses within communities that face potential floods can greatly mitigate the impacts of a future flood and might even eliminate the risk.

Data from EM-DAT, the Office of US Foreign Disaster Assistance – Centre (OFDA) – Centre for Research on the Epidemiology of Disasters (CRED) International Disaster Database show that the number of natural disasters reported rose markedly between 1970 and 2013, due mainly to a sustained rise in climate-related events, mainly floods and storms, combined with the increase in the population of the world, forcing people to occupy more marginal and riskier habitats. In recent years, there has been a decline in the average number of people affected which CRED ascribes, at least in part, to population growth. Death rates in disasters, on the other hand, increased over the same period, being about three times greater in low-income countries than in high-income nations. The role of disaster mitigation activities in the declines reported is not clear and CRED and UNISDR note that more research into this topic is urgently needed (CRED, 2015; CRED & UNISDR, 2015).

Disaster risk reduction involves a number of disciplines of study and work, including disaster mitigation, disaster management and disaster preparedness. Disaster mitigation is defined by UNISDR as, 'the lessening or minimizing of the adverse impacts of a hazardous event'. It notes that the adverse impacts of hazards, in particular natural hazards, often cannot be prevented fully, but their scale or severity can be substantially lessened by various strategies and actions. Mitigation measures include engineering techniques and hazard-resistant construction as well as improved environmental and social policies and public awareness. Mitigation measures include disaster management and disaster preparedness.

Disaster Management

Disaster management is the organisation, planning and application of measures preparing for, responding to and recovering from disasters (UNISDR, 2016). Disaster management may not completely avert or eliminate the threats; it focuses on creating and implementing preparedness and other plans to decrease the impact of disasters and 'build back better'. Failure to create and apply a plan could lead to damage to life and assets, and to lost revenue. The term 'emergency management' is also used, sometimes interchangeably, with the term 'disaster management', particularly in the context of biological and technological hazards, and for health emergencies. While there is a large degree of overlap, an emergency can also relate to hazardous events that do not result in serious disruption of the functioning of a community or society.

Disaster Preparedness

Disaster preparedness involves taking actions to prepare for, and mitigate, the effects of disasters. Records of potential and actual disasters and responses in a region, and response data from elsewhere, make it possible to predict likely problems and to put in place preventive measures. Measures of this kind should be as simple and straightforward as possible, and it is vital to include the members of potentially affected communities in the process as well as local and national governments. People should be trained to deal with the expected types of disaster. The communities can take ownership of the preparation and risk reduction process, thus building local relationships and interactions. As an example, communities should advise the responsible authorities to position supplies for disaster response where they are not likely to be affected seriously by a disaster but are easily accessible by communities if and when they are affected. Post-disaster recovery is an integral part of this planning.

This type of local involvement can greatly help to mitigate the psychosocial impacts of disasters on persons and communities and to prevent the disintegration of communities when disasters do strike, and it can contribute to system and community resilience. Indeed, there is strong evidence of the importance to recovery and people's health of supporting people's and communities' agency in the process of recovery and, once again, we make connections with the dimensions of the human condition described in Chapter 2. But, there is a risk of misinterpreting this finding to imply that governments and the responsible authorities might limit their interventions to supporting communities. The lesson is more about how communities and the people in them are supported, how their recovery is propelled, and how community leaders and persons are afforded respect by everyone who intervenes.

It is also vital to ensure that organisations which respond, inside and outside potentially affected communities, are aware of what might be the psychosocial impacts of the disaster they face and how they might be mitigated. Experiences in the UK indicate just how it is possible to make assumptions about the levels of knowledge that agencies have, and that affects the priority they afford to this task. Once again, involving and empowering communities in planning and preparing for disasters is likely to reduce the psychosocial impacts by allowing people to retain a measure of control over their lives, even when the worst occurs.

How People are Affected by Disasters

The needs of populations that are struck by disasters, which may raise extraordinary challenges and stress, reflect the kinds of problems that communities ordinarily experience. To these are added the needs that arise from the impact of the disaster on the people who are affected. Thus, for example, affected populations have health and social care needs that arise in most similar populations. Added to these problems are the exacerbations of need that result from the changes to people's care and the adjustments that disasters may bring. In addition, there are new needs that may result from the event and changes in social support and circumstances that are faced by people who are directly and indirectly affected.

Some of these pre-existing, exacerbated and new sets of needs may lead to long-term problems for a proportion of the affected population that do not necessarily resolve when communities return to a more ordinary pattern of activity and functioning.

In order to illuminate this theme, we draw together in this section observations, from science and from experience gained during our work with populations that were affected by disasters, of a selection of the ways in which people experience and cope with events and their needs, and link them with the themes in this book.

People at Greatest Risk

Generally, the people who are at greatest risk of many of the potential impacts of disasters are those who are poor. An International Monetary Fund working paper, produced in 2012, reported (based on data produced by CRED) that, since the 1960s, about 99 per cent of the world population affected by disasters has lived in developing countries, and that 97 per cent of all deaths have occurred in developing countries (Laframboise & Loko, 2012). CRED (2015) noted that, on average, more than three times the number of people died per disaster in low-income countries than in high-income countries, in 1994–2013.

People who are poor and disadvantaged are at greater risk of being involved in many types of disaster, often due to having to live in marginal habitats or poorly constructed dwellings, and they have fewer social connections, lesser capacities and fewer resources available to them. As a result, they are also at greater risk of the direct and indirect physical and psychosocial consequences. Richer people can move out of disaster-prone areas or can attempt to mitigate the impact of hazards by, for example, constructing earthquake-resistant buildings. Poorer people get left behind in areas that face more hazards, and in unsafe dwellings. Moreover, they usually have fewer resources and receive less support from families, communities, financial recovery systems and social safety nets to prevent, cope and adapt. Women and children can be particularly vulnerable. In addition, older people, persons who are ill before events and people whose mental health is poor are often at greater risk (Centers for Disease Control and Prevention, 2012; Pan American Health Organisation, 2017).

These features were in evidence when FMTs (Foreign, now called Emergency, Medical Teams) went into the Philippines in 2013 in the wake of Typhoon Haiyan. Typhoons in that part of the world follow a fairly predictable route, albeit with some variation. The major well-developed urban areas are outside the usual typhoon pathway and people who are rich enough and educated enough to live or find jobs there move out of the way of the typhoon track. It is the poorest and most vulnerable people who are left behind and they are, therefore, more likely to be affected by these phenomena.

There was great altruism shown within the affected areas in the Philippines. As the FMTs got closer to the effects of the typhoon their members noticed local fundraising and aid operations, that were absent from richer areas, unaffected by the typhoon, where life appeared to be carrying on as normal. Thus, even poorer communities may respond altruistically to untoward events.

Communities: Tensions Between Sage Advice and Residents' Needs and Preferences

The extent to which communities disintegrate following disasters greatly increases the impact, both physical and psychosocial, on the people involved. The degree to which this impact is mitigated depends, in a large part, on the speed and effectiveness with which communities are re-established or, possibly temporary, substitute communities are established. It may also depend on the extent of external assistance, and the sensitivity with which it is provided. Heavy-handed or inappropriate provision of assistance, particularly if it is seen to undermine or denigrate the efforts of local providers, is likely to delay or even prevent communities being re-established. There is a fine balance between doing too little, enough, or too much, and that may be mediated by the attitudes of the people who intervene.

The Lockerbie air disaster, in December 1988, was the biggest terrorist attack on UK soil, killing 243 passengers, 16 air crew and 11 people on the ground. The experience of one of us (AR) as a medical officer at the site was that many of the local people coped with the immediate aftermath of the disaster by trying to force normality onto this highly abnormal situation. Many were seen queuing at the local shop as dawn broke, angrily demanding to know why the shop was closed and how were they supposed to get their newspapers and milk. Immediately behind them was the fuselage, embedded in a row of houses.

That situation illustrates the differences in priorities that can occur between different groups of people who are affected by a disaster. In that event, there was also the tension between the importance of recovering human remains with dignity, and the need to preserve forensic evidence. Rescuers were told to leave bodies *in situ*, to be photographed and filmed the following morning to support the investigation. Local people and some of the responders found this hard to accept. Great concern was expressed about what would happen to body parts that were left exposed in the fields overnight. A matter that caused particular distress was that a victim of the crash was still strapped in a seat that had become lodged in the roof of a house where it was clearly visible. The external authorities required that the body be left in place while the local people asked for the person's remains to be treated respectfully and to be removed. The local police did not stop actions to remove the dead person's body.

Unanticipated Impacts

Furthermore, certain types of disaster may have wide and complicated effects on affluence, communities and social life within them. The Ebola outbreak, which occurred in West Africa in 2013–2016, provides an example of how disasters affect communities. Based on the case numbers reported by the World Health Organization (WHO, 2016), only a very small proportion (around 0.13 per cent) of the estimated population in Guinea, Liberia and Sierra Leone (Central Intelligence Agency, 2016), the three countries that were mainly involved, actually caught the disease.

However, there were many serious effects on populations as a whole of the countries involved. Several studies have shown that breakdowns in the health services, which were already overstretched, led to marked increases in the numbers of cases of, and deaths from, other diseases, such as malaria, and conditions, such as maternal mortality (e.g. Helleringer & Noymer, 2015; Parpia et al., 2016; VSO and the Liverpool School of Tropical Medicine, 2015; Walker et al., 2015). In addition, people who catch and survive Ebola can suffer from a legacy of poor health and after-effects of the infection (Clark et al., 2015), a situation that is occurring in the three countries most affected by the outbreak (Vetter et al., 2016).

Second, there were dramatic effects on the economies of those countries and the World Bank estimates that economic losses may have exceeded $2.2 billion (World Bank Group,

2015). The population was affected by rising costs of basic necessities, increased unemployment and job losses, inflation, reduced agricultural output, food shortages and loss of foreign investment. Thus, we see evidence of the impacts of the disease, the primary stressor, and the many secondary stressors (Lock et al., 2012).

Third, and of great importance, were the social changes resulting from the outbreak, which were nationwide. Control of the outbreak required members of the affected populations to make changes in deeply held and valued traditional burial practices, and normal patterns of highly tactile greeting behaviour had to be abandoned. People became unwilling to engage in activities such as trade, schooling, sports and attendance at health centres, which might expose them to infection. Attitudes towards people who had recovered from the disease, and towards those combatting the disease (healthcare workers, burial workers) became, and in many instances remained, hostile and some people were rejected by their communities. There are many orphans, who are receiving variable standards of support and care (Evans & Popova, 2015).

Displacement

One of the most serious outcomes of disasters on the physical and mental health of the people affected is population displacement. Losses of homes and possessions, breakdown of communities and, all too often, separation of families, puts immense strain on people. Furthermore, it threatens the social identities and social support that this book has already shown as important to so many aspects of our lives.

Displacement affects physical health. Several authors have pointed out that the risk factors for outbreaks of communicable disease after disasters are associated primarily with population displacement (Noji, 1997; Watson et al., 2007). Displaced persons may:

- Have reduced or no access to healthcare services;
- Have increased susceptibility to infection if their immune systems are compromised by stress and poor diet;
- Have increased exposure to novel organisms to which they have no resistance if they move to new areas; and
- Find themselves in overcrowded accommodation with poor sanitation and contaminated water or food.

Awareness of the make-up of a displaced population is vital to planners, to ensure that appropriate help can be given. Watson et al. (2007) showed that four groups of people are at particular risk within displaced populations:

- Children (especially those who are less than five years old and who are unaccompanied);
- Women (especially pregnant women and nursing mothers);
- Older people; and
- Disabled people.

Displacement puts a great strain on those affected. People who have to leave their homes and communities as the result of floods, for example, may be severely stressed and disconnected from their friends, families, social care and healthcare services. Thus, not only are their needs for social support increased by events but their social connectedness may be reduced at the very time they need it most.

If survivors and families can remain in their homes they may be able to retain a measure of agency over their lives, and communities can be re-established. This means that people who are involved in the rescue, immediate aftermath and the recovery phases may have to make difficult decisions about the advice they give to people who are affected in which displacement for their physical safety has to be balanced with the established risks that stem from displacement. This emphasises the importance of trying to help people to sustain their social connectedness when they are displaced.

The ability to become involved in restoring a community, following a disaster, is most important, because it restores and reinforces agency. After flooding, concerns about health, problems with relationships and loss of items of sentimental value have been shown to be associated with poorer mental health outcomes (Tempest et al., 2017). None of this should deter responders from intervening decisively if people are at risk, but anyone who recommends displacement of people in the face of disasters should be aware of the importance of minimising the unintended consequences by making sure that people take with them items that they require, such as medication, address books, mobile phones and objects of sentimental value. Furthermore, items that could easily be seen as trivial by a third party should not be dismissed lightly as they may have a deep and important meaning to their owners. People who are displaced should also, for example, be assisted in remaining in contact with relatives and friends and connected to primary healthcare. These things are important components of our social identities. Furthermore, displacement threatens the social support that this book has already shown as important to so many aspects of our lives.

Communities that act as hosts to people who are displaced by disasters are often affected. They may be damaged or destroyed by the experience or they may be strengthened. Examples come from the conflicts in the former Yugoslavia, in the 1990s. In Bosnia Hercegovina alone, over half the population of 4.4 million was displaced, with an estimated 1.3 million internally displaced and 1.2 million refugees (Young, 2001). About 50 per cent of them were displaced within the borders of the former Yugoslavia and most were placed with host families rather than in refugee camps. This placed great strains on the communities that acted as hosts due to overcrowding and loss of privacy, overstretching services, such as healthcare, that were already limited, and contributing to shortages of items such as food (Black & Healing, 1993; Healing et al., 1996).

Responding to Disasters

In her seminal exploration of five disaster scenarios, Solnit, a writer, historian and activist, reflects on the social meaning of disasters. Her work is an interesting juxtaposition of apocalypse and utopia – hence her title, *A Paradise Built in Hell*. She challenges the oft-stated notion of people who are involved being helpless or out of control. Relating to the San Francisco earthquake of April 1906, Solnit (2010, p. 15) says, '... the people were for the most part calm and cheerful, and many survived the earthquake with gratitude and generosity ... Disaster requires an ability to embrace contradiction'.

Solnit asserts that, 'People know what to do in a disaster. [But] ... loss of power [is] the disaster in the modern sense ... [though] ... solidarity, altruism, and improvisation are within most of us and reappear at these times. This is the paradise entered through hell' (Solnit, 2010, p. 10). If Solnit's assertions are broadly true, the question about how best to respond to people's social and psychological needs might be reframed as:

- How can we best recognise, respect and use people's knowledge about what to do in the local context?
- How can we restore the agency of people who have been affected?

- How can we best support people in sustaining, restoring and creating their social connectedness?
- How can we best enable people who have been affected to improvise, show altruism and use their solidarity with others to benefit other people and themselves?

Psychological first aid (PFA) is intended to reduce people's initial distress in the immediate aftermath of severe events and to foster their adaptive functioning. It is not a single intervention or treatment, but an evidence-informed modular approach that is designed to respond to people's psychosocial needs after emergencies. It is one such articulation of how to respond to these four questions (Brymer et al., 2006). It provides principles for immediate responses to the psychosocial needs of survivors of, and responders to, disasters. Forbes et al. (2012) provide a summary of the core components of PFA: ensuring people are safe and cared for; helping people to normalise their experiences by providing calm, compassionate support that enhances how people cope; enabling people by providing social support; helping them to restore their agency and perceptions of themselves as effective persons; being aware that some people develop mental disorders; and enabling people to seek further help by signposting access to other welfare and health services and enabling access to more specialised healthcare are core elements (Hobfoll et al., 2007; Williams & Kemp, 2016).

People affected by disasters can feel isolated and forgotten. Local doctors and nurses were asked by one author of this chapter (AR), at a technical debriefing session at the end of the Bosnian conflict, what was the most important, most significant and most welcome programme that had been carried out. Immediately and unanimously they said, 'You came'. They did not feel isolated and they knew that they were not forgotten as long as the aid workers kept coming back.

More information on the psychosocial and mental health needs of affected populations, including children, and on delivering psychosocial and mental health programmes is available in a report (Williams et al., 2014a) and several chapters (Williams et al., 2014b Williams & Kemp, 2016, 2018).

Sudden-Onset Disasters

The acute medical needs of populations of people immediately after a sudden-onset disaster almost always have to be met by local services. It takes time for international aid to deploy. The nature of some disaster scenarios results in more fatalities than injuries; for example, tsunamis. In these circumstances, people's acute medical needs are very limited and can usually be met by local capacity, if it remains intact. However, there can be huge pressures on international aid agencies to respond, and they may be subjected to severe criticism if they do not. Nevertheless, responding inappropriately is not without consequence and the Asian tsunami provided a number of examples of both good and bad practice (Grunewald et al., 2007; Roy, 2006).

Probably, the first large-scale international response to a sudden-onset disaster was after the Armenian earthquake in 1988. The lessons recognised from this are:

- Outsiders are highly likely to want to help and, therefore, to turn up.
- If not invited, external agencies and persons can be seen by local people as a burden.
- If invited, but they do not do what they are invited to do by local people, external agencies are still likely to be seen as a burden.

- Local people affected by the disaster look more easily to local rather than national authorities (Noji et al., 1990).

These points should be borne in mind when planning responses to large-scale disasters.

Conflicts

Most of the needs of the affected populations in conflicts are similar to those of persons affected by natural disasters or sudden-onset, human-made disasters (safe food, clean water, secure shelter, healthcare, etc.) but there are some marked differences too. In conflicts, the time scale tends to be much longer, with the affected populations exposed to extended periods of danger, and aid programmes can be seriously compromised by political pressures and, due to the security situation, by the inability of aid workers to reach many people who are in need. In addition, whereas in acute-onset natural disasters trauma is the main immediate cause of morbidity and mortality (outbreaks of or increases in the incidence of communicable disease may occur later), in many wars, more people die from illness than trauma. Estimates of mortality in the war in Darfur (2004–2008), for example, suggested that more than 80 per cent of ca. 300,000 deaths were due to disease (Degomme & Guha-Sapir, 2010). Damage to and destruction of key infrastructures in conflict, allied to break-downs of medical services, can greatly increase the prevalence of communicable diseases (Puvacic & Weinberg, 1994).

The affected population(s) are also likely to suffer long-term physical and mental health problems, which may extend long beyond the period of the war itself, due to long-term chronic exposure to risk (Ghobarah et al., 2004; Pedersen, 2002; Vulic et al., 2012). Children may be especially at risk (Chriman & Dougherty, 2014).

The constant uncertainty and fear that can exist during conflicts may undermine faith in governments and social structures. It is just this type of situation that terrorists attempt to create by repeatedly performing violent acts with the intention of ensuring that the population suffers constant tension and a continuing sense of threat.

Impacts on Responders

Disasters also have impacts upon people who provide assistance. Responding to disasters is a highly stressful activity. At first sight, responders do appear to manage their experiences relatively well compared with people in affected communities, and particularly so if they are trained professional staff who are cared for well by their employers.

Nonetheless, responders may find themselves attempting to deal with overwhelming health or other needs, in situations that are insecure and in which accommodation and food are of poor quality, and where they may be far from home. In conflicts, responders are faced with the additional stresses of being exposed to the general hazards of war and, increasingly, of finding themselves at risk of becoming specific targets (Stoddard et al., 2017).

If responders are not properly supported, their mental health and social functioning may be significantly impaired (Alexander & Klein, 2009; Morganstein et al., 2016). Chronic exposure to risk can affect both mental and physical health (Cardozo et al., 2012; McFarlane, 2004; Vulic et al., 2012). It is notable that professional healthcare first responders are more likely than the general population and other health workers to take early retirement (Sterud et al., 2006). Those who lead teams in the field, and the aid agencies involved, have a key role to play in ensuring the wellbeing of their staff (see also Chapters 28 and 29 of this book). Brooks et al. (2015) provide a summary of the risk factors that affect the psychosocial wellbeing of people deployed in humanitarian relief roles after disasters that they found in a systematic review of the literature. Information on meeting the needs of responders is available from a report (Williams et al., 2014a) and several chapters (Williams & Greenberg, 2014).

The healthcare workers who went to West Africa in 2014 and 2015 to help combat the Ebola outbreak found themselves in a situation in which they were trying to provide care for patients under very taxing and stressful conditions. Working in tropical heat in Personal Protective Equipment (PPE) was very demanding, and the people involved rapidly became physically exhausted. In addition, they were faced with the constant fear of developing a highly lethal disease. Fortunately, only a few of them developed the disease, and most recovered although with serious long-term sequelae in several cases, but almost all of the people who went were affected by the experience (Van Bortel et al., 2016). The commonest reported stressor on their return home was stigmatisation by colleagues (Redmond et al., 2016).

Proper Planning Prevents Poor Performance

The effectiveness of any response to a disaster can be improved and the impact of working in a disaster can be mitigated by proper preparation and planning. Responses to disasters should be planned, prepared and practised.

Lessons from Experience about Planning and Preparation

We identify in Table 16.1 a number of principles for humanitarian aid that are derived mainly from our experience. These lessons reflect the ideas in this book strongly and show that managing the implications of events in all sorts of settings can benefit from the messages in this book. Vice versa, applying them in practice in more ordinary circumstances can benefit from the hard-edged lessons gleaned from working in disasters.

Humanitarian aid work is complex and multifaceted. Failure to apply any of these key principles increases the risk of failure of a programme, with consequences for the client population and for the responders. It is particularly important to try to avoid reacting unusually to unusual circumstances. The experience of AR in deploying teams to major emergencies for 30 years is that people function best when they are doing things with which they are familiar.

The impacts cannot be removed, but by giving responders a frame of reference, which is reflected in their social identity as members of humanitarian aid teams, the negative impact of events is likely to be reduced. Usual activities can be created for unusual circumstances by training, preparing and practising an agreed plan. This has been done, for example, by setting up the UK-Med Register (www.uk-med.org) and the associated training pathway. The Register actively seeks people who might look to volunteer to work after a disaster (in the aftermath of an earthquake, for example) to volunteer now. This creates time in which professional healthcarers can prepare for what they might experience.

Building Back Better

Much work has been done to address the physical and infrastructure aspects of post-disaster recovery, including restoration of government, restoration of the physical infrastructure,

Table 16.1 Lessons from experience and science

Item	Principle	Detail	Social implications
1	Disasters are unusual events but many aspects are predictable.	Knowledge of local conditions, and of previous disasters and near disasters in the area informs planning and preparation.	Reduction of risk by activities to prevent disaster provides local people with self-determination and agency.
2	Involve local people, leaders and authorities in planning.	Ideally, responses should be led locally. Foreign aid workers should support, train and work behind the scenes.	This builds capacity.
3	Understand the society affected by each disaster.	Brief aid workers on local culture and behaviours before deployment.	Improves effectiveness, and reduces stress on responders. Reduces misunderstandings.
4	There should be a presence in the affected country(ies).	Aid is delivered most effectively by organisations with a presence in the country before the disaster or working under the umbrella of such an organisation.	Involving local people and understanding their needs and preferences improves effectiveness of responses.
5	There should be an exit strategy.	Include an exit strategy in planning for an intervention from the beginning.	Staff should be trained in affected areas in order to ensure programme continuity.
6	Aid workers should be trained in advance.	Train team members in: • specialised techniques in their fields of expertise; • understanding humanitarianism and working in the sector; • ways of coping and adapting to field environments.	Training provides opportunities for aid workers to meet future colleagues before deployment. This increases team effectiveness at all levels and enables teams to develop supporting social identities.
7	There should be specialists and support staff.	Teams should include the specialists and the support staff needed to meet their terms of reference.	This approach increases effectiveness of response and supports team integration and morale.
8	There should be non-medical specialists.	Social anthropologists and social communicators (for example) can ensure that	This improves effectiveness, and reduces stress on the responders.

Table 16.1 (cont.)

Item	Principle	Detail	Social implications
		aid programmes are acceptable to the affected population, and can open channels of communication.	
9	Security and health of team members are important.	Aid agencies must have in place mechanisms to ensure: • the security and health of team members; • evacuation when required (for reasons of injury, ill health, deterioration of security); • communication with home.	There is a maintenance of morale and effectiveness of aid workers.
10	Team leaders are needed.	Leadership is a difficult but vital task and it includes: • ensuring that the programme is carried out; • regular briefings and feedback to the team; • dealing with possible problems for members of their teams and conflicts within the team; • liaison with local and national authorities; • contact with HQ.	Advice is available about leading, training and supporting people who intervene (Williams & Greenberg, 2014). OP94 contains checklists of actions for leaders in preparing staff before, during and after deployments (Williams et al., 2014a).
11	Psychologically safe work environments should be provided.	Team members must believe that others will not resent, penalise or think less of them for asking for help, information or feedback.	This improves staff wellbeing and welfare; there are fewer mistakes/errors of judgement.
12	Staff should be supported when they return home.	Welcome returning staff from a deployment whether returning on their own or with a team. Reunite team after an interval for a review.	There may be a need to continue follow-up and support activities for 18 months or more.

reconstruction of urban and rural housing, development of agriculture, re-establishment of healthcare, etc. However, restoring communities to these aspects of normality is likely to be insufficient. The modern UN requirement is to 'build back better' (UNISDR, 2015a).

The psychosocial element of disasters was neglected by the humanitarian aid world for many years. Efforts are now being made to address these needs. Priority 4 of the Sendai Framework for Disaster Risk Reduction (UNISDR, 2015b) calls on states 'To enhance recovery schemes to provide psychosocial support and mental health services for all people in need'. This includes responders to disasters.

People's psychosocial recovery after disasters is a multidimensional process that is linked to preventative measures that are taken before disasters occur, their social and economic circumstances, reconstruction of built environments and societal infrastructure, restoration of assets and services provided after events. The ability to become involved in restoring and developing a community or area, following a disaster, is most important to restoring and reinforcing agency. Experience has shown that survivors of disasters look to restore their view of normality as soon as possible, and people who wish to help can achieve better results by finding ways of helping them to do so.

After World War II, restoring economies to countries damaged by the conflict probably did more to establish and maintain peace and much to reduce overall psychological damage than many other interventions. The greatest example of this was the Marshall Plan for Europe (http://marshallfoundation.org/marshall/the-marshall-plan/). Similarly, it was deliberate policy to restore the economy following the conflict in Kosovo in the 1990s. Many micro-loans were made to communities to allow them to set up businesses so that life could be resumed as soon as possible (Ahmeti, 2014).

Concerns about standards of care, provided by foreign medical teams following the earthquake in Haiti (Redmond et al., 2011) led to the WHO establishing the Emergency Medical Teams (EMTs) initiative, designed to ensure that incoming medical response teams (Foreign Medical Teams – FMTs) follow the classification and minimum standards set by WHO and its partners, and come trained and self-sufficient so as not to burden the national system (WHO, 2013). These recommendations were implemented very successfully for the first time in the aftermath of Typhoon Haiyan in the Philippines. They enabled the government there to have much closer control over the aid that it accepted into the country and also to deploy that aid more efficiently on the basis of knowledge of the teams' capabilities.

Just as has been shown by research in Haiti, communities in the Philippines were not helpless, but were more organised, and they were agents of their own assistance and manipulators of the aid that was coming in (Redmond et al., 2011). Recognising these matters, and the key roles and authority of community leaders, resulted in FMTs being immediately accepted and, consequently, they were able to gain immediate access to these communities.

Conclusions: Disasters and the Six Features of the Human Condition

Smith sets out six features of the human condition in Chapter 2 of this book. Disasters are capable of upsetting each one. The danger and destruction of disasters can affect our physical wellness, bring us face-to-face with death, destroy social groupings, force us to act in ways that do not appear cognitively logical, reduce our existence to basic survival and remove our ability to exercise free will and to control our destinies. People who are directly affected by a disaster, and those who respond and bring aid, are affected. Their worlds are turned upside down.

Programmes that are designed to provide help for communities affected by disasters and to help people to recover from disasters and return to a way of life that is acceptable to them, and agencies that support aid workers, should address all of the six features. It is not enough to provide safe food, clean water, security and shelter, although this is a good start. Aid programmes must address the whole spectrum of physical and psychosocial need and Smith's six features of the human condition provide a good framework for planning, preparation and review.

References

Ahmeti, F. (2014). Microfinance as a tool for economic development in transitional countries: Experience from Kosovo. European Scientific Journal, **10**: 269–287.

Alexander, D. A. & Klein, S. (2009). First responders after disasters: A review of stress reactions, at-risk, vulnerability, and resilience factors. Prehospital Disaster Medicine, **24**: 87–94.

Black, M. E. & Healing, T. D. (1993). Communicable diseases in former Yugoslavia and in refugees arriving in the United Kingdom. Communicable Disease Report, **3**: R87–90.

Brooks, S. K., Dunn, R., Sage, C. A. M. et al. (2015). Risk and resilience factors affecting the psychological wellbeing of individuals deployed in humanitarian relief roles after a disaster. Journal of Mental Health, **24**: 385–413; doi: 10.3109/09638237.2015.1057334.

Brymer, M., Jacobs, A., Layne, C. et al. (2006). Psychological First Aid: Field Operations Guide, 2nd edition. Durham, NC: National Child Traumatic Stress Network and National Center for PTSD.

Cardozo, B. L., Crawford, C. G., Eriksson, C. et al. (2012). Psychological distress, depression, anxiety, and burnout among International humanitarian aid workers: A longitudinal study. PLoS One, September 12; doi.org/10.1371/journal.pone.0044948.

Centers for Disease Control and Prevention (2012). Emergencies and the elderly: Taking care of older adults during a disaster. See https://blogs.cdc.gov/publichealthmatters/2012/09/emergencies-and-the-elderly/.

Central Intelligence Agency (2016). World factbook. See www.cia.gov/library/publications/download/download-2016/index.html

CRED (2015). The Human Cost of Natural Disasters. 2015. A Global Perspective. Louvain: Université Catholique de Louvain.

CRED–UNISDR. (2015). The Human Cost of Weather Related Disasters 1995–2015. Louvain: Université Catholique de Louvain.

Chriman, A. K. & Dougherty, J. G. (2014). Mass trauma: Disasters, terrorism, and war. Child and Adolescent Psychiatric Clinics of North America, **23**: 257–279.

Clark, D. V., Kibuuka, H., Miljard, M. et al. (2015). Long-term sequelae after Ebola virus disease in Bundibugyo, Uganda: A retrospective cohort study. The Lancet Infectious Diseases, **15**: 905–912.

Degomme, O. & Guha-Sapir, D. (2010). Patterns of mortality rates in Darfur conflict. The Lancet, **375**: 294–300.

Evans, D. K. & Popova, A. (2015). Orphans and Ebola. Estimating the Secondary Impact of a Public Health Crisis. Washington, DC: World Bank Group, Africa Region, Office of the Chief Economist.

Forbes, D., Creamer, M. & Wade, D. (2012). Psychological support and recovery in the aftermath of natural disasters. International Psychiatry, **9**: 15–17.

Ghobarah, H. A., Huth, P. & Russett, B. (2004). The post-war public health effects of civil conflict. Social Science and Medicine, **59**: 869–884.

Grünewald, F., Boyer, B., Maury, H. & Pascal, P. (2007). Indian Ocean Tsunami 2004: 10 Lessons

Learnt from the Humanitarian Response Funded by the French State. Paris: Ministère des Affaires Etrangères et Européennes. See http://www.diplomatie.gouv.fr/IMG/pdf/430_Int_Tsunami-2.pdf.

Healing, T. D., Drysdale, S. F., Black, M. E. et al. (1996). Monitoring health in the war affected areas of the former Yugoslavia 1992–1993. European Journal of Public Health, **6**: 245–251.

Helleringer, S. & Noymer, A. (2015). Magnitude of Ebola relative to other causes of death in Liberia, Sierra Leone, and Guinea. The Lancet Global Health, **3**: e255–256.

Hobfoll, S. E., Watson, P., Bell, C. C. et al. (2007). Five essential elements of immediate and mid-term mass trauma intervention: Empirical evidence. Psychiatry, **70**: 283–315.

Laframboise, N. & Loko, B. (2012). IMF Working Paper. Natural Disasters: Mitigating Impact, Managing Risks. Washington, DC: International Monetary Fund, External Relations Department & Western Hemisphere Department.

Lock, S., Rubin, G. J., Murray, V. et al. (2012). Secondary stressors and extreme events and disasters: A systematic review of primary research from 2010–2011. PLoS Currents Disasters, 29 October; doi: 10.1371/currents.dis.a9b76fed1b2dd5c5bfcfc13c87a2f24.

McFarlane, C. A. (2004). Risks associated with the psychological adjustment of humanitarian aid workers. Australasian Journal of Disaster and Trauma Studies, 2004-1.

Morganstein, J. C., Benedek, D. M. & Ursano, R. J. (2016). Post-traumatic stress in disaster first responders. Disaster Medicine and Public Health Preparedness, **10**: 1–2; doi: 10.1017/dmp.2016.10.

Noji, E. K, editor (1997). The Public Health Consequences of Disasters. Oxford: Oxford University Press.

Noji, E. K., Kelen, G. D., Armenian, H. K. et al. (1990). The 1988 earthquake in Soviet Armenia: A case study. Annals of Emergency Medicine, **19**: 891–897.

Pan American Health Organisation. (2017). Care of Mentally or Physically Challenged Persons and the Elderly. Geneva: World Health Organization.

Parpia, A. S., Ndeffo-Mbah, M. L., Wenzel, N. S. et al. (2016). Effects of response to 2014–2015 Ebola outbreak on deaths from malaria, HIV/AIDS and tuberculosis, West Africa. Emerging Infectious Diseases, **22**: 433–441; doi: 10.3201/eid2203.150977.

Pedersen, D. (2002). Political violence, ethnic conflict, and contemporary wars: Broad implications for health and wellbeing. Social Science and Medicine, **55**: 175–190.

Puvacic, Z. & Weinberg, J. (1994). Impact of war on infectious disease in Bosnia-Hercegovina. British Medical Journal, **309**: 1207–1208.

Redmond, A. D., Mardel, S., Taithe, B. et al. (2011). Qualitative and quantitative study of the surgical and rehabilitation response to the earthquake in Haiti, January 2010. Prehospital and Disaster Medicine, **26**: 1–8.

Redmond, A. D., Tubb, P., Alcock, R. et al. (2016). The UK-Med Response to Ebola in Sierra Leone. Manchester: Manchester University.

Roy, N. (2006). The Asian tsunami: PAHO disaster guidelines in action in India. Prehospital and Disaster Medicine, **21**: 310–315.

Solnit, R. (2010). A Paradise Built in Hell. New York, NY: Penguin Books.

Sterud, T., Ekeberg, Ø. & Hem, E. (2006). Health status in the ambulance services: A systematic review. BMC Health Services Research, **6**: 82–92.

Stoddard, A., Harmer, A. & Czwarno, M. (2017). Aid worker security report. Behind the attacks: A look at the perpetrators of violence against aid workers. See https://aidworkersecurity.org/sites/default/files/AWSR2017.pdf.

Tempest, E. L, English National Study on Flooding and Health Study Group, Carter, B., Beck, C. R. & Rubin, G. J. (2017). Secondary stressors are associated with probable psychological morbidity after flooding: A cross-sectional analysis. European Journal of Public Health, **27**: 1042–1047; https://doi.org/10.1093/eurpub/ckx1822017.

UNISDR (2015a). Annual report 2015. See https://reliefweb.int/sites/reliefweb.int/files/resources/48588_unisdrannualreport2015evs.pdf.

UNISDR (2015b). Sendai framework for disaster risk reduction 2015–2020. See www.unisdr.org/files/43291_sendaiframeworkfordrren.pdf.

UNISDR (2016). Open-ended Intergovernmental expert working group on indicators and terminology relating to disaster risk reduction. See www.unisdr.org/we/inform/publications/51748.

Van Bortel, T., Basnayake, A., Wurie, F., et al. (2016). Psychosocial effects of an Ebola outbreak at individual, community and international levels. Bulletin of the World Health Organization, **94**: 210–214.

Vetter, P., Kaiser, L., Schibler, M., Ciglenecki, I. & Bausch, D. G. (2016). Sequelae of Ebola virus disease: The emergency within the emergency. The Lancet Review, **16**: e82–e91; https://doi.org/10.1016/S1473-3099(16)00077-3.

VSO and The Liverpool School of Tropical Medicine. (2015). Report. The Impact of Ebola on Maternal Health in Sierra Leone. Sierra Leone and Liverpool: Voluntary Service Overseas and The Liverpool School of Tropical Medicine.

Vulic, D., Secerov-Zecevic, D., Tasic, I. & Burgic-Radmanovic, M. (2012). War trauma factors and cardiovascular risk. Current Cardiovascular Risk Reports, **6**: 141–145.

Walker, P. G. T., White, M. T., Griffin, J. T. et al. (2015). Malaria morbidity and mortality in Ebola-affected countries caused by decreased health-care capacity, and the potential effect of mitigation strategies: A modelling analysis. The Lancet Infectious Diseases, **15**: 825–832.

Watson, J. T., Gayer, M. & Connolly, M. A. (2007). Epidemics after natural disasters. Emerging Infectious Diseases, **13**: 1–5; doi: 10.3201/eid1301.060779.

WHO (2013). Classification and minimum standards for foreign medical teams in sudden onset disasters. See www.who.int/hac/global_health_cluster/fmt_guidelines_september2013.pdf.

WHO (2016). Ebola situation report – 16 March 2016. See http://apps.who.int/ebola/current-situation/ebola-situation-report-16-march-2016.

Williams, R. & Greenberg, N. (2014). Psychosocial and mental health care for the deployed staff of rescue, professional first response and aid agencies, NGOs and military organisations. In Ryan, J., Hopperus Buma, A., Beadling, C., Mozumder, A. & Nott, D. M., editors. Conflict and Catastrophe Medicine. New York, NY: Springer, pp. 395–432.

Williams, R. & Kemp, V. (2016). Psychosocial and mental health before, during and after emergencies, disasters and major incidents. In Sellwood, C. & Wapling, A., editors. Health Emergency Preparedness and Response. Wallingford: CABI, pp. 83–98.

Williams, R. & Kemp, V. (2018). Principles for designing and delivering psychosocial and mental healthcare. Journal of the Royal Army Medical Corps; doi: 10.1136/jramc-2017-000880.

Williams, R., Bisson, J. & Kemp, V. (2014a). OP 94. Principles for Responding to the Psychosocial and Mental Health Needs of People Affected by Disasters or Major Incidents. London: The Royal College of Psychiatrists.

Williams, R., Kemp, V. J & Alexander, D. A. (2014b). The psychosocial and mental health of people who are affected by conflict, catastrophes, terrorism, adversity and displacement. In Ryan, J., Hopperus Buma, A., Beadling, C., Mozumder, A. & Nott, D. M., editors. Conflict and Catastrophe Medicine. New York, NY: Springer, pp. 805–849.

World Bank Group (2015). Update on the Economic Impact of the 2014–2015 Ebola Epidemic on Liberia, Sierra Leone and Guinea. Washington, DC: World Bank Group.

Young, K. (2001). UNHCR and ICRC in the former Yugoslavia: Bosnia Hercegovina. International Review of the Red Cross, **83**: 781–806.

Chapter **17**

Shared Social Identity in Emergencies, Disasters and Conflicts

John Drury and Khalifah Alfadhli

Introduction

This chapter builds on previous chapters, on crowds (Chapter 15) and emergencies and disasters (Chapter 16), to show the relationship between the two. It describes a programme of research that has examined the extent to which shared social identity determines collective behaviour in emergencies and disasters.

We recognise that engagement and action by the public is necessary when communities and agencies in them plan for emergencies. The increased threat of major incidents, disasters and terrorist attacks means that professional responders will not always be in place in time or in sufficient number to help (Cole et al., 2011; see Chapter 16).

The social identity approach is relevant here because it explains the conditions under which crowds and groups of people can operate as psychological communities that support their members in times of danger and stress. This chapter also describes how social identity principles have been applied to understanding informal psychosocial support among some refugees of war.

We recognise that shared social identity is not the only psychological process operating in disasters and, while existing interpersonal bonds between family members can explain much of the pattern of social support observed in these events, the concept of social identity is required to make sense of the strong evidence for strangers providing each other with support.

'Mass Panic'?

Part of the context of the programme of research described here was the pervasiveness of 'mass panic' as an explanation for behaviour in emergencies. 'Mass panic' can be considered as a pattern of related ideas about how crowds respond in major incidents and emergencies. It can be found in popular discourse, early academic research and some of the guidance on emergency response. As a concept, the core feature of 'mass panic' is the notion of collective overreaction – that is, that behaviour in an emergency will be unreasonable in response to threat because of the psychology of the crowd. We briefly trace the development of research in the scientific literature that has employed the concept of 'mass panic' and explain why a different kind of approach – indeed a different *discourse* – is needed to understand the psychology of mass emergency behaviour.

Some of the first research on the behaviour of crowds in response to threat was from military sources. The research arose as a response to the practical problem of troops losing discipline and scattering when coming under fire (Bendersky, 2007). This work suggested that extreme threat caused existing social bonds between people to dissolve, leading to individualistic and disorganised behavioural responses. Further, 'irrational' beliefs and behaviours were said to spread easily through a crowd by a process of 'contagion'.

The field developed through studies of fires in civilian settings such as nightclubs. The received wisdom became that, in emergencies, the 'panicking' crowd causes many more fatalities than the fire or other threat that the crowd was seeking to escape from through, for example, people jamming doors, trampling each other or otherwise abandoning the normal rules of social conduct. Particular tragic cases were cited repeatedly as paradigmatic examples of how crowd panic can turn an emergency into a disaster. One such case is the Cocoanut Grove nightclub fire of 1942, in Boston, Massachusetts, in which 492 people died.

A closer look at this case, however, suggests a rather different story than 'crowd panic' as the cause of the deaths (Chertkoff & Kushigian, 1999). The venue suffered from a lack of emergency exits. There were no exit signs. The main door jammed as people tried to escape. The windows were nailed shut to prevent patrons from sneaking out without paying for their tab. The bar-staff tried to lead people to safety but were unable, not unwilling, to do so. Indeed, while there was some trampling and pushing, there was no evidence that people in the crowd caused most of the deaths. Despite the blame-attributing function of 'panic' in this case, it was the managers who were successfully prosecuted for manslaughter and neglect of the laws regulating buildings.

From the 1950s onwards, there were an increasing number of research reports in which the authors stated that there was little evidence of crowd panic. Cases included the atomic bombing of Japan at the end of World War II (Janis, 1951), and, in more recent times, the King's Cross underground fire of 1987 (Donald & Canter, 1992) and the evacuation of the World Trade Center in 2001 (Connell, 2001). A similar conclusion was drawn in reviews of the collated evidence (Fritz & Williams, 1957). As well as these empirical problems, conceptual problems were raised. Quarantelli (1960) questioned how, from outside an emergency, it could be judged that a behaviour is an overreaction. What are the criteria for judging that behaviour in an emergency is reasonable or unreasonable? In an emergency, information is limited and the most reasonable way to behave often is not clear. Others have argued similarly that whether or not behaviour is rational in an emergency is not a useful question and instead the focus should be on the predictors of specific behaviours, such as pushing or trampling (Chertkoff & Kushigian, 1999).

When we shift the focus away from the question of rationality to that of behaviours, we find that social support and social coordination are more common in emergencies and disasters than pushing and trampling (Fritz & Williams, 1957), which only occur rarely in certain constrained physical circumstances (Chertkoff & Kushigian, 1999). Helping among those caught up in an emergency has been found to take place even in the most difficult circumstances; people often try to maintain order even as they struggle to survive. For example, an investigation into the fatal crush at one of The Who's concerts in the USA, in 1979, found that many fans helped each other if they were able, and those who could not physically do so nevertheless expressed the desire to help (Johnson, 1987).

Given this kind of evidence, the research question in our own programme of research changed from, 'Why do people panic?' to 'What explains social support in emergencies and disasters?'

Norms, Roles and Existing Relationships

Explanations for the prevalence of social support in emergencies have focused on roles, rules and relationships. Thus, sociologists have stressed the importance of the concept of *social norm*. For example, in his study of the Beverley Hills supper club fire in 1977, Johnson (1988) noted that, as people tried to evacuate, they helped others up when they fell; and elderly people were given more help than others, reflecting a general societal norm to help the people who are perceived as being most at risk. Rather than 'unregulated competition' in emergencies, there is a continuity with everyday life through conformity to the same norms that structure behaviour normally, Johnson argued. Moreover, people do not simply conform individually; they also collectively regulate the behaviour of others in their group through reference to norms, as was observed, for example, during the World Trade Center evacuation when people admonished the few who pushed in front instead of waiting their turn (Connell, 2001).

A second explanation for social support in emergencies is that of existing interpersonal bonds among people in the crowd. Thus Mawson (2007), drawing upon Bowlby's attachment theory (Bowlby, 2012), suggests that people have a need to be close to the familiar in threatening situations, and that being close to existing affiliates has a calming effect. Support for this idea comes from Jonathan Sime's study of the fire at the Summerland leisure complex, on the Isle of Man, in 1973 (Sime, 1983). This study found that very often people tried to stay together in family groups, and that these groups were often delayed in their escape by the slowest member, such as a child or elderly person. Thus, turning around the idea in the notion of 'panic' that people die in emergencies because of others' selfishness, Mawson's argument and Sime's study suggest, instead, that people die out of love: they prefer to be together, and even die together sometimes, rather than escape alone.

There is considerable evidence for the role of existing interpersonal relationships between family members and friends in producing social support in emergencies and disasters. But, in emergencies and disasters, people find themselves among strangers as well as familiar people (Clarke, 2002). If existing social bonds between individuals was the only factor determining social support among survivors in an emergency, then we should expect that the greater the number of strangers, the less social support there is. Yet in reviews of the evidence, and across a range of different emergencies, social support among strangers has been observed frequently (Chertkoff & Kushigian, 1999; Fritz & Williams, 1957; Sime, 1983). In relation to the evacuation of the World Trade Center, Connell (2001) states that 'helping (including carrying others' jackets or briefcases, offering others bottles of water) was most common . . . between strangers' (p. 13). What is particularly interesting about social support among strangers in emergencies is, first, that it can carry a personal cost or risk from the point of view of the 'rational maximiser': it may be safer to leave others to their fate and simply try to escape oneself. Second, help in emergencies is sometimes more frequent than in everyday life. The phenomenon is, therefore, on the surface, a psychological puzzle. The concept of social identity was applied to mass emergency behaviour to resolve this apparent puzzle.

A Social Identity Analysis of Crowd Behaviour in Novel and Unstructured Situations

In order to understand how social support becomes a collective phenomenon in a crowd of strangers, we drew on theory developed through the study of behaviour in riots (Reicher, 1984). Like the crowd in an emergency, in many riots, the crowd involved is in a novel and unstructured situation. Crowds in riots and most crowds in emergencies both display social coherence in their behaviour. Their behaviour is spontaneous and yet also patterned and limited by shared definitions of appropriate conduct (i.e. norms).

Research on riots showed that people were able to act as one, that is, they became a *psychological* crowd rather than simply a physical one, through a shift in salience from their disparate personal identities to a single shared social identity. In Reicher's study of the St Pauls' riot in 1980 (Reicher, 1984), the shared social identity was that of St Pauls' residents. This shared understanding of 'who we are' among participants meant that the crowd selected common targets, and that, even though emotions ran high and the event was characterised by both violence to people, mostly the police, and damage to property, there were clear limits to that behaviour. Certain people and property – other residents, local shops, homes – were not touched and, indeed, were actively protected, suggesting coordination and collective self-regulation.

Social Identity Processes in a Simulated Emergency

In a first set of studies to examine the extent to which social identity determined the behaviour of crowds involved in an emergency, we designed a laboratory experimental paradigm. This used a visualisation, or virtual reality animation, of a fire in an underground railway station, to enhance engagement in a role-play (Drury et al., 2009c). The task for each participant was to manoeuvre an avatar to safety through the crowd, with the option to push others aside, as well as four opportunities to stop and help fallen people. We manipulated salience of social identification by presenting this scenario in differing ways. In a version intended to make a personal identity salient in a physical crowd, subjects were told that they were part of a crowd of shoppers; and in a version intended to make a shared social identity salient, subjects were told they were part of a crowd of fellow football fans on their way back from a match. In line with predictions, shared social identity predicted more helping and less pushing than did personal identity across a number of studies.

Through their ability to isolate variables, experimental studies like these can indicate that social identity processes might be operating in emergencies. But ecological validity is obviously low given that participants did not genuinely feel in danger even if they did not know that their avatar would survive. Moreover, it was not simply the danger of death that was missing from this experimental paradigm. Many of the people who are affected by disasters report a change in how they perceive or feel about their relationships with others in the affected group. Thus, they often describe a new feeling of 'we-ness' with fellow survivors (Connell, 2001), and a sudden 'closeness' or 'togetherness' with other people caught up in the disaster (Johnson, 1988). Therefore, shared social identity among survivors may be created by the disaster itself, either transcending whatever group identities are salient, or bringing otherwise disconnected people together. Therefore, we hypothesised that a disaster can create a sense of *common fate*, which functions as a form of comparative fit (Drury et al., 2009a) in the terms of *self-categorization theory* (Turner et al., 1987). The sense of common fate can enhance perceptions of within-group similarity and the clarity of group boundaries (Turner, 1981, p. 91), thus augmenting identification with other survivors as a category.

The July 7 London Bombings: Social Support in a Crowd of Strangers

In a second study, we examined accounts of social support, psychological unity and common fate among survivors of the London bombings on 7 July 2005 (Drury et al., 2009b). The bombings took place on three underground trains and one bus and killed 56 people, including the four bombers, and caused injuries, many of them serious, to over 700 other people. Those who were in the underground trains were left literally in the dark for some time before the emergency services reached them. We interviewed 19 of the survivors and gathered accounts in the form of secondary data from media interviews and from witness statements in the Report of the London Assembly 7 July Review Committee from 90 others.

First, then, we examined their accounts of behaviour, both their own and the behaviour they observed in others, in the period immediately after the explosions. The helping behaviours reported included giving reassurance, sharing bottles of water, physically supporting others and tying tourniquets. We found that survivors reported carrying out and observing many more instances of helpful behaviour towards fellow survivors than personally selfish behaviours. Of our 19 interviewees, 13 reported helping someone else at least once. Those people who did not report helping said that they were not themselves in a position to help: two were not near any survivors, one was in plaster and the other attributed his behaviour to shock. Seven said they were helped by other people; the eighth did not give enough information. All of our interviewees (except two who did not give enough information) reported witnessing people helping others, and, in most cases, this helping was described as widespread, despite difficult conditions that included darkness, injury and pain.

Some of the supportive behaviour took the form of simple courtesy, such as allowing others to go first, but it seemed to be very important to the people who experienced it. The importance of courtesy was also practical, however, for queuing and comporting themselves in an orderly manner can mean the difference between life and death for survivors attempting to evacuate a difficult or narrow exit route.

We then examined two factors that could plausibly account for the high levels of help displayed. First, we looked at whether or not people felt in danger. It is possible that the reason that help was so common was because it was not perceived to carry a personal risk or cost. Perhaps people did not feel in danger. Importantly, however, most of the people in our study who mentioned it said they were in fear of death: they feared a second explosion, the tunnel collapsing, being hit by another train or being electrocuted on a live rail. Second, we looked at whether people were with family members or friends. It is possible that levels of help were so high because people were helping people they knew. But most people in our data set said that they were among strangers. The bombing took place during rush hour; most people were commuters on their way to work.

In the interviews, we asked people whether or not they 'felt any sort of bond or any sort of unity with others who were there'. In the pattern of responses, there was clear evidence that the perception of common danger or fate created a strong sense of unity. Indeed, among our interviews, the vocabulary of psychological togetherness was extremely rich and indicative of a powerful new relationship with the strangers around them: 'unity', 'together', 'similarity', 'affinity', 'part of a group', 'everybody, didn't matter what colour or nationality', 'you thought these people knew each other', 'warmness', 'vague solidity', 'empathy'. There was also evidence of a connection between this sense of shared identity and behaviour, in that most of the people who reported feeling unity also reported helping. Indeed, for some survivors, observations of others' helping also reinforced a sense of togetherness.

A Comparative Analysis

While the data from the London bombings case study were consistent with the social identity explanation for social support in a mass emergency, we also sought to carry out a study with a comparative design, so we could examine more systematically the process we hypothesised. To this end, we interviewed 21 survivors of 11 different emergencies, including the Hillsborough disaster of 1989, two sinking ships, a hotel fire and two office block evacuations (Drury et al., 2009a).

Again, we asked people about the behaviours they engaged in and witnessed and whether or not they felt a sense of unity with those around them. An independent judge divided responses into those in which people's replies showed that they had a sense of psychological unity with other people in the crowd affected, and those people who reported little sense of unity, or whose responses were unclear. We found that the people who reported feeling unity were slightly more likely than the others to report a sense of common fate, whereas those who reported no common fate tended to report little unity with the rest of the crowd. Reports of helping, whether having engaged in it, experienced it or witnessed it, were high for almost all interviewees. But, importantly, reports of own helping were higher for those people who reported shared social identification.

A Social Identity Model of Collective Resilience

The evidence from the studies we have described, together with the basic principles of crowd psychology described in Chapter 15, are the basis of a social identity model of collective resilience as introduced in Chapter 11. The term 'collective resilience' here refers to a group *process*, not to a state, disposition or outcome. We have defined it as 'the way a shared social identification allows people in a crowd to express solidarity and cohesion, and thereby to coordinate and draw upon collective sources of support and other practical resources, to deal with adversity' (Drury et al., 2009a, p. 502). Emergencies and disasters create common needs in a crowd of survivors, such as getting to safety, preventing further injury or trauma, reducing distress, but they also affect different social groups differentially (see Chapter 16). Here, we explain how social identity processes are a resource for the crowd affected as a whole.

As explained in Chapter 15, moving from 'me' to 'we' entails a shift to socially shared values and goals, and the consequent *relational* transformation includes the understanding that the people around us have these same values and goals: we are 'the same' so we see the world in the same way. Shared goals in a crowd can be essential in an emergency. If there are competing definitions of the situation and of how to respond, the result can be disorganised and self-defeating. For example, there was a choice between the shared goal of removing a carriage door together versus efforts to escape independently (and perhaps less effectively), for some survivors of the London bombings (Drury et al., 2009b).

The relational transformation also entails trusting others around us to act appropriately, that is, in the group's interests, in response to the emergency. It means expecting them to give emotional support and practical help where needed, and to cooperate with each other as they attempt to evacuate and combat the threat or protect themselves in other ways. It also means that people have the *motivation* to provide social support for others in the group, as described in Chapter 15: people care about the fate of others because they are now 'us'.

Where there is sufficient coordination, cooperation and support, the crowd provides its members with greater collective efficacy and feelings of safety and less anxiety, compared to a crowd in which shared identification is low and people are divided. The sense of agency provided by psychological membership of a crowd means that crowd members are more able to act together to reach safety and to organise the prevention of further trauma. In the evacuation of Tower 1 of the World Trade Center on 11 September 2001, it was essential for the crowd to move as one down the packed staircase, coordinating their behaviour, moving at the same pace in order for everyone to get safely out of the building before it collapsed. When some people did disrupt the flow by acting as individuals by, for example, pushing in or using their phones, others in the crowd had the confidence to pull them back into line (Connell, 2001).

In summary, the social identity model describes a process whereby a common fate creates a group in which people identify with each other. This identification creates the motivations and expectations that make social support, cooperation and coordination possible in response to the emergency. The nature and role of social support needs a little more unpacking, however.

Different Forms of and Pathways to Social Support

In the interview studies we have described (Drury et al., 2009a, b) the social support people referred to took different forms, including giving practical help, emotional support (e.g. reassurances) and coordination or cooperation among survivors. Whereas practical help entails someone who is able-bodied helping someone less able, coordination or cooperation involves two equals acting together in some way for their or the collective good. Examples of the latter include allowing the other to go first, holding doors open, making space for others or participating in activity in which two or more people are required, such as removing a heavy door together or joining a search party. In many emergencies, most survivors are able-bodied and need to cooperate to get to safety, rather than requiring 'help' as such. The evacuation of Tower 1 of the World Trade Center is an example. Since cooperation is a form of joint action, the process is slightly different than for helping. Helping might be predicted from shared social identification: we help others because our shared identification means that we see their interests and suffering as our own. In the case of cooperation, however, what is required on top of this sense of identification and consequent motivation is the *expectation* that others will also be acting and that they will be supportive or cooperative. Emotional support conveys the sense of being cared for, which is known to contribute to recovery (Shultz, 2014); small acts, including acts of practical support, can convey caring and contribute to recovery in this way.

We were able to test some of these ideas about social support with a large representative sample in a study carried out with colleagues from Pontificia Universidad Católica de Chile (Drury et al., 2016). In February 2010, a large earthquake took place off the coast of Chile, around 360 km south-west of Santiago. It resulted in a tsunami, which hit the coast 35 minutes after the earthquake and caused flash floods. The earthquake itself led to over 500 fatalities, while over 100 more were due to the tsunami, with many more people being seriously injured. Around 500,000 buildings were severely damaged, and 9 per cent of the population in the affected areas lost their homes. With the emergency services overwhelmed, solidarity among the people affected by these events was essential for survival and recovery.

We designed a questionnaire, which was distributed to 1,240 adults in the affected regions. As we hypothesised, survivors' reported sense of common fate (e.g., 'We all shared the same fate') predicted social identification with other people affected by the disaster. Social identification predicted both emotional support being given (e.g., 'Giving emotional support') and expectations of social support (e.g., 'I came to expect other people to be cooperative'). As expected, there was a significant mediation such that social identification predicted coordinated social support (e.g., 'I participated in groups that organised to find help/survivors/supplies, etc.') through increased expectations of social support. In addition, survivors' perceptions that others were acting supportively increased the likelihood that they too gave social support. Importantly, this effect of observing social support on one's own social support was significantly greater for people who were high in emergent social identification.

Extending the Model of Collective Resilience: The Social Identity Basis of Psychosocial Support among Refugees of Conflict in a Developing Country

The situation faced by refugees of war and conflict resembles that of people affected by a disaster, in a number of ways. First, both disasters and war cause death, injury and loss of homes and possessions to large numbers of people at once. Second, both types of event can mean that survivors face many months, if not years, of trying to cope with *secondary stressors* (Lock et al., 2012) – that is, stressors not directly due to the disaster or war itself but operating through the societal response, or lack of societal response, to the events. We have previously shown the nature and operation of secondary stressors in flooding, and how shared social identities can mitigate some of their effects (Ntontis et al., 2017). In recent research, we sought to apply the same concepts to examine how refugees drew upon social resources (shared social identities), to deal with some of the stressors that are consequent upon their displacement in a developing country.

The research comprised an ethnography, based in the Jordanian city of Irbid, close to the Syrian border, followed by a series of questionnaire surveys of Syrian refugees in Turkey and Jordan. A thematic analysis of interviews and a factor analysis of a survey (Alfadhli & Drury, 2018a) suggested that secondary stressors took three forms for Syrian refugees: financial stressors (which were found to be the most important); stressors to do with the environment (stressors that are circumstantial either in the structure of the exile environment, such as services and legal requirements, or feelings such as lack of familiarity in this environment); and stressors arising from social relations (including discrimination by people in the host country). The ethnographic study (Alfadhli & Drury, 2018b) enabled us to identify the processes through which the refugees sought to cope with these stressors. We found many examples of support among refugees, on both personal and collective levels. Examples included teaching after-school classes to Syrian children, running extra-curriculum activities and organising aid caravans to the refugee tents on the outskirts of the city. While some of the examples of support were based on existing networks or interpersonal relations, others were based on a new network of social relations that were formed in exile. This new network was characterised by the identity of 'refugee', which stemmed from a sense of common fate, despite the stigma attached to the refugee identity.

In our questionnaire surveys (Alfadhli & Drury, 2017), we found a pattern of results that was very similar to the findings from the Chile earthquake (Drury et al., 2016). In the survey carried out among Syrian refugees in Turkey ($n = 222$), shared social identity with other refugees predicted participation in coordinated support; shared social identity also predicted expected support, which in turn predicted collective efficacy. Our survey of Syrian refugees in Jordan (n = 156) tested a more complex model, examining the extent to which both secondary stressors and social identity processes impacted on refugees' wellbeing. The analysis suggested, first, that secondary stressors increased stress, which in turn reduced wellbeing. Second, we showed the buffering effect of shared social identity. As in the previous studies, common fate predicted shared social identity with other refugees, which in turn predicted expected support and coordinated support. Expected support increased collective efficacy and this latter effect contributed positively to wellbeing.

The current situation of refugees of conflict in developing countries, where the United Nations High Commissioner for Refugees (UNHCR) Syrian crisis response plan funds only half of the budget required (UNHCR, 2016), should make us consider all available resources to help refugees. One source is the refugees' own informal social support capacities, a notion suggested by the concept of collective resilience, as described earlier in this chapter and in Chapter 11. The present research, which indicates that group-based psychosocial support operates among refugees in similar ways to that in crowds in disasters, therefore suggests a role for shared social identities. Refugees depend on external help, but they can make better use of the resources they have if they identify and act as social groups. These findings are in line with the literature on secondary stressors in disasters (Lock et al., 2012), showing the significant impact these stressors have on wellbeing (see Chapter 11). In addition to lowering the exposure to secondary stressors, these findings provide policymakers and practitioners with additional means to counter the adverse effects of secondary stressors on the wellbeing of refugees in developing countries.

Conclusions

This chapter argues that we need the concept of social identity to explain the pattern of social support that is commonly found among strangers who are involved in emergencies and disasters. Not all crowds in emergencies are characterised by social support and order, but, if the response is disorganised and chaotic, there are better explanations than 'mass panic'. Some crowds are divided, and some crowds are physical crowds, not psychological crowds. Problems can occur when large numbers of people are co-located in space but too many of them act as individual persons (see Chapter 15). The evidence in this chapter indicates some of the conditions required for shared social identity (versus personal identity salience) and coordination (versus individualism) to occur, even in difficult events such as emergencies and disasters. It shows that similar patterns can also occur among refugees of conflict in developing countries. These conditions include a sense of common fate among survivors.

Acknowledgements

The research described in this chapter was collaborative and involved the following colleagues: Rupert Brown (University of Sussex); Chris Cocking (University of Brighton); Roberto González (Pontificia Universidad Católica de Chile); Daniel Miranda (Pontificia Universidad Católica de Chile); and Steve Reicher (University of St Andrews). We acknowledge financial support from the following funders: Pontificia Universidad Católica de Chile and the Interdisciplinary Center for Social Conflict and Cohesion Studies (Ref. CONICYT/FONDAP/15130009); the Economic and Social Research Council (Ref. RES-000–23-0446); and a scholarship from King Saud University, Saudi Arabia, to the second author.

References

Alfadhli, K. & Drury, J. (2017). Psychosocial support among Syrian refugees in Jordan: An ethnographic exploration of the role of shared identity. Paper presented at 18th General Meeting of the EASP, Granada, Spain, July.

Alfadhli, K. & Drury, J. (2018a). A typology of secondary stressors among refugees of conflict in the Middle East: The case of Syrian refugees in Jordan. PLoS Currents Disasters, 10 May; doi: 10.1371/currents.dis.4bd3e6437bff47b33ddb9f73cb72f3d8.

Alfadhli, K. & Drury, J. (2018b). The role of shared social identity in mutual support among refugees of conflict: An ethnographic study of Syrian refugees in Jordan. Journal of Community and Applied Social Psychology, **28**; doi: 10.1002/casp.2346.

Bendersky, J. (2007). 'Panic': The impact of Le Bon's crowd psychology on US military thought. Journal of the History of the Behavioral Sciences, **43**: 257–283.

Bowlby, J. (2012). The Making and Breaking of Affectional Bonds. London: Routledge.

Chertkoff, J. M. & Kushigian, R. H. (1999). Don't Panic: The Psychology of Emergency Egress and Ingress. Westport, CT: Praeger.

Clarke, L. (2002). Panic: Myth or reality? Contexts **1**: 21–26.

Cole, J., Walters, M. & Lynch, M. (2011). Part of the solution, not the problem: The crowd's role in emergency response. Contemporary Social Science, **6**: 361–375.

Connell, R. (2001). Collective Behavior in the September 11, 2001 Evacuation of the World Trade Center. University of Delaware, Disaster Research Center. Preliminary paper #313.

Donald, I. & Canter, D. (1992). Intentionality and fatality during the King's Cross underground fire. European Journal of Social Psychology, **22**: 203–218.

Drury, J., Brown, R., González, R. & Miranda, D. (2016). Emergent social identity and observing social support predict social support provided by survivors in a disaster: Solidarity in the 2010 Chile earthquake. European Journal of Social Psychology, **46**: 209–223.

Drury, J., Cocking, C. & Reicher, S. (2009a). Everyone for themselves? A comparative study of crowd solidarity among emergency survivors. British Journal of Social Psychology, **48**: 487–506.

Drury, J., Cocking, C. & Reicher, S. (2009b). The nature of collective resilience: Survivor reactions to the 2005 London bombings. International Journal of Mass Emergencies and Disasters, **27**: 66–95.

Drury, J., Cocking, C., Reicher, S. et al. (2009c). Cooperation versus competition in a mass emergency evacuation: A new laboratory simulation and a new theoretical model. Behavior Research Methods, **41**: 957–970.

Fritz, C. E. & Williams, H. B. (1957). The human being in disasters: A research perspective. Annals of the American Academy of Political and Social Science, **309**: 42–51.

Janis, I. (1951). Air War and Emotional Stress. New York, NY: McGraw-Hill.

Johnson, N. R. (1987). Panic at 'The Who concert stampede': An empirical assessment. Social Problems, **34**: 362–373.

Johnson, N. R. (1988). Fire in a crowded theatre: A descriptive investigation of the emergence of panic. International Journal of Mass Emergencies and Disasters, **6**: 7–26.

Lock, S., Rubin, G. J., Murray, V. et al. (2012). Secondary stressors and extreme events and disasters: A systematic review of primary research from 2010–2011. PLoS Currents Disasters, 29 October; doi: 10.1371/currents.dis.a9b76fed1b2dd5c5bfcfc13c87a2f24.

Mawson, A. (2007). Mass Panic and Social Attachment: The Dynamics of Human Behaviour. Aldershot: Ashgate.

Ntontis, E., Drury, J., Amlôt, R., Rubin, G. J & Williams, R. (2017). Emergent social identities in a flood: Implications for community psychosocial resilience. Journal of Community and Applied Social Psychology, 26 July: 1–12; https://doi.org/10.1002/casp.2329.

Quarantelli, E. L. (1960). Images of withdrawal behaviour in disasters: Some basic misconceptions. Social Problems, **8**: 68–79.

Reicher, S. D. (1984). The St. Pauls' riot: An explanation of the limits of crowd action in terms of a social identity model. European Journal of Social Psychology, **14**: 1–21.

Shultz, J. M. (2014). Perspectives on disaster public health and disaster behavioral health integration. Disaster Health, 2: 69–74.

Sime, J. D. (1983). Affiliative behavior during escape to building exits. Journal of Environmental Psychology, 3: 21–41.

Turner, J. C. (1981). The experimental social psychology of intergroup behaviour. In Turner, J. C. & Giles, H., editors, Intergroup Behaviour. Oxford: Blackwell, pp. 66–101.

Turner, J. C., Hogg, M. A., Oakes, P. J., Reicher, S. D. & Wetherell, M. C. (1987). Rediscovering the Social Group: A Self-Categorization Theory. Oxford: Blackwell.

UNHCR (2016). UNHCR Syria regional refugee response 2016. See https://data2.unhcr.org/en/situations/syria.

Chapter 18

Complex Trauma and Complex Responses to Trauma in the Asylum Context

Cornelius Katona and Francesca Brady

Introduction

Both the authors are clinicians who work at the Helen Bamber Foundation (HBF), a human rights charity that works with asylum seekers and refugees who have experienced extreme violations of their human rights.

Since she entered the Bergen Belsen concentration camp in May 1945, only a few weeks after its liberation, our Founder, Helen Bamber, worked continuously for nearly 70 years as a pioneer in the documentation of extreme human cruelty and in assessing the needs and providing comprehensive care for survivors of extreme cruelty. Helen's overwhelming sense of mission and of duty were closely linked to her early experiences at Bergen Belsen, which also provided a starting point for her notion of integrated care. She spoke of bearing witness, through the detailed documentation of the mental and physical evidence of the cruelty to which her clients had been subjected, which are cornerstones of the model of integrated care.

The HBF is committed to honouring and maintaining Helen Bamber's legacy by delivering and refining the model of integrated care for survivors of extreme human cruelty that she pioneered, and which we describe in this chapter.

The Main Client Groups We Work with at the Helen Bamber Foundation

Helen had founded the Medical Foundation for the Care of Victims of Torture, now known as Freedom from Torture, in 1985. One of the main reasons why, at the age of 80, she left it to set up a new organisation was her growing realisation that the lived experience of having extreme cruelty imposed upon a person, and the damage that resulted from that cruelty, was similar irrespective of whether or not the perpetrator was an agent of the state (a key element in the standard definition of 'torture'). Her new organisation, HBF, was and remains small in size but broad in remit in that it offers comprehensive assessment and integrated care to survivors of all forms of extreme human cruelty.

The main groups we work with are victims of torture, human trafficking, domestic violence, gender-based violence and violence related to sexual orientation.

The Main Commonalities Between Client Groups

What we have observed is that there are striking similarities across these groups from a clinical point of view, not only in the symptoms they describe but also in the problems they experience in coming to terms with what had happened to them; and in 'moving on' from their identity as dependent victims and re-integrating into society. Although many of the people we see have not experienced major trauma in childhood, their clinical presentation is often strikingly reminiscent of that of victims of prolonged childhood abuse.

As Helen Bamber realised, this is hardly surprising. Almost all of our clients have been subjected to repeated and multiple acts of cruelty, usually over a prolonged period. Almost invariably, they have had severe and repeated physical pain inflicted upon them. They have also experienced multiple losses. This may include loss of close family members, loss of their previous identity, roles and status, and loss of dignity and pride. They often see themselves as having been betrayed, and may also feel that they have betrayed others, by the very fact of having left, but, sometimes, also because of what they were forced to do in order to escape. In our clinical experience, sexual abuse and the sense of betrayal are particularly closely linked to a sense of shame and self-revulsion. Also, they are often associated with prominent dissociative behaviours. One of the key similarities is the continuing propensity of many of our clients to experience further exploitation or abuse. Like people who have been abused in childhood, they become more vulnerable to future cruelty, rather than learning from their past experiences to generate rational strategies to ensure their future safety.

We also often see people who take repeated and inappropriate risks. This may involve risky sexual behaviour that often also reflects their vulnerability to exploitation, repeated impulsive self-harm (often by cutting or head-banging), self-medication with alcohol or illicit drugs, and petty crime.

Victims of torture, trafficking and domestic violence have all too often experienced prolonged periods of being subjected to very close control. It is, therefore, unsurprising that they lose agency and develop persisting difficulties in making even relatively mundane choices.

Another feature we often see following both torture and other forms of extreme cruelty is profound loss of trust. This can lead not only to difficulty in forming relationships but also to problems in working with health and social care professionals and in day-to-day interactions with housemates, acquaintances or strangers.

Most clients present with numerous health problems. In respect of their mental health, we see people with a wide range of diagnoses, including anxiety, depression, substance misuse and psychoses, as well as comorbid personality disorders. In terms of physical health problems, many clients complain of chronic pain and headaches. The ubiquity of pain seems to apply whatever the forms of cruelty to which they have been subjected, though it must also be borne in mind that the physical ill-treatment they have suffered, or which they have subsequently inflicted on themselves, may be contributing directly as well as indirectly to the pain they currently experience. In addition to this, clients may present with other physical health problems that may result from the poor conditions in which they are living (e.g. damp or unhygienic accommodation) or which may become chronic due to a lack of access to healthcare and resultant lack of treatment.

Common Perpetuating Factors

The other key commonality uniting asylum-seeking survivors of human cruelty is the wide range of post-migration factors that they are likely to experience, which are likely to maintain or aggravate their mental health problems.

Perhaps, it is all too obvious that people who leave their country, seeking protection, anticipate that they will be welcomed and protected. Unfortunately, the reality is often very different. In our collective clinical experience at HBF, post-migration experiences often act to perpetuate the mental and physical health difficulties that people experience as well as aggravating their practical problems in rebuilding their lives.

Asylum-seeking victims of human cruelty have, by definition, been separated from their country. They have very often also been separated from their families and other support networks and may not know where their families are or what has happened to them. This is often a major source of additional anxiety and distress. As we have described, many of our clients at HBF have significant issues with trust as a result of their histories of ill-treatment. This is likely to hinder them in forming new relationships and support networks, and it leaves many of our clients feeling isolated and lonely.

Further to this are the practical challenges that come with being in a new country, such as understanding and accessing healthcare, housing and benefits. Asylum seekers may have great difficulty in understanding and navigating these systems in order to meet their basic welfare needs and access medical care and legal support. Most asylum seekers do not speak the language of their host country, making this process even more challenging. Others face racism or other forms of discrimination. It is widely acknowledged that a 'culture of disbelief' pervades the asylum and welfare systems in the UK, which leads to many clients experiencing what feels to them as repeated rejections or accusations of lying.

Many of our clients remain in immigration limbo for several years during which time they are unable to work. As access to accommodation and, extremely limited, financial assistance is dependent on the status of their asylum claim, it is common for asylum seekers to experience repeated or extended periods of homelessness and destitution (Masocha & Simpson, 2012). An additional preoccupation for many asylum seekers is the risk of their being detained in an immigration removal centre (IRC). The IRCs exist for administrative purposes to facilitate deportation or monitor people who are considered to be at risk of absconding. In reality, many people are detained who do not pose a flight risk, and whose asylum case is not at a point where imminent removal is likely or appropriate. Detention in IRCs is indefinite, i.e. individuals are given no indication of for how long they might be held or whether they will be released back to the community in the UK or removed from the UK.

There is robust clinical evidence that both immigration detention and prolonged immigration uncertainty have adverse mental health effects (Robjant et al 2009a, b). Furthermore, rates of non-affective psychosis as well as depression, anxiety and post-traumatic stress disorder (PTSD) are higher among detained asylum seekers than in other migrant groups.

Many asylum seekers had previously been in regular work in their country of origin. Finding themselves not permitted to work during the, often prolonged, period of waiting for a decision on their asylum claim can lead to further problems. A person's skills degrade and, in turn, this can engender feelings of hopelessness, helplessness and dependence on others, which only reinforces feelings of alienation and low self-esteem. Even if people are granted refugee status, it can often be a long journey to gaining the language skills and qualifications they need to work and support themselves independently, aside from any mental or physical health problems that may impact on their ability to work.

The Diagnostic Concept of Complex PTSD

Herman (1992) introduced the concept of 'complex PTSD' to describe response to chronic or repetitive trauma resulting in a loss of a sense of safety, trust in others and of self-worth. This diagnostic concept has recently been recognised in the 11th Edition of the International Classification of Diseases which came out in 2018 (ICD-11, 2018).

The International Society for Traumatic Stress Studies (Cloitre et al., 2012) further highlights additional problems that these people present, including emotional dysregulation, attention and consciousness problems, dissociative symptoms and marked impairments in their interpersonal functioning. Dissociative responses among survivors of sexual violence (particularly from childhood) have been widely reported. The UK Psychological Trauma Society (2017) provides a useful summary of the challenges relating to diagnosing and treating people who have complex PTSD.

The Key Components of the Model of Integrated Care

In view of the multiple, repeated and prolonged trauma our clients have experienced, their ongoing uncertainty about immigration and their associated difficulties in securing their basic needs and maintaining their skills, clients referred to the HBF almost invariably have multiple and complex care needs. In this context, it is noteworthy that the guidelines of the National Institute for Health and Care Excellence for PTSD (NICE, 2005, 2018) recommend that 'clinicians working with refugees should not only have knowledge of the complexity of the emotional reaction that many experience (going well beyond PTSD in many cases) but should also have an awareness of immigration law, welfare rights and cultural and political diversities'.

The first step in addressing the complexity and multiplicity of our clients' needs is to carry out a comprehensive initial needs assessment. Each client is assisted through discussion to identify their health, practical and social needs and is supported to think about how these needs might be prioritised or addressed, taking into account their own skills, strengths and future aspirations. This indicates HBF's potential roles while also establishing the client's autonomy and agreeing a realistic set of goals and expectations. In our experience, this is helpful in overcoming the trust issues that can otherwise impede therapeutic and practical progress. Subsequent multi-professional team discussion enables formulation and delivery of a care plan. Regular monitoring of outcomes and progress towards goals establishes any emerging issues that must also be addressed while also facilitating each client's movement towards community reintegration.

We are in the process of developing a monitoring and evaluation system that incorporates regular review of the needs and care plans for each client. In future, this is likely to enable us to monitor both clients' overall progress, in terms of key outcomes such as mental distress and social functioning, and their progress with respect to the specific goals of each component of the model of integrated care.

The key, and closely coordinated, elements of integrated care that HBF provides directly are summarised in Figure 18.1. Next, we describe each one in turn.

Legal Protection and Medico-Legal Reports

Legal protection of our clients is one of HBF's most important roles. While we do not provide legal representation for them, we recruit and train clinical experts to prepare independent medico-legal reports (MLRs) in accordance with the Manual on Effective Investigation and Documentation of Torture and Other Cruel, Inhuman or Degrading Treatment or Punishment, commonly known as the Istanbul Protocol. These reports document the physical and psychological sequelae of torture and other forms of cruel, inhumane or degrading treatment.

Late disclosure of trauma, and particularly sexual trauma, disorientation and memory impairment regarding key facts (e.g. specific dates and locations) as a result of the impact of

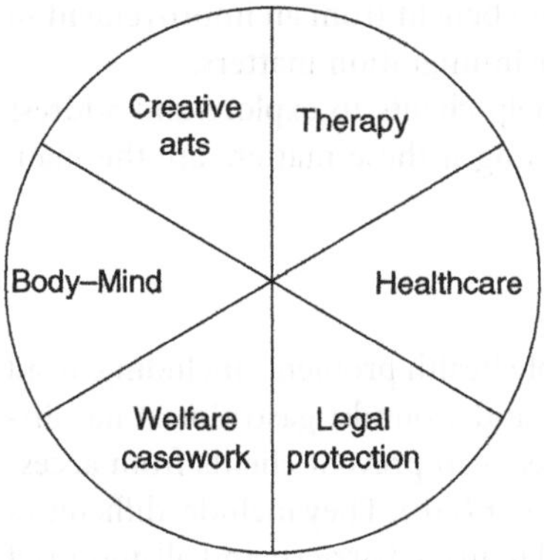

Figure 18.1 Key components of the model of integrated care.

trauma are often interpreted as lack of credibility and can result in refusal of a survivor's application for legal protection (Bogner et al., 2007). We use our experience in working with survivors to provide expert evidence to facilitate the legal system's understanding of the psychological matters that affect the people with whom we work.

Navigating the asylum system in the UK can be a challenge for clients and professionals alike. The legal protection team offers crucial support and guidance for clients and the staff team throughout this process. Clinicians and legal advisors work together closely to promote a wider understanding of the external agencies of the issues that face our clients.

Psychological Therapies

Recognition of the mental health and therapeutic needs of survivors of ill-treatment has always been at the forefront of HBF's work. Following a detailed assessment and collaborative decision-making process, clients are offered a psychotherapeutic intervention that is best suited to their needs.

The majority of our clients complain of symptoms of PTSD or 'complex PTSD', although few understand their terrifying symptoms as being a common or understandable consequence of severe ill-treatment. We run psychoeducation groups about PTSD symptoms and how to manage them while clients are awaiting their individual therapy sessions to normalise these problems and help them to regain their sense of agency regarding their mental health problems.

All clients who have PTSD are offered a trauma-focused intervention, in line with NICE guidelines (NICE, 2005, 2018). Depending on clients' preferences and the presenting issues, this is, typically, a course of trauma-focused cognitive therapy (Ehlers & Clark, 2000), narrative exposure therapy (NET; Schauer et al., 2011) or eye movement desensitisation and reprocessing (EMDR; Shapiro, 1989).

Unfortunately, many clients of uncertain immigration status have been denied treatments within statutory National Health Services in the UK on account of a lack of sufficient current stability, which was once considered a prerequisite before undertaking trauma-focused therapy. NET was developed to be delivered within refugee camps to provide treatment for survivors of multiple trauma in a setting in which safety and certainty about the future could not be guaranteed. At HBF, many clients receive NET and other trauma-focused interventions. They engage well and often benefit from an improvement in their symptoms in spite of, often, lengthy delays in their immigration matters.

We also offer a range of other psychotherapies to help clients to explore and address existential crisis or disruption in interpersonal functioning if these matters are the main presenting problems.

Physical Healthcare

Often, survivors of torture and ill-treatment have multiple health problems including: head injuries; neurological disorders; badly healed fractures and wounds; gastrointestinal disorders; and sexually transmitted infections. Many barriers can prevent clients from accessing effective healthcare from their local general practitioner (GP). They include: difficulties presenting the right documents to register at a surgery; language barriers; and all-too-brief appointments in which their numerous and complex problems can only be touched on before the time is up. Our in-house GPs provide a specialist advisory clinic. They offer extended appointments with experienced interpreters to allow clients enough time to discuss their histories and concerns in full. Following an in-depth assessment, the GPs at HBF offer specialist advice to our clients' GPs and other healthcare providers.

Welfare and Housing Casework

Asylum seekers and survivors of ill-treatment often experience socio-economic deprivation. They may lack permanent or safe-place accommodation and face financial destitution. As a result of their past experiences and current mental health problems, our clients remain at risk of further abuse and exploitation, particularly when they lack sufficient resources to meet their basic needs. HBF has a Housing and Welfare Caseworker who supports clients to access stable accommodation and financial support. Clients are also supported in gaining access to education, training and employment opportunities, when appropriate.

The Creative Arts Programme

A lack of trust in others and social deprivation leave many of our clients facing isolation and loneliness, and most lack the financial resources or confidence to access social activities in their communities. HBF volunteers provide free creative arts and skills groups, including English and computer classes. These groups offer vital opportunities for survivors to explore their independence, reconnect with their pre-trauma identity and learn new skills to improve their future employment prospects. Crucially, they also offer the opportunity to socialise and develop supportive peer relationships.

The Mind–Body Programme

Many survivors of torture and human cruelty experience chronic physical pain or have other difficulties in 'connecting' to their bodies as a result, for example, of the severe dissociative symptoms we have described. The specialist physical rehabilitation programme at HBF includes group activities such as pilates and yoga, as well as individual sessions of osteopathy and acupuncture, where appropriate. These interventions support clients in learning to manage their pain and rebuild their physical strength, and to develop a more positive relationship with their bodies.

Summary and Conclusions

At the HBF, we see victims of a wide range of human rights abuses, including torture, human trafficking, domestic abuse and violence relating to gender or sexual orientation. What the victims have in common is the experience of complex, repeated and prolonged trauma and high vulnerability to further trauma, which is all too often enhanced by protracted immigration uncertainty, loss of status and skills, lack of medical and legal support, and a culture of rejection and disbelief.

Clinical responses to complex trauma and its aftermath include feelings of loss, pain and shame, loss of trust or a sense of agency, and dissociative behaviour. These experiences all impair the ability of survivors to tell their story clearly and consistently, which, in turn, perpetuates the disbelief and rejection they experience.

An integrated approach to client care is crucial in ensuring that their key needs, including those related to legal protection and to welfare and housing issues, are identified and addressed. Statutory and non-governmental agencies should work together to ensure a holistic approach to assessing clients' needs comprehensively – even where they extend beyond the range of needs that a particular service can meet. Signposting and inter-agency communication and joint working is crucial to the care of survivors of human rights abuses, and it facilitates their sustained recovery.

References

Bogner, D., Herlihy, J. & Brewin, C. R. (2007). Impact of sexual violence on disclosure during Home Office interviews. The British Journal of Psychiatry, **191**: 75–81.

Cloitre, M., Courtois, C. A., Ford, J. D. et al. (2012). The ISTSS expert consensus treatment guidelines for Complex PTSD in adults. See www.istss.org/ISTSS_Main/media/Documents/ISTSS-Expert-Concesnsus-Guidelines-for-Complex-PTSD-Updated-060315.pdf.

Ehlers, A. & Clark, D. M. (2000). A cognitive model of posttraumatic stress disorder. Behaviour Research and Therapy, **38**, 319–345.

Herman, J. L. (1992). Trauma and Recovery: From Domestic Abuse to Political Terror. New York, NY: Basic Books (reprinted in 2010).

ICD-11 (2018). ICD-11 for mortality and morbidity statistics. See https://icd.who.int/browse11/l-m/en#/http%3a%2f%2fid.who.int%2ficd%2fentity%.

Masocha, S. & Simpson, M. K. (2012). Developing mental health social work for asylum seekers: A proposed model for practice. Journal of Social Work, **12**: 423–443.

NICE (2005). Post-traumatic stress disorder: The management of PTSD in adults and children in primary and secondary care (CG26). See https://www.nice.org.uk/guidance/ng116/evidence/march-2005-full-guideline-pdf-6602623598.

NICE (2018). Post-traumatic stress disorder. NICE Guideline [NG116]. See https://www.nice.org.uk/guidance/ng116.

Robjant, K., Hassan, R. & Katona, C. (2009a). Mental health implications of detaining asylum seekers: A systematic review. The British Journal of Psychiatry, **194**: 306–312.

Robjant, K., Robbins, I. & Senior, V. (2009b). Psychological distress amongst immigration detainees: A cross-sectional questionnaire study. British Journal of Clinical Psychology, **48**: 275–286.

Schauer, M., Neuner, F. & Elbert T. (2011). Narrative Exposure Therapy: A Short Term Treatment for Traumatic Stress Disorders, 2nd edition. Cambridge, MA: Hogrefe Publishing.

Shapiro, F. (1989). Efficacy of the eye movement desensitisation procedure in the treatment of traumatic memories. Journal of Traumatic Stress, **2**: 199–223.

UK Psychological Trauma Society (2017). Guideline for the treatment and planning of services for complex post-traumatic stress disorder in adults. See www.ukpts.co.uk/links_6_2920929231.pdf.

Chapter 19

The Mental Health of Veterans: Ticking Time Bomb or Business as Usual?

Deirdre MacManus, Anna F. Taylor and Neil Greenberg

Introduction

Military personnel operate within the relatively closed environment of the Armed Forces (AF), which has a distinct culture that is broadly separate from the rest of society (Bergman et al., 2014). They are required to carry out duties that may lead to them being injured or killed and, often, the decision about whether to risk one's life is not in the hands of the individual whose life is being risked. The social bonds between military personnel and their colleagues and their families, and with wider society, are worthy of some scrutiny. There is plenty of evidence that slightly less than 200,000 UK regular and reserve personnel are able to carry out the most arduous and dangerous of duties at least in part because of the close-knit and, in the main, supportive social networks that are characteristic of the AF. However, while the strength of social bonds during active service are likely to sustain operational resilience, it is less clear how well military personnel may fare when they transition out of service, back into the 'real' world, where the rules of social engagement are different and where trustworthiness and reliability are not necessarily core components of civilian life.

The Iraq and Afghanistan conflicts have led the media, public and, at times, politicians, to speculate on the resultant impact on the mental health of the UK AF. Evidence from past conflicts has established a relationship between the rate of physical casualties, which has been considerable, and levels of psychiatric morbidity (Kang & Hyams, 2005). Military personnel, especially those in combat roles, are a group of people who are at high risk for developing a range of mental health disorders including post-traumatic stress disorder (PTSD), depression, anxiety disorders, alcohol misuse and aggressive behaviour (Sundin et al., 2011). Furthermore, it is estimated that around a quarter of military personnel returning from the 1991 Gulf War reported symptoms of physical ill health, sometimes severe, which became colloquially known as 'Gulf War Syndrome' (Iversen et al., 2009).

After the 2003 invasion of Iraq, UK troops were part of a difficult counterinsurgency and reconstruction effort, which resulted in the numbers of troops deployed and casualties sustained being greater than had been anticipated. Soon afterwards, the intensity and scope of the conflict in Afghanistan increased, with UK troops opposing a violent and protracted insurgency, along with the challenges of dealing with the widespread use of improvised explosive devices (IEDs) and other forms of asymmetric threat, such as snipers and suicide bombers.

While there were, inevitably, numerous psychological casualties, contrary to many people's expectations, the recent Iraq and Afghanistan operations has not led to an overall increase in mental health problems among UK AF personnel (Sundin et al., 2011). Data gathered in 2007–2009 from UK troops, who are part of a representative sample of the entire UK military, show that the rate of probable PTSD has remained low although deployed reservists and combat personnel have greater levels of mental health symptoms upon return home (Iversen et al., 2009). Furthermore, alcohol misuse continues to be a common concern among regulars and, to a lesser degree, among reservists (Fear et al., 2007).

In light of evidence of significant mental health morbidity among US veterans of Iraq and Afghanistan (Hoge et al., 2006), this chapter aims to appraise the evidence and possible explanations for the seemingly high levels of resilience among UK compared to US troops.

Mental Health of Regular UK Military Personnel

The bulk of research into the mental health of the UK AF in the last 15 years has been undertaken by the research group based at King's Centre for Military Health Research (KCMHR) at King's College London. That group set up a large prospective cohort study, coinciding with the beginning of the 2003 Iraq War, to follow up the health and wellbeing of troops who were deployed compared with those who were not (Hotopf et al., 2006). The first phase of the KCMHR cohort study (data collection 2004–2006) found both that overall the mental health of deployed troops did not differ from non-deployed personnel and that there was no evidence of a new 'Gulf War Syndrome' (Horn et al., 2006). As the wars went on, research carried out with American troops deployed to Iraq showed rising rates of mental ill health (Hoge et al., 2004) while phase 2 of the KCMHR cohort (data collection 2007–2009) found that the mental health of regular troops who did and did not deploy to Iraq or Afghanistan remained similar (Fear et al., 2010).

In comparison with US research findings, the prevalence of symptoms of probable PTSD among UK regulars, following return from deployment, remained low with estimates ranging between 1.3 and 4.8 per cent (Rona et al., 2007). A study of mental health among UK regulars during deployment found that 3.8 per cent reported symptoms of probable PTSD (Mulligan et al., 2010). These figures compare favourably to PTSD rates in the UK general population, which have been found to be approximately 3 per cent (Jenkins et al., 2009), and a meta-analysis of studies of UK military personnel did not find an increase in prevalence of PTSD over time since return from deployment (Rona et al., 2016).

Symptoms of common mental disorders, such as depression and anxiety, were the most frequently reported mental health problems among UK military personnel who were deployed to Iraq or Afghanistan. Based on the 12-item General Health Questionnaire, 16.7–19.6 per cent reported symptoms of common mental disorders (Hotopf et al., 2006; Rona et al., 2006; Fear et al., 2010) and 27.2 per cent when using the Patient Health Questionnaire (Iversen et al., 2009). However, there was no evidence that deployment to Iraq or Afghanistan increased the risk of common mental disorder among regular personnel (Hotopf et al., 2006). Of note, however, is that the risk of common mental disorder in this sample of UK military personnel was found to be twice that of people in other occupations in the UK general population, after adjustment for sex, age, social class, education and marital status (Goodwin et al., 2015). However some caution is needed in interpreting this finding as data from the general population and AF were collected differently and other evidence has shown that data collection methods can affect the way that people respond to questionnaires.

Mild traumatic brain injury (mTBI) is a condition that is characterised by short-term loss of consciousness (LOC) and/or altered mental state (AMS) as a result of a head injury or blast explosions. mTBI has emerged as an important concern in the US military (Warden et al., 2006; Hoge et al., 2008) and US studies have described it as a 'signature injury' of the recent Iraq and Afghanistan conflicts (Jones et al., 2007). A large survey of US infantry who were deployed to Iraq found that 15 per cent of US troops reported persistent symptoms of mTBI, post deployment (Hoge et al., 2008). Other US studies have reported estimates from 12 per cent to 23 per cent (Pietrzak et al., 2009; Schneiderman et al., 2008; Tanielian et al., 2008), rising to around 40 per cent among injured personnel who had been exposed to a blast (Okie, 2005). However, rates of mTBI in UK troops appear to be much lower as demonstrated by a large representative sample study of UK regular personnel, which found that 4.4 per cent of troops reported mTBI symptoms, although troops in combat roles reported a higher rate of 9.5 per cent (Rona et al., 2012). Another UK study found rates of about 1 per cent in troops who were still deployed to Afghanistan (Jones et al., 2014), suggesting that recall bias may substantially affect studies of mTBI carried out post deployment.

Alcohol misuse (defined as drinking at a level likely to cause physical or psychological harm) has consistently been found to be much more of a problem for the UK military than PTSD. Between 11 per cent and 22 per cent of troops report alcohol misuse (Fear et al., 2010); the highest rates have been found among combat troops. Furthermore, unlike PTSD, rates of alcohol misuse are higher in deployed (16 per cent) compared to non-deployed personnel (11 per cent) (Fear et al., 2010). Comparison of alcohol misuse, in the same age and gender groups, in the general population in England and Wales and the UK AF shows that both servicemen and women are more likely to misuse alcohol than their general population counterparts (Fear et al., 2007), and their pattern of use has been shown to persist over the longer term and to impact negatively on their mental health (Goodwin et al., 2017).

Mental Health Status of Combat Troops

Unlike the majority of regular personnel, combat exposure has been consistently identified as a risk factor for PTSD. The intensity of traumatic exposures experienced in theatre has been shown to have a greater effect than most pre-trauma risk factors, such as a history of childhood adversity (Ozer et al., 2003). KCMHR studies have shown that combat troops show a small but significant increase in the risk of symptoms of PTSD compared to non-combat troops (7 per cent versus 4 per cent) (Fear et al., 2010).

However, not all combat troops are at increased risk of PTSD. Elite forces such as Royal Marines and Army Airborne personnel report fewer mental health problems compared with other infantry after deployment to Iraq (Iversen et al., 2008; Sundin et al., 2010). This may be because of differences in selection and training, and indeed compared with other infantry, elite forces report fewer pre-deployment risk factors, such as a history of childhood adversity, as well as higher levels of unit cohesion, which has been found to protect against mental health problems (Sundin et al., 2010).

Violent Offending

Aggression and violence shown by soldiers post deployment, and who have recently returned from combat missions, has been a long-standing issue (Allport, 2009). US Vietnam era research first found a statistical association with combat exposure and aggression among returning troops (Calvert & Hutchinson, 1990; Yager et al., 1984). MacManus et al. (2012) found that almost 13 per cent of UK troops reported having assaulted someone in the weeks following return from their deployment to

Iraq. However, the risk of assaulting someone post deployment was higher in troops who were deployed in a combat role; deployment by itself was not a risk factor. A further study, which linked the KCMHR cohort (almost 14,000 participants) with their official criminal records (MacManus et al., 2013), confirmed that the risk of increased violent offending was associated with having served in a combat role on deployment, and it highlighted that male military personnel had a greater lifetime risk of violent offending than a similarly aged sample of men from the general population. Interestingly, over their lifetime, military personnel were less likely to have committed a non-violent offence than a similarly aged sample from the general population. This implies that, while military service, in particular serving in a combat role, can increase propensity for violent offending, it may also serve to decrease the risk of other offending.

Self-Harm and Suicide

In the USA, death by suicide is a leading cause of death in the military personnel over recent years (Kang & Bullman, 2008; Black et al., 2011; Armed Forces Health Surveillance Center, 2012). In spite of universal access to healthcare services, mandatory suicide prevention training and other preventive efforts, rates have risen sharply and exceed combat and deployment deaths. The situation is, however, different in the UK where research, examining mortality data from Defence Statistics between 1984 and 2007, showed that AF personnel were statistically significantly less like to commit suicide than comparable age-banded groups of the UK general population (Fear et al., 2009). Official statistics on military suicide continue to be published each year and lower military rates continue to be reported each year. The exception to this findings is for Army males under 20 years of age, who were 1.5 times as likely to die by suicide than expected (standardised mortality ratio (SMR) = 150, 95% CI (confidence interval) 118 to 190; 68 deaths) (Fear et al., 2009). It is likely that childhood adversity that was experienced before joining the services is the cause for this exception given that the SMR for older Army personnel is also below that of comparably aged members of the general population, and there is evidence of increased risk of suicide in early service leavers (Buckman et al., 2012). However, while official statistics show that UK military suicide SMRs are somewhat reassuring, media reporting does not always take account of the factual evidence. One example of this are the flawed statements often made about an epidemic of suicide in veterans of the 1982 Falklands War. The evidence shows that this claim is wholly untrue since the SMR for Falklands veterans is lower than expected (Holmes et al., 2013).

UK data estimate that self-harm in the UK military varies between 1 per cent and 5.6 per cent compared with 4.9 per cent in the general UK population (Hines et al., 2013). Contrary to predictions, self-harm in the UK military was not associated with deployment, but was linked to available social support in childhood and adulthood (Hines et al., 2013). However a telephone interview study found ex-service personnel were twice as likely to report having harmed themselves during their lifetime compared to still serving personnel (10.5 per cent versus 4.2 per cent, respectively) (Pinder et al., 2012). Once again, this finding is likely to be related to childhood adversity and the presence of mental disorders, which are more common in early service leavers who, in the main, have not even passed out of basic training (Hines et al., 2013; Pinder et al., 2012). Importantly, it appears that suicide and self-harm in the UK military has not been directly linked to deployment experiences and, where higher rates are found, often among younger men, the risk appears to be more to do with pre-military risk factors and difficulties associated with life after leaving the service.

Mental Health of Reserve Forces Personnel

Reserve forces include volunteer reserves and those with a residual commitment, post regular service. The studies from KCMHR have shown that UK reservists report more negative outcomes and are twice as likely to report common mental disorders and probable PTSD after deployment compared with regular personnel (Fear et al., 2010). Empirical studies, based both in the USA and UK, have repeatedly demonstrated that, compared with regular military personnel, reservists have an increased prevalence of mental illness post deployment (Fear et al., 2010; Hoge et al., 2006; Rona et al., 2006; Thomas et al., 2010).

The reasons for the differences between regulars and reservists post deployment have been the source of much debate. It is possible that reservists may find reintegrating into civilian life after coming home more difficult compared with regular personnel (Browne et al., 2007). Reservists are more likely to report feeling unsupported by the military, and to have difficulties with social functioning during the homecoming period (Harvey et al., 2011). The study by Harvey et al. (2012) also found that a perceived lack of support from the military was associated with increased reporting of probable PTSD and alcohol misuse. What appears to be of greater concern is that many of these difficulties appear to persist. A longitudinal study which compared deployed (n = 552) and non-deployed (n = 391) UK reservists found that, five years post deployment, the deployed group were more than twice as likely to suffer from probable PTSD. The deployed group also report more actual or serious consideration of separation from their partners. While the authors concluded that the majority of mental health and social problems among reservists following deployment are transient, they remained at increased risk of PTSD and relationship problems, five years after returning home (Harvey et al., 2012). Further research has also highlighted that UK reservists who were deployed to Iraq and Afghanistan were at increased risk of violent behaviour on return compared to those who did not deploy (Kwan et al., 2017) although, day to day, non-deployed reservists are more like civilians than military personnel. This impact of deployment on the risk of violent behaviour was not shown among regular personnel, though being deployed in a combat role increased the risk of violent behaviour among both regulars and reserves.

Resilience among UK Military Personnel Compared to Their International Counterparts?

In summary, research has consistently found that the majority of UK military personnel, including those returning from recent deployment, report good mental health. This finding is contrary to reports by much of the media and by some military charities. There are, unsurprisingly, some exceptions to this; most importantly, alcohol misuse and violence is more common in the post-deployment period. Research has also highlighted the vulnerability of certain groups of at-risk personnel; in particular, troops with a combat role and reserve forces personnel. It has also revealed certain groups which demonstrate increased resilience, such as the elite forces.

While directly comparing mental health status between nations is challenging, there has been an abundance of research over the last 20 years that has consistently found mental health problems are more frequently reported by service personnel and veterans from the USA as compared with troops from the UK, Canada, Germany and Denmark (Richardson et al., 2010). Hoge et al. (2006) reported PTSD rates among returning US troops of between 5 per cent and 10 per cent (Hoge & Castro, 2006) while studies based on data from the US veterans administration have found PTSD rates between 21 per cent and 29 per cent (Wells et al., 2011). Comparable UK rates have been between 2 per cent and 7 per cent (Fear et al., 2010; Sundin et al., 2011).

There have been numerous possible explanations suggested for the differences. First, US personnel tend to be younger and of lower socio-economic background than their UK counterparts. Second, the majority of US troops have undertaken 12-month deployments whereas six-month tours of duty are routine for UK forces. Third, the US military deploys a greater proportion of reservists who, as we have shown, suffer with poorer mental health post deployment. Fourth, entitlement to healthcare and benefits for veterans is markedly different in the USA and UK; the lack of a free at the point of contact national health service in the USA being the starkest variation. Fifth, although earlier US studies reported that US troops were engaged in more dangerous duties than UK troops, combat exposure has been similar for both nations' troops, based on the proportion of deployed personnel killed or seriously injured since 2006. So, this is unlikely to be a major explanatory factor. Sixth, US culture may be more receptive to psychological disorder. US national studies, for example, consistently report higher rates of whole-population PTSD than the rates found within the UK (Kessler et al., 2005). Last, assessing the true prevalence of symptoms of mental disorder is challenging because of an unwillingness of military personnel to declare symptoms as a consequence of stigmatising beliefs about mental health. Although psychiatric stigma among UK forces appears to be reducing with time (Osório et al., 2013a), it still persists (Osório et al., 2013b). Thus, it might be that US troops are less reticent than personnel from other nations about revealing their true state of mental health. However, this explanation is not substantiated by a recent study, which found comparable rates of reported stigma between US, UK, Australian and Canadian troops, shortly after leaving Afghanistan (Gould et al., 2010).

Might Military Leadership and Management-Related Factors Increase the Resilience of Military Personnel?

Studies of military resilience have shown that the risk of developing mental health problems is mitigated by unit cohesion, morale and leadership (Jones et al., 2012). UK troops serving in Afghanistan ($n = 1{,}471$) in 2010 completed a self-report survey about aspects of their current deployment, including their perceptions of levels of cohesion, morale, leadership and combat exposure, as well as their mental health status. Overall, 17.1 per cent reported probable common mental disorder and 2.7 per cent, probable PTSD; both outcomes were higher in troops who had experienced more combat exposure. Interestingly, high levels of self-reported unit cohesion, morale and perceived good leadership reported in the deployed environment were all associated with lower levels of poor mental health. Although the study was cross-sectional in nature, the results suggest that all three factors help to modulate the effects of combat exposure on developing mental health symptoms. This study provides support for the hypothesis that, within organisations such as the military, resilience is better envisaged as lying between persons rather than within them.

Another important difference between US and UK Armed Forces is that UK troops routinely spend around 36 hours at a third location decompression (TLD) facility before returning to their home bases. TLD is a social, supportive and educational intervention, following prolonged operational deployment, which aims to smooth people's transitions between operations and returning home. Research into the effects of TLD found that it had a positive impact upon mental health outcomes (PTSD and multiple physical symptoms) and harmful alcohol use (Jones et al., 2010a, 2013). Interestingly, when the samples were stratified by combat exposure, personnel with low and moderate levels of combat exposure experienced the greatest positive mental health effects. While the study used propensity scores to mimic some of the characteristics of a randomised controlled trial (RCT), the true value or otherwise of TLD can only be properly ascertained by an RCT. However, it appears that TLD, primarily an opportunity to informally interact with colleagues with whom one had deployed, can, in some cases, positively influence the mental health of troops returning from deployment.

The UK military has established a post-incident peer support system called Trauma Risk Management (TRiM), which has been widely used by the Royal Marines since the late 1990s (Jones et al., 2003) and has been in widespread use by the rest of the Armed Forces since 2007 (Greenberg et al., 2008). TRiM aims to provide military units with an integral peer support process that is designed to assess the psychological risk in personnel exposed to traumatic events and engage them with helping services, when and if needed. Studies of the effects of TRiM have shown that: it is highly acceptable to those who may benefit from it; it is capable of detecting changes in post-incident mental health; it helps to mobilise social support (Frappell-Cooke et al., 2010); and improves organisational function while not causing harm (Greenberg et al., 2010). Of note is that TRiM is not routinely used by the US military and this is another potential pro-resilience factor that works to ensure that military personnel who are operating in highly challenging environments can properly support each other.

Conclusions

The evidence presented in this chapter suggests that, in the main, UK military personnel have remained resilient in spite of having suffered significant numbers of fatalities and casualties during operational duties in the past 15 years. There are, however, still some areas of concern. Alcohol misuse remains a widespread problem for the UK Armed Forces. There is evidence of increased violence and PTSD among combat troops. Reserves have shown particular vulnerability to the negative impacts of deployment on their mental health and behaviour. However, the majority of the research indicates that, compared to US troops at least, the majority of UK personnel are facing fewer problems as a result of prolonged combat missions in the Middle East.

The sustained resilience of UK service personnel is likely to be substantially influenced by the high degree of social support found in UK troops. The high levels of leadership, cohesion and morale among troops who have been deployed to Iraq and Afghanistan over recent years is likely to have acted as social glue, bonding personnel together into close-knit teams that function well even in the most austere of environments. Thus, the mutual support required for military teams to be operationally effective is equally as likely to have mitigated, to a great degree, the potentially detrimental effects of deployed military service. What is much less clear is how well the bonds formed within service remain beneficial once military personnel transition to become veterans.

Also, within the AF, personnel have access to high-quality mental health services (Jones et al., 2010b) as well as a number of evidence-based mitigation measures such as TLD and TriM. It is only in the past five years that the National Health Services in the UK have developed coherent mental health service provision for veterans. Prior to that, the gap was filled by third-sector military mental health charities, and their provision was not consistent across the UK. Hopefully, future research will elucidate just how extensive the impact of deployment is on service personnel and their families. However, what is also required is a more detailed understanding of just what are the longer-term costs for society of deploying troops to conflict zones. Only with a proper understanding of the true costs of deployment can the nation properly plan for proper provision of healthcare services post deployment that are required to ensure that Armed Forces personnel suffer no disadvantage as a result of their military service.

Disclosure

Neil Greenberg is an ex-serving full-time member of the UK Armed Forces, and is currently employed by King's College London. Deirdre MacManus is Lead Consultant Psychiatrist for the London and the South East National Health Service Veterans' Mental Health Transition, Intervention and Liaison Service.

References

Allport, A. (2009). Demobbed: Coming Home After the Second World War. Newhaven, CT: Yale University Press.

Armed Forces Health Surveillance Center (2012). Deaths by suicide while on active duty, active and reserve components, US Armed Forces, 1998–2011. Medical Surveillance Monthly Report, **19**: 7.

Bergman, B. P., Burdett, H. J. & Greenberg, N. (2014). Service life and beyond–institution or culture? The RUSI Journal, **159**(5), 60–68.

Black, S. A., Gallaway, M. S., Bell, M. R. & Ritchie, E. C. (2011). Prevalence and risk factors associated with suicides of Army soldiers 2001–2009. Military Psychology, **23**: 433.

Browne, T., Hull, L., Horn, O. et al. (2007). Explanations for the increase in mental health problems in UK reserve forces who have served in Iraq. The British Journal of Psychiatry, **190**: 484–489.

Buckman, J. E., Forbes, H. J., Clayton, T. et al. (2012). Early Service leavers: A study of the factors associated with premature separation from the UK Armed Forces and the mental health of those that leave early. The European Journal of Public Health, **23**: 410–415.

Calvert, W. E. & Hutchinson, R. L. (1990). Vietnam veteran levels of combat: Related to later violence? Journal of Traumatic Stress, **3**: 103–113.

Fear, N. T., Iversen, A., Meltzer, H. et al. (2007). Patterns of drinking in the UK Armed Forces. Addiction, **102**: 1749–1759.

Fear, N. T., Jones, M., Murphy, D. et al. (2010). What are the consequences of deployment to Iraq and Afghanistan on the mental health of the UK armed forces? A cohort study. The Lancet, **375**: 1783–1797.

Fear, N. T., Ward, V., Harrison, K. et al. (2009). Suicide among male regular UK Armed Forces personnel, 1984–2007. Occupational and Environmental Medicine, **66**: 438–441.

Frappell-Cooke, W., Gulina, M., Green, K., Hacker Hughes, J. & Greenberg, N. (2010). Does trauma risk management reduce psychological distress in deployed troops? Occupational Medicine, **60**: 645–650.

Goodwin, L., Norton, S., Fear, N. T. et al. (2017). Trajectories of alcohol use in the UK military and associations with mental health. Addictive Behaviors, **75**: 130–137; https://doi.org/10.1016/j.addbeh.2017.07.010.

Goodwin, L., Wessely, S., Hotopf, M. et al. (2015). Are common mental disorders more prevalent in the UK serving military compared to the general working population? Psychological Medicine, **45**: 1881–1891; doi: 10.1017/S0033291714002980.

Gould, M., Adler, A., Zamorski, M. et al. (2010). Do stigma and other perceived barriers to mental health care differ across Armed Forces? Journal of the Royal Society of Medicine, **103**: 148–156.

Greenberg, N., Langston, V. & Jones, N. (2008). Trauma risk management (TRiM) in the UK Armed Forces. Journal of the Royal Army Medical Corps, **154**: 124–127.

Greenberg, N., Langston, V., Everitt, B. et al. (2010). A cluster randomized controlled trial to determine the efficacy of Trauma Risk Management (TRiM) in a military population. Journal of Traumatic Stress, **23**: 430–436.

Harvey, S. B., Hatch, S. L., Jones, M. et al. (2011). Coming home: Social functioning and the mental health of UK reservists on return from deployment to Iraq or Afghanistan. Annals of Epidemiology, **21**: 666–672.

Harvey, S. B., Hatch, S. L., Jones, M. et al. (2012). The long-term consequences of military deployment: A 5-year cohort study of United Kingdom reservists deployed to Iraq in 2003. American Journal of Epidemiology, **176**: 1177–1184.

Hines, L., Jawahar, K., Wessely, S. & Fear, N. T. (2013). Self-harm in the UK military. Occupational Medicine, **63**: 354–357.

Hoge, C. W. & Castro, C. A. (2006). Post-traumatic stress disorder in UK and US forces deployed to Iraq. The Lancet, **368**: 837.

Hoge, C. W., Auchterlonie, J. L. & Milliken, C. S. (2006). Mental health problems, use of mental health services, and attrition from military service after returning from deployment to Iraq or Afghanistan. Journal of the American Medical Association, **295**: 1023–1032.

Hoge, C. W., Castro, C. A., Messer, S. C. et al. (2004). Combat duty in Iraq and Afghanistan, mental health problems, and barriers to care. New England Journal of Medicine, **351**: 13–22.

Hoge, C. W., McGurk, D., Thomas, J. L. et al. (2008). Mild traumatic brain injury in US soldiers returning from Iraq. New England Journal of Medicine, **358**: 453–463.

Holmes, J., Fear, N. T., Harrison, K., Sharpley, J. & Wessely, S. (2013). Suicide among Falkland war veterans. British Medical Journal, **346**; https://doi.org/10.1136/bmj.f3204.

Horn, O., Hull, L., Jones, M. et al. (2006). Is there an Iraq war syndrome? Comparison of the health of UK service personnel after the Gulf and Iraq wars. The Lancet, **367**: 1742–1746.

Hotopf, M., Hull, L., Fear, N. T. et al. (2006). The health of UK military personnel who deployed to the 2003 Iraq war: A cohort study. The Lancet, **367**: 1731–1741.

Iversen, A. C., Fear, N. T., Ehlers, A. et al. (2008). Risk factors for post-traumatic stress disorder among UK Armed Forces personnel. Psychological Medicine, **38**: 511–522.

Iversen, A. C., van Staden, L., Hughes, J. H. et al. (2009). The prevalence of common mental disorders and PTSD in the UK military: Using data from a clinical interview-based study. BMC Psychiatry, **9**: 68.

Jenkins, R., Meltzer, H., Bebbington, P. et al. (2009). The British Mental Health Survey Programme: Achievements and Latest Findings: New York, NY: Springer.

Jones, E., Fear, N. T. & Wessely, S. (2007). Shell shock and mild traumatic brain injury: a historical review. American Journal of Psychiatry, **164**: 1641–1645.

Jones, N., Burdett, H., Wessely, S. & Greenberg, N. (2010a). The subjective utility of early psychosocial interventions following combat deployment. Occupational Medicine, **61**: 102–107.

Jones, N., Fear, N. T., Jones, M., Wessely, S. & Greenberg, N. (2010b). Long-term military work outcomes in soldiers who become mental health casualties when deployed on operations. Psychiatry: Interpersonal and Biological Processes, **73**: 352–364.

Jones, N., Fear, N. T., Rona, R. et al. (2014). Mild traumatic brain injury (mTBI) among UK military personnel whilst deployed in Afghanistan in 2011. Brain Injury, **28**: 896–899.

Jones, N., Jones, M. & Fear, N. T. (2013). Can mental health and readjustment be improved in UK military personnel by a brief period of structured postdeployment rest (third location decompression)? Occupational and Environmental Medicine, ;**70**: 439–445; doi: 10.1136/oemed-2012-101229.

Jones, N., Roberts, P. & Greenberg, N. (2003). Peer-group risk assessment: a post-traumatic management strategy for hierarchical organizations. Occupational Medicine, **53**: 469–475.

Jones, N., Seddon, R., Fear, N. T. et al. (2012). Leadership, cohesion, morale, and the mental health of UK Armed Forces in Afghanistan. Psychiatry: Interpersonal and Biological Processes, **75**: 49–59.

Kang, H. & Bullman, T. (2008). Risk of suicide among US veterans after returning from the Iraq or Afghanistan war zones. Journal of the American Medical Association, **264**: 2241–2244.

Kang, H. K. & Hyams, K. C. (2005). Mental health care needs among recent war veterans. New England Journal of Medicine, **352**: 1289.

Kessler, R. C., Chiu, W. T., Demler, O. & Walters, E. E. (2005). Prevalence, severity, and comorbidity of 12-month DSM-IV disorders in the National Comorbidity Survey Replication. Archives of General Psychiatry, **62**: 617–627.

Kwan, J., Jones, M., Somaini, G. et al. (2017). Post-deployment family violence among UK military personnel. Psychological Medicine, 1–11; doi: 10.1017/S0033291717003695.

MacManus, D., Dean, K., Al Bakir, M. et al. (2012). Violent behaviour in UK military personnel returning home after deployment. Psychological Medicine, **42**: 1663–1673.

MacManus, D., Dean, K., Jones, M. et al. (2013). Violent offending by UK military personnel deployed to Iraq and Afghanistan: A data linkage cohort study. The Lancet, **381**: 907–917.

Mulligan, K., Jones, N., Woodhead, C., et al. (2010). Mental health of UK military personnel while on deployment in Iraq. The British Journal of Psychiatry, **197**: 405–410.

Okie, S. (2005). Traumatic brain injury in the war zone. New England Journal of Medicine, **352**: 2043–2047. doi: 10.1056/NEJMp058102.

Osório, C., Jones, N., Fertout, M. & Greenberg, N. (2013a). Changes in stigma and barriers to care over time in UK armed forces deployed to Afghanistan and Iraq between 2008 and 2011. Military Medicine, **178**: 846–853.

Osório, C., Jones, N., Fertout, M. & Greenberg, N. (2013b). Perceptions of stigma and barriers to care among UK military personnel deployed to Afghanistan and Iraq. Anxiety, Stress and Coping, **26**: 539–557.

Ozer, E. J., Best, S. R., Lipsey, T. L. & Weiss, D. S. (2003). Predictors of posttraumatic stress disorder and symptoms in adults: A meta-analysis. Psychological Bulletin, **129**: 52.

Pietrzak, R. H., Johnson, D. C., Goldstein, M. B., Malley, J. C. & Southwick, S. M. (2009). Posttraumatic stress disorder mediates the relationship between mild traumatic brain injury and health and psychosocial functioning in veterans of Operations Enduring Freedom and Iraqi Freedom. The Journal of Nervous and Mental Disease, **197**: 748–753.

Pinder, R. J., Iversen, A. C., Kapur, N., Wessely, S. & Fear, N. T. (2012). Self-harm and attempted suicide among UK Armed Forces personnel: Results of a cross-sectional survey. International Journal of Social Psychiatry, **58**: 433–439.

Richardson, L. K., Frueh, B. C. & Acierno, R. (2010). Prevalence estimates of combat-related post-traumatic stress disorder: Critical review. Australian and New Zealand Journal of Psychiatry, **44**: 4–19.

Rona, R. J., Burdett, H., Bull, S. et al. (2016). Prevalence of PTSD and other mental disorders in UK service personnel by time since end of deployment: A meta-analysis. BMC Psychiatry, **16**: 333; doi: 10.1186/s12888-016-1038-8.

Rona, R. J., Fear, N. T., Hull, L. et al. (2007). Mental health consequences of overstretch in the UK armed forces: First phase of a cohort study. British Medical Journal, **335**: 603.

Rona, R. J., Hooper, R., Jones, M. et al. (2006). Mental health screening in armed forces before the Iraq war and prevention of subsequent psychological morbidity: Follow-up study. British Medical Journal, **333**: 991.

Rona, R. J., Jones, M., Fear, N. T. et al. (2012). Mild traumatic brain injury in UK military personnel returning from Afghanistan and Iraq: Cohort and cross-sectional analyses. The Journal of Head Trauma Rehabilitation, **27**: 33–44.

Schneiderman, A. I., Braver, E. R. & Kang, H. K. (2008). Understanding sequelae of injury mechanisms and mild traumatic brain injury incurred during the conflicts in Iraq and Afghanistan: Persistent postconcussive symptoms and posttraumatic stress disorder. American Journal of Epidemiology, **167**: 1446–1452.

Sundin, J., Forbes, H., Fear, N. T., Dandeker, C. & Wessely, S. (2011). The impact of the conflicts of Iraq and Afghanistan: A UK perspective. The International Review of Psychiatry, **23**: 153–159.

Sundin, J., Jones, N., Greenberg, N. et al. (2010). Mental health among commando, airborne and other UK infantry personnel. Occupational Medicine, **60**: 552–559.

Tanielian, T., Haycox, L. H., Schell, T. L. et al. (2008). Invisible wounds of war. Summary and recommendations for addressing psychological and cognitive injuries. See www.rand.org/pubs/monographs/MG720z1.html.

Thomas, J. L., Wilk, J. E., Riviere, L. A., et al. (2010). Prevalence of mental health problems and functional impairment among active component and National Guard soldiers 3 and 12 months following combat in Iraq. Archives of General Psychiatry, **67**: 614–623.

Warden, D. L., Gordon, B., McAllister, T. W. et al. (2006). Guidelines for the pharmacologic treatment of neurobehavioral sequelae of traumatic brain injury. Journal of Neurotrauma, **23**: 1468–1501.

Wells, T. S., Miller, S. C., Adler, A. B. et al. (2011). Mental health impact of the Iraq and Afghanistan conflicts: A review of US research, service provision, and programmatic responses. The International Review of Psychiatry, **23**: 144–152.

Yager, T., Laufer, R. & Gallops, M. (1984). Some problems associated with war experience in men of the Vietnam generation. Archives of General Psychiatry, **41**: 327–333.

Chapter 20

Violent Radicalisation: Relational Roots and Preventive Implications

Kamaldeep S. Bhui and Rachel Jenkins

Introduction and Background

Terrorism is attracting a great deal of attention in the national and international media, and is now becoming the subject of scientific discourse in a number of academic and practice disciplines. Formerly, most studies were undertaken on convicted terrorists, under some level of secrecy, for fear that public disclosure might compromise counter-terrorism efforts; the data might be seen as sensitive or restricted to a small number of actors. This makes it difficult for the public to appreciate the reasoning for public measures that aim to prevent radicalisation and terrorism.

Media reporting of many recent incidents focuses largely on religious rhetoric that is expressed in order to justify political aspirations, including establishing a new state, challenging perceived discrimination and international foreign policies, which are seen to attack or target particular religious groups or communities. Media reports also show that people with mental illnesses, acting violently in public spaces, are likely to be considered as posing a terrorist threat first, and especially so if their expressed motivations refer to terrorist movements. Notably, this is the case if they suggest justifications based on political ideologies of extreme religious movements in Syria and Iraq.

This has led to more discussion about the so-called 'lone wolf' effect. People who have mental illnesses are more vulnerable to persuasion; they might be exposed to terrorist narratives that excite and engage them in supporting extremist movements and in committing a violent offence (Gill et al., 2014).

Of course, this influence of terrorist propaganda may take hold in people without mental illnesses, suggesting that the justification given for violence drives the labelling of the offence as terrorist or not. And this can occur irrespective of the real justifications, actual contact with terrorist groups and acts that are resourced and driven by terrorist groups.

If we take this to the extreme, justifications for homicide and any offending are likely to be very context- and person-specific. If, following a violent incident, mental illness influences the content of the perpetrator's beliefs and they include political statements or terrorism-related statements, even in the absence of any previous or direct link with terrorist groups, the person or people may be mistakenly labelled as a terrorist.

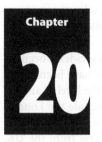

The majority of deaths around the world due to terrorist incidents are, in fact, of people of Muslim heritage. The national contexts, local actors, specific narratives and sources of conflict are likely to differ in high-income western democracies, when contrasted with other parts of the world, so challenging efforts to come up with a unified theory of terrorism. Despite this, historians have identified factors that are common to terrorists, pursuing different objectives in different continents and at different times. These shared factors include the need to: belong; be part of a powerful group; love the group; and be loved by it (McCauley & Moskalenko, 2011). The importance of group identity and activation, and crowds acting in unison, is also emphasised as a source of potential conflict in Chapters 15 and 17 by Drury et al., and in Chapter 21 by Alderdice.

According to the Global Terrorism Database, 80 per cent of all world incidents occur in just five countries: Pakistan, Nigeria, Iraq, Afghanistan and Syria. There have been recent incidents in France, Belgium, Canada, the USA and the UK. This raises the level of anxiety in the respective governments and populations. In the UK, examples include the London bombings in 2005; the murder of Fusilier Lee Rigby in Woolwich by two men of Nigerian heritage; and, more recently, over 500 men and women travelling to Syria from the UK, either in order to join the fighting or, if media reports are to be believed, to become brides and provide a family life for men who are perceived to be heroic soldiers. Even more recently there have been deaths due to knife and gun attacks, and driving into pedestrians in London; significant attacks in Paris, Belgium, Nice and in Manchester; alongside many other bombings and incidents in Syria, Libya, Iraq, Afghanistan, Turkey and Paraguay.

Radicalisation

Since 9/11 and 7/7, the USA, Canada and European Governments have put forward theories about radicalisation to explain why some of their citizens have committed terrorist attacks. The attackers were born and brought up in western democracies, with all the benefits of education, security and better employment prospects than in many regions of the world, and with opportunities for ascending social status. Nonetheless, they turn against their country and, in the process, kill other citizens and sometimes themselves.

The definitions of radicalisation that are found in both academic and public sources tend to emphasise that radicalisation is either one of two processes:

(1) A political ideology that makes use of religious rhetoric and in so doing draws on the value of religious beliefs to unite people who otherwise support disparate causes. Thus, they then identify outgroups as enemies, encouraging increasingly extreme actions against the outgroup. Like all political or social movements, these groups form and re-form around new aspirations, political ideologies and manifesto pledges, to persuade new followers; often there is significant conflict and competition between these groups.

(2) A more rational expression of grievances among those people who feel disadvantaged, discriminated against and willing to move to social activism; this process selects people whose motivation is very high to secure a political change such that they are willing to take up violence and commit crimes.

This broad typology is captured in definitions of violent radicalisation, provided by the US Department of Homeland Security and by definitions from sociological analyses as, for example, found in Wikipedia, and is presented in Box 20.1.

Box 20.1 Definitions of radicalisation

- The US Department of Homeland Security: the process of adopting an extremist belief system, including the willingness to use, support or facilitate violence, as a method to effect societal change.
- Wikipedia' definition, based on social theories: an individual (person) changes from passiveness or activism to become more revolutionary, militant or extremist.

Radicalisation is often associated with youth, adversity, alienation, social exclusion, poverty or the perception of injustice to self or others.

Given that not all people who are radicalised become terrorists, and some terrorists cannot be said to have been transformed by persuasion, the term 'violent radicalisation' was coined. This term originated in EU policy circles after the Madrid bombing of 11 March 2004, and refers to a process of socialisation leading to the use of violence (European Commission's Expert Group on Violent Radicalisation, 2008). One of the problems with the concept is that it is not built on notions of prevention but on conviction of terrorists. Thus, there is little empirical data on how to prevent violent radicalisation. We quote a systematic review and report from the Youth Justice Board in the UK (Christmann, 2012):

> The review found that ... despite a prolific output of research, few studies contained empirical data or systematic data analysis. Furthermore, ... the weight of that literature is focused upon terrorism rather than radicalisation. As such, the evidence is concerned with that smaller cohort of individuals who, once radicalised, go on to commit acts of violence in the pursuit of political or religious aims and objectives. This introduces a systematic bias in the literature, away from the radicalisation process that precedes terrorism.

Whether radicalisation represents a political ideology to challenge states or a social movement, born of grievances due to mistreatment or injustice, it is clear that social processes and relational networks are critical to why people take up radical causes, become motivated by extremist rhetoric and progress along the pathway to violent action. Yet violent action is not the only outcome. We know that many supporters of terrorism assist with digital media or communications and planning; or some just assist with domestic chores.

If there is violence, in some instances, social isolation and impotence in the face of perceived oppression may be offered as justification for the acts of some, so-called, lone wolves. Social capital is often associated with better health and social cohesion, but recent work has shown that good social capital can also be associated with more terrorist organisations, as people with social capital tend to have more resources, networks, trust in those resources, feel secure in themselves and, therefore, are in a good position to start a new movement (Helfstein, 2014).

By contrast, in conflict zones, for example, the Israel–Palestine conflict, terrorist activity is more associated with perceived injustice and discrimination in the wider context of nearby war and conflict, established around religious identities but influenced by deeper social and economic imbalance (Victoroff et al., 2010). Indeed, the range of types of people and contexts is so great that it becomes very difficult to consider terrorists, terrorism and the profiles of persons who are vulnerable to violent radicalisation, as a single group from a similar demographic or socio-economic background or psychological make-up (Christmann, 2012). Understanding local societies, belonging, the strains placed on relationships and cohesion, and the political economy that offers security and hope to all, become important.

An understanding of who is convicted and their preceding trajectories, and how this helps us to consider vulnerability of otherwise ordinary people to support terrorist and extremist causes, is needed, in order to prevent others from taking the same pathway. Vulnerability is not used as a term to excuse or mitigate the acts of terrorists, but to indicate that the progression into this pathway is not inexorable, predictable or linear, and that the destinies, of young people in particular risk, can be influenced. There are many accounts of people leaving these movements, regretting their involvement and recognising with hindsight what influences led them to follow terrorist movements.

Thus, vulnerability here means, first, the inability to challenge persuasive conversation, media or other encouragement to take up a political cause that is associated with violence. Second, it refers to progress along the pathway towards violence. It is useful to characterise which persons can resist this and which ones can choose alternatives as they increasingly come under pressure to believe social and political causes that sanction extreme actions. This chapter is geared towards the vulnerable group, trying to understand who becomes involved in violent radicalisation, not because that is how they have always thought, but because it offers them solutions for transient and immediate concerns. Violence and violent causes seem to be an attractive option through which to address threats in the face of few alternative ways of securing safety, friendship, group belonging and religious certainty.

Vulnerability or Susceptibility?

Case Study 1

Three young women, aged 15, travel to Turkey, and then through to Syria, without border agencies stopping them, and without friends or their families becoming aware of the actions they intend. These young women were performing well in their school studies, had friends and seemed to be living well. The parents are unable to comprehend what has happened and are grief struck; and, at the same time, angry with people who have encouraged their daughters to go to Syria.

On presenting the plight of young people, many strong reactions are heard; that they be criminalised, stripped of citizenship rights and not allowed to return to the UK. The justification is that they made decisions to travel to another part of the world and engage in conflict. Journalistic terms are applied to men and women irrespective of their ages or the sense of maturity that they might be expected to show. The term 'Jihadi brides', for example, was specifically applied to the three 15-year-olds who travelled to Syria, through Turkey, after contact with a known recruiter, Aqsa Mahmood, a young woman who went to Syria to marry an Isil fighter. The construction of this romanticised notion is clearly a function of the digital age and news constructions rather than real information about who are these young people and what drives these behaviours (Ibrahim, 2017).

Might other young people in difficulty be subject to the same alienation and social condemnation, including, for example, young people involved in crime, such as theft, or in gangs, using drugs, engaging in premarital sex or being subject to sexual abuse or exploitation? Immaturity, flawed judgement and poor decision-making are part of the adolescent process, and many public health programmes attempt to tackle these matters. Seeing extremism as one potential hazard during maturation through adolescence, and not giving it special status as a totally alien foreign experience, would enable more open conversations with young people, early in their lives. That approach could assist them to become aware about these perils, learn to indicate that they need help and provide information about where to get it in the future.

In recent years, border agencies did not intervene to stop underage women travelling alone. Yet, a cohort of young men and women becoming involved in these affairs might be better understood as vulnerable, given that they are open to exploitation in many ways. Indeed, the parallels with grooming in child sexual abuse cases has been made in the media by Sara Khan, who runs a charity to empower women to identify radicalisation and to offer a counter-narrative.[1] Groomed victims of abuse do not recognise the dangers and often think they are in a real relationship, only to learn with hindsight that they have been violated and misdirected, and that the relationship they perceived as a special relationship was, in fact, exploitative.

What drives this behaviour? An approach which allows us to apply knowledge of specific processes that afford protection from identified risk factors, and which uses tested types of socialisation, draws on public health models of prevention for young people who take drugs, become obese or take up smoking (Slobada & Petras, 2014). This means using influences from parents, teachers, wider society, clubs, religious and social institutions, which offer certain attitudes and behaviours that are considered normative. There are personal factors related to age, maturation, personality, intellectual and reflective ability, as well as contexts that shape particular expectancies. For example, early conduct disorder and hyperactivity are implicated in later crime (Murray et al., 2015). Parents and partners can influence future criminality (Meeus et al., 2004). Boys in adolescence are more likely to be perpetrators of homicide than girls (Rice, 2015). The process of socialisation is not uniform, but varies not only by individual personality and the ways in which people integrate the personal and contextual influences on them, but also by the ability of each person to respond successfully to the challenges of development, depending on their emotional, cognitive and intellectual capacities. People who adapt unsuccessfully risk making faulty choices or using maladaptive patterns of coping, as well as being unemployed and offending (Zagar et al., 2009).

Interventions that promote socialisation are at the heart of many public health programmes, and might be applied to radicalisation. The loss of positive influences, or lack of them, and the natural separation from parents during adolescence is a critical period, which may lead to weakening of positive and protective ties. These transitions offer an opportunity for more unorthodox influences to emerge as a critical factor in shaping future decisions made by young people at greater risk. Public health models of intervention have been successfully applied to other areas of public health, such as smoking cessation and drug use and violence prevention (Cozens, 2007).

Studies from the USA emphasise minority youth as being especially at risk of criminalisation (Velis et al., 2010). Much has been written on cultural identity and the weakening of the relationships of young people who are children of immigrants with their perceived culture or origin. The term 'perceived culture' is invoked because young children of immigrants born in the UK may not have had exposure to the authentic original culture, but its features are presented through social and peer networks and through family influences.

Any breakdown in communication between parents and their children may lead to a lesser, unorthodox or reconstructed version of religious belonging, practice and culture being transmitted. This influence is weighted and limited by, perhaps, parental understandings and their own levels of literacy, and their engagement with their culture of origin and the new host culture. Our previous study of cultural integration in boys and girls aged 11 to 14 has shown that cultural integration, when assessed longitudinally by friendship choices, produces a healthier trajectory than other forms of acculturation such as

[1] http://www.wewillinspire.com/author/sara-khan/

assimilation, traditionalism or marginalisation (Bhui et al., 2012b). Through cross-sectional studies, we have also shown that traditionalism, especially for young girls when measured by their clothing choices, can be a protective factor; delays in biological and psychological development due to social protections may be one explanation for a good health outcome (Bhui et al., 2008). And so the overall picture is how to assist young people to move from traditionalism to a stage of cultural integration, but, nonetheless, to avoid encountering charismatic figures, offering risky narratives that are attractive because of promises of religious orthodoxy and salvation. If these beliefs are marketed as more orthodox and true to religious and sacred purpose, they may be appear to be closer to parental values or perhaps even ideologically superior.

So, the question is why do some people, often intelligent, high-performing students in school or university, commit themselves to such a fatal trajectory of violence? As well as considering the variables of intelligence and cognitive strain due to delays in emotional maturation, it is also important to consider 'pull' factors, which promise religious rewards or sacred rewards in the afterlife, which may be presented as 'paradise'. This seems to be an additional drive to that of seeking justice or redressing grievances due to the actions of international foreign policies.

Case Study 2

On 22 May 2013, a British Army soldier, Fusilier Lee Rigby, was attacked and killed by Michael Adebowale and Michael Adebolajo. They ran down the soldier in their car and then used knives to stab and hack him to death. Both were of Nigerian heritage, raised as Christians, who converted to Islam. The incident was remarkable as the attackers stayed on the scene, talking to passers-by, appearing on YouTube videos taken on the spot, and one of them spoke to the camera, while holding a knife with blood-stained hands. The argument presented was that Muslims were being killed by British soldiers, and that Muslims were not permitted to live by Sharia despite living in Muslim lands. Swearing by Allah, they said that they would not stop fighting. The rhetoric was argumentative, attacking international foreign policy, and it seemed to be a well-rehearsed script, given the pace and flow. Adebolajo gave a bystander a two-page note, setting out his justification for the attack. Both men were known to British security services, and Adebolajo was linked to previous demonstrations against extremist right-wing parties. Both were said to be involved in radicalised networks over a considerable period of time, and yet both were from stable backgrounds, and university careers, although links to British universities were questioned and unverified.

The biographies in these two case studies have interesting differences. In Case 1, intelligent young women with great potential were somehow persuaded to pursue a radical path; whereas, in Case 2, the two men were less successful, with longer histories of exposure to radical thought, with less investment in a future career or potential, although all were from stable family backgrounds. The men presented a clear message they had absorbed and were relaying.

Communications theorists consider the process of recruitment to radical movements as a conventional marketing exercise, persuading people that what they buy into is what they want and that their life will be better for it (O'Shaughnessy & Baines, 2009). Having studied Al Qaeda marketing DVDs, O'Shaugnessy and Bains consider that the exploitation of masculinity and the invitation to fantasy in a male group, along with sanction from religious authorities and appeal to military-like action, together offer a potent mix of desires for young men. Dramatic devices, charismatic leaders and persuasive appeals to excitement and taking part in a bigger cause attract young men. These persuasive technologies are not unlike those deployed by the armed forces when offering young people a new career, identity and purpose in life (O'Shaughnessy & Baines, 2009).

Indeed, there are similarities with the arguments deployed by successive popes and heads of state to wage medieval Crusades. The religious beliefs that were crucial to warfare of this nature placed enormous significance on imagined awesome but reassuring supernatural forces of overwhelming power and proximity, which were nevertheless expressed in hard concrete physical acts: prayer; penance; giving alms; attending church; pilgrimage; and violence. Crusading reflected social mentality that was grounded in war as a central force of protection, arbitration, social discipline, political expression and material gain. The Crusades confirmed a communal identity, comprising aggression, paranoia, nostalgia, wishful thinking and invented history. Understood by participants at once as a statement of Christian charity, religious devotion and godly savagery, the wars of the cross helped fashion for adherents a shared sense of belonging to a Christian society (Christopher, 2007).

By contrast, the attraction for the young women in Case Study 1 was a female gender role of wife and supporter, and not a fighter. The gendered expression of radicalisation suggests that the process that we are collectively still trying to understand obeys many ordinary rules of socialisation; including, indeed, those psychosocial processes and phenomena that are covered in this book. Yet, this is a form of socialisation that has fatal outcomes and which leads to political violence and terrorist activity. As observed by other authors, members of groups may share identities that are associated with positive outcomes or with impacts that are not.

Why can religious belief be such a force for good and evil? Apart from the religious meaning that a conflict might endorse, Hedges has argued that war and conflict generally makes the world understandable, giving meaning while suspending self-critical thought, such that the suffering associated with war is justified as a higher good (Hedges, 2014). We have seen the human need for meaning in Chapter 4. Religiosity may offer the definition of potential good, defending the ingroup from perceived threat. In the West, we see religion as a coherent set of obligatory beliefs, institutions and rituals, sealed off from secular life. Of course, it is not so sealed off, but religiosity of others around the word is recognised for being closely associated with socialisation and a whole way of life (Armstrong, 2014).

Preventive Targets

Designing preventive interventions requires a better understanding of aetiology, and time points in people's life-courses at which the interventions offered may be effective. Our knowledge of violent behaviour invokes the interaction between early experiences of life, adversity, and the absence of a sufficiently containing, constraining or nurturing environment, be that provided by parents or wider society. Any future interventions require a better understanding of these processes and points of intervention, and it was the commitment to this understanding that led to our studies of radicalisation in young men and women of Pakistani and Bangladeshi origin, living in the community in two cities of the UK (Bhui et al., 2014a, b).

The findings were counterintuitive in that discrimination and adversity, in the form of life events, appeared not to be associated with people developing sympathies for violent radicalisation and terrorism. Indeed, in a later paper, we show that life events are, in fact, associated with a lower risk of people showing sympathies for extreme actions (Bhui et al., 2016). We found that 2–2.5 per cent of our subjects had sympathies for violence, and 1–1.5 per cent sympathised with the most extreme acts of terrorism. Their sympathies were associated with youth, full-time education and not being poor. These findings contrast with studies in Germany, suggesting that unequal social status is important; and studies in conflict zones also suggest power relationships are important. We also found that migrants (i.e. those not born in the UK) were more likely to condemn such acts, as were those people who have multiple physical health problems and people who have larger social networks. In a further analysis, a cluster analysis classified individuals into one of three groups: most sympathetic, the most condemning and a large intermediate group. Depressive symptoms and youth were more likely to be associated with more sympathetic attitudes. Low social capital was not associated with more sympathies and we found global measures of political engagement also to be unhelpful indicators. Of course, better measures of social capital and engagement are needed in further research, as well as larger samples, and the inclusion of other types of extremism.

Approaches to intervening might tackle people's ideologies and belief systems directly, by challenging them, and might draw on cognitive behaviour techniques. But, so far, use of these techniques in deradicalisation programmes has not been that successful because of rather psychologically isolated sets of beliefs and ideologies (psychoanalytic theories suggest a psychic retreat, or split off, of part of the mind that is not amenable to rational new evidence or re-negotiation, and that is isolated from the external world). In these circumstances, the only interventions that might be helpful are those that promote positive relations and alternative pathways, integration in society and social activism, leading to a better sense of identity, purpose, meaning and belonging. Programmes of this nature commonly make use of positive psychology and wellbeing, in order to attack people's deficits through positive relationships. Gang members from the favelas, for example, have been trained to use music and dance as a positive employment opportunity, and to improve skills. With these activities comes status, see examples from the favelas of Brazil being used to reduce gang membership in Hackney.[2]

In addition to considering direct interventions at the sharp end of radicalisation, it is helpful to consider a public health-oriented multisectoral approach to reducing the likelihood of vulnerability, and promoting resistance to radicalisation (Bhui et al., 2012a; Weine et al., 2017). Such an approach would consider the potential for intervention in political, community, religious, educational, social, criminal justice and health sectors, both separately and collaboratively.

Public health interventions for prevention have been classified as universal (those applicable to the whole population), selective (those applicable to a major subgroup of the population) and indicated (those that are necessary for people who are at high risk). This framework can be used to classify potential interventions to prevent radicalisation.

Universal Interventions

Public health interventions to promote resilience and prevent radicalisation include social engagement with communities and developing more positive networks to prevent people entering trajectories into adverse outcomes over time. These approaches have been used

[2] See www.peoplespalaceprojects.org.uk/en/projects/from-the-favela-to-the-world-2009-2012/

with people who are violent or members of gangs, who smoke or are obese, and they can be applied to radicalisation. Many of these interventions may share aetiological targets and positive outcomes with a number of other interventions and programmes. For example, generic parenting interventions, violence prevention, and child protection. So, all the existing 'healthy growing', 'healthy ageing', and 'lifelong learning' approaches, as ways of promoting population health, remain essential. Specific to radicalisation, the essential ingredients for students in schools and colleges seem to be managing and negotiating intergroup conflict from an early age, understanding discrimination and the origins of violence and terrorism. Such programmes are recommended for public services, and for schools. This is controversial as teachers struggle with multiple demands of an academic curriculum, and how to make such interventions more age-appropriate. There are anxieties about levels of information that might be either traumatic, comforting, frightening or outside of students' world views. Yet, following the new Counter Terrorism and Security Act in the UK (2015), all public institutions, including universities, have greater responsibilities to notice and prevent extremism. The schools' inspectorate in England (called OFSTED) has mandated school teaching curricula that help combat extremism.[3] These requirements may seem unprecedented but there is good evidence of school-based and school-wide interventions improving risky health behaviours among youth (Bond et al., 2004, 2007; Patton et al., 2006). The chapters by Drury et al. on crowds, identity and behavioural activation offer further potential explanations on how radicalisation influences groups. Amongst these influences are shared motivations and ideas, thus recommendating group-based or school-based interventions (Chapters 15 and 17).

England is currently moving towards creating healthy communities, by encouraging GPs to work in collaboration with other sectors and agencies, and by creating Health and Wellbeing Boards to provide opportunities for joint intersectoral planning. Including extremism within these measures would be helpful and closely ally efforts for health societies with those for safer societies. This would mean that local government planning becomes context-specific, more likely to succeed and work in closer collaboration with local communities.

Community interventions include multiple organisations participating in the shared narratives of intervention and seeing common causes to jointly protect society, families and individuals, while protecting safety and democracy. The building blocks of resilient relationships require promotion, so young people can question, negotiate beliefs and difference, debate without conflict or perceived survival threats, feel empowered to challenge injustice and dismiss the need for violence that is born of anxiety and pessimism.

Selective Interventions

There is a role for public services to be equipped with basic knowledge to support awareness and of the importance of safeguarding, should they come into contact with young individuals who they think are susceptible as well as those who are promoting extremist ideology.

Interventions might target gangs and gang culture in general, and masculinity for men coping with low self-esteem, powerlessness and questions about their potency. Plans for training professionals who are in contact with higher-risk people are already unfolding; this includes, for example, training for teachers, police officers, social workers and prison officers. EU-wide initiatives are also ensuring health professionals and those staff who

[3] www.preventforschools.org/?category_id=40

work closely with people suffering mental distress, who are suggestible or vulnerable to group pressures, are also better informed and have a pathway to prevention.[4]

It has been argued that violent radicalisation of young people is a child-protection issue as is suggested by our first case study.[5,6] If so, this would imply that radicalisation by other people is a form of abuse, and that all adults have a responsibility to prevent its occurrence and to protect young people from it. This means that public sector workers might acquire statutory responsibilities to prevent it and report it, and to follow appropriate procedures. This also is contentious.

Some radicals, but not all, emerge from gangs. The National Institute for Health Research (NIHR) and the Maurice & Jacqueline Bennett Charitable Trust funded a study that included a survey of 4,664 men aged 18 to 34 in Britain (Coid et al., 2013). The survey covered measures of psychiatric illness, violence and gang membership. It is the first time that research has looked into whether gang violence is associated with psychiatric illness, other than substance misuse. The survey sample was weighted to include significant numbers from areas that have high levels of gang membership (e.g. Hackney and Glasgow East), lower social classes and with a higher than average population of ethnic minority residents. Of the total sample, 3,284 (70.4 per cent) reported that they had not been violent in the past five years; 1,272 (27.3 per cent) said they had assaulted another person or been involved in a fight, and 108 (2.1 per cent) claimed membership of a gang. Using these results, the participants were split into three groups for the analysis: gang members, violent men and non-violent men. Both violent men and gang members were found to be younger than non-violent men, more likely to have been born in the UK and more likely to be unemployed. In respect of their mental health, gang members and violent men were significantly more likely to suffer from a mental disorder and to use psychiatric services than non-violent men. The exception was depression, which was significantly less common among gang members and violent men. Violent, ruminative thinking, violent victimisation and fear of further victimisation were significantly higher in gang members and believed to account for high levels of psychosis and anxiety disorder in gang members. Of the 108 gang members surveyed: 86 per cent had an antisocial personality disorder, two thirds were alcohol-dependent, 25 per cent screened positive for psychosis, 57 per cent per cent were drug-dependent, 34 per cent had attempted suicide and 59 per cent had an anxiety disorder.

This research demonstrates very high levels of mental disorder among this group and this identifies a complex public health problem at the intersection of violence, substance misuse and mental illnesses in young men. It is probable that high levels of anxiety disorder and psychosis among gang members were explained by post-traumatic stress disorder (PTSD), which is the most frequent psychiatric outcome of exposure to violence. However, this could only partly explain the high prevalence of psychosis, which warrants further investigation. The authors suggest that the higher rate of suicide attempts among gang members may be associated with other psychiatric illnesses, but could also correspond with the notion that impulsive violence may be directed both outwardly and inwardly. Street gangs are concentrated in inner urban areas characterised by socio-economic deprivation,

---

4 http://ec.europa.eu/dgs/home-affairs/what-we-do/networks/radicalisation_awareness_network/index_en.htm

5 http://www.saferinternet.org.uk/Content/Childnet/SafterInternetCentre/downloads/Online_Safety_-_LSCB_bulletin_-_Radicalisation.pdf

6 http://www.theguardian.com/politics/2014/mar/03/boris-johnson-radicalisation-child-abuse

high crime rates and multiple social problems. The authors report that around one per cent of 18–34-year-old men in Britain are gang members. The level rises to 8.6 per cent in the London borough of Hackney, where one in five black men reported gang membership.

Indicated Interventions: the Criminal Justice Agencies

There are a number of cases of young men who become radicalised in prisons, and there is much that could be done to prevent exposure to radical beliefs, and to improve the rehabilitation aspects of prison so that people leave prison as more committed and responsible citizens. Recent cuts in prison funding have probably exacerbated this situation. While indicated interventions in specialist forensic settings are not the focus of this chapter, there is a rich literature on deradicalisation programmes for offenders (Dugas & Kruglanski, 2014).

Conclusions

Countering violent extremism and terrorist offending requires the synthesis of a vast amount of research on the influence of culture and religion in group identity formation, knowledge about perceived injustices, formation of grievance and anger, and consequential decisions to either act socially, politically or through violence. Specialist efforts in mental healthcare, including those with youth in schools and among workers in public institutions and public office, must sit alongside more population-based efforts to counter violent offending within a population health framework. In approaches of this kind, the substance of cause and prevention lies in communities, shared identities, a sense of connection and belonging, and a commitment to a shared and fair society.

Lessons can be learnt across sectors, populations and from different types of offending. This can help to ensure that fear, the essential element of the strategy of terrorism, does not drive isolation and fragmentation in counter-terrorism responses. Terrorist offending is very rare, is carried out by both right- and left-wing extremist movements and can be related to many religious and political ideologies over the centuries.

Our responses must be acutely and intensely cognisant of societal and identity-related drivers of criminality, offending and violence, and of the sources of societal malaise that can be invoked as justifications for violence. A broader approach to countering violence is likely to be more successful, and this should not overlook more common and closely related acts and behaviours such as violence more generally and violence related to racism.

References

Armstrong, K. (2014). Fields of Blood: Religion and History of Violence. London: Bodley Head.

Bhui, K., Everitt, B. & Jones, E. (2014a). Might depression, psychosocial adversity, and limited social assets explain vulnerability to and resistance against violent radicalisation? PLoS One, **9**: e105918; doi: 10.1371/journal.pone.0105918.

Bhui, K., Khatib, Y., Viner, R. et al. (2008). Cultural identity, clothing and common mental disorder: A prospective school-based study of white British and Bangladeshi adolescents. Journal of Epidemiology and Community Health, **62**: 435–441; doi: 10.1136/jech.2007.063149.

Bhui, K., Silva, M. J., Topciu, R. A. et al. (2016). Pathways to sympathies for violent protest and terrorism. The British Journal of Psychiatry, **209**: 483–490; doi: 10.1192/bjp.bp.116.185173.

Bhui, K., Warfa, N. & Jones, E. (2014b). Is violent radicalisation associated with poverty, migration, poor self-reported health and common mental disorders? PLoS One, **9**: e90718; doi: 10.1371/journal.pone.0090718.

Bhui, K. S., Hicks, M. H., Lashley, M. et al. (2012a). A public health approach to understanding and preventing violent radicalization. BMC Medicine, **10**: 16; doi: 10.1186/1741-7015-10-16.

Bhui, K. S., Lenguerrand, E., Maynard, M. J. et al. (2012b). Does cultural integration explain a mental health advantage for adolescents? International Journal of Epidemiology, **41**: 791–802; doi: 10.1093/ije/dys007.

Bond, L., Butler, H., Thomas, L. et al. (2007). Social and school connectedness in early secondary school as predictors of late teenage substance use, mental health, and academic outcomes. The Journal of Adolescent Health: Official Publication of the Society for Adolescent Medicine, **40**: 357 e9-18; doi: 10.1016/j.jadohealth.2006.10.013.

Bond, L., Patton, G., Glover, S. et al. (2004). The Gatehouse Project: Can a multilevel school intervention affect emotional wellbeing and health risk behaviours? Journal of Epidemiology and Community Health, **58**: 997–1003; doi: 10.1136/jech.2003.009449.

Christmann, K. (2012). Preventing Religious Radicalisation and Violent Extremism. London: Youth Justice Board.

Christopher, T. (2007). God's War: A New History of the Crusades. London: Penguin.

Coid, J. W., Ullrich, S., Keers, R. et al. (2013). Gang membership, violence, and psychiatric morbidity. The American Journal of Psychiatry, **170**: 985–993; doi: 10.1176/appi.ajp.2013.12091188.

Cozens, P. (2007). Public health and the potential benefits of crime prevention through environmental design. New South Wales Public Health Bulletin, **18**: 232–237.

Dugas, M. & Kruglanski, A. W. (2014). The quest for significance model of radicalization: Implications for the management of terrorist detainees. Behavioral Sciences and the Law, **32**: 423–439; doi: 10.1002/bsl.2122.

European Commission's Expert Group on Violent Radicalisation (2008). Radicalisation Processes Leading to Acts of Terrorism. Brussels: European Commission.

Gill, P., Horgan, J. & Deckert, P. (2014). Bombing alone: Tracing the motivations and antecedent behaviors of lone-actor terrorists. Journal of Forensic Science, **59**: 425–35; doi: 10.1111/1556-4029.12312.

Hedges, C. (2014). War is a Force that Gives Us Meaning. New York, NY: PublicAffairs.

Helfstein, S. (2014). Social capital and terrorism. Defence and Peace Economics, **25**: 363–380; doi: 10.1080/10242694.2013.763505.

Ibrahim, Y. (2017). Visuality and the 'Jihadi-bride': The re-fashioning of desire in the digital age. Social Identities, published online: 26 Sep; doi: 10.1080/13504630.2017.1381836.

McCauley, C. & Moskalenko, M. (2011). Friction: How Radicalization Happens to Them and Us. Oxford: Oxford University Press.

Meeus, W., Branje, S. & Overbeek, G. J. (2004). Parents and partners in crime: A six-year longitudinal study on changes in supportive relationships and delinquency in adolescence and young adulthood. Journal of Child Psychology and Psychiatry, and Allied Disciplines, **45**: 1288–1298; doi: 10.1111/j.1469-7610.2004.00312.x.

Murray, J, Menezes, A. M., Hickman, M. et al. (2015). Childhood behaviour problems predict crime and violence in late adolescence: Brazilian and British birth cohort studies. Social Psychiatry and Psychiatric Epidemiology, **50**: 579–589; doi: 10.1007/s00127-014-0976-z.

O'Shaughnessy, N. & Baines, R. (2009). Selling terror: the symbolisation and positioning of Jihad. Marketing Theory, **9**: 14.

Patton, G. C, Bond, L., Carlin, J. B. et al. (2006). Promoting social inclusion in schools: A group-randomized trial of effects on student health risk behavior and well-being. American Journal of Public Health, **96**:1582–1587; doi: 10.2105/AJPH.2004.047399.

Rice, T. R. (2015). Violence among young men: The importance of a gender-specific developmental approach to adolescent male suicide and homicide. International Journal of Adolescent Medicine and Health, **27**: 177–181; doi: 10.1515/ijamh-2015-5008.

Slobada, Z. & Petras, H. (2014). Defining Prevention Science. New York, NY: Springer.

Velis, E., Shaw, G. & Whiteman, A. S. (2010). Victim's profile analysis reveals homicide affinity for minorities and the youth. Journal of Injury and Violence Research, **2**: 67–74; doi: 10.5249/jivr.v2i2.50.

Victoroff, J., Quota, S., Adelman, J. R. et al. (2010). Support for religio-political aggression among teenaged boys in Gaza. Part I: Psychological findings. Aggressive Behavior, **36**: 219–231; doi: 10.1002/ab.20348.

Weine, S. M., Stone, A., Saeed, A. et al. (2017). Violent extremism, community-based violence prevention, and mental health professionals. Journal of Nervous and Mental Disease, **205**: 54–57; doi: 10.1097/NMD.0000000000000634.

Zagar, R. J, Busch, K. G., Grove, W. M. et al. (2009). Looking forward in records of young adults who were convicted of homicide or assault as youth: Risks for reoffending. Psychological Reports, **104**: 129–154; doi: 10.2466/PR0.104.1.129-154.

Chapter 21

Ways Out of Intractable Conflict

John, Lord Alderdice

Introduction

With some exceptions, people who grew up in the 1960s in the USA and Western Europe became used to a world on a fairly continuous trajectory of economic development, political stability and physical security. They were then joined by an increasing number of other states in the old Soviet bloc, in South Asia and in Latin America, which were becoming more democratic, stable, prosperous, peaceful and relatively free. It has been a profound shock to see all of this change. Questions about what creates and sustains intractable violent conflict and how it may be possible to find ways out of it, have not been so relevant in the lifetime of most of the people reading this book as they are now.

I summarise in this chapter the kinds of questions that I have asked and continue to ask about the resolution of intractable conflict, in the anticipation that some of my experiences, tempered by those of others to whom I turn in my account, may assist other authors of this book to draw these thoughts into the commentary on the importance of social relationships to people's health and the progress of communities that are, ordinarily, faced with challenges. In turn, I hope that readers will find this contribution to the diverse topics of this book helpful in thinking through what might be their contributions to the communities in which they live. I ask four rhetorical questions.

Why and Under What Circumstances Do Some Conflicts Persist and Defy Resolution for Long Periods?

There is a sense in which all of life involves conflict. Where there are relationships, there are diverse wishes, and, even within an individual, there is a degree of conflict about whether to go this way or that. However, when people speak about intractable conflict they are generally not thinking about the inevitable personal struggles represented by the human condition (see Chapter 2), but rather about violent political conflict. In the democratic world, disagreements can usually be addressed without resorting to violence, terrorism and war, so it is often a puzzle to observers from stable parts of the world that some conflicts not only turn violent but seem so resistant to resolution for very long periods. Why is it not possible to negotiate a mutually acceptable outcome?

Self-evidently, conflicts come to an end when one side is defeated and destroyed. There can be no conflict when 'the other' no longer exists. In the past, destruction of a nation or even a whole civilization was not uncommon. For someone with a sense of history, it is like moving to stand on the top of the ancient Crusader fort in Byblos to look down at the excavated remains of no less than 17 separate civilizations, many of which are not only gone, but largely forgotten by the mass of people. The same can be seen in other parts of the world;

even the memory of some conflicts is gone because there is no-one left from the defeated people.

Famously this principle of defeat and destruction was the advice from Niccolo Machiavelli in *The Prince* (Wisehouse Classics, p. 19):

> men ought either to be well treated or crushed, because they can avenge themselves of lighter injuries, of more serious ones they cannot; therefore the injury that is to be done to a man ought to be of such a kind that one does not stand in fear of revenge.

This combination of defeat and destruction is a long-standing principle of war, from early passages of the Bible (e.g. Joshua, Chapter 6:21) through to our own time with treatment of the Jews by the Nazis, where the aim was not defeat but annihilation.

In a sense, therefore, intractable conflicts arise either when it proves impossible for one side to defeat the other, or where there is victory but not destruction, and the defeated people live to fight another day. Sun Tzu was very aware of this and wrote in *The Art of War* (Chiron Academic Press, translated by Lionel Giles) about how to treat an enemy in defeat so that they were less motivated to come back for revenge. When a body of people is defeated, and especially if, in that defeat, they perceive themselves to be humiliated, as is almost inevitably the case, there remains a toxic core of resentment and a profound desire to 'right the wrong'. Where a direct confrontation with the overwhelming power of the majority government of the incomers is manifestly impossible, for example in the case of First Nation people in Australia or North America, the anger and bitterness tends to be turned in on the community itself, leading to domestic violence, sexual abuse, drug and alcohol addiction, and social chaos. However, even when a restitution of the status quo ante seems utterly impossible and the community is split up and dispersed far from its home, the feelings remain. The return of the Jewish Diaspora to Israel, for example, is a remarkable demonstration that, after almost two millennia, those sentiments survived strongly enough in a dispersed community to lead ultimately to a violent reversal of fortunes.

The combination of humiliation, a sense of deep unfairness and the inability to resolve the causes of these feelings through peaceful, democratic development, provides the vulnerability for a violent explosion. These three elements contribute to a sense of existential threat to the survival of the identity of the community that cannot be accepted with equanimity, indeed, it actually results in a change in the way of thinking of the community under threat. In a fairly peaceful, stable community, the thinking of the group is relatively rational and guided by the best socio-economic-power interests of the community. When under threat, we see the appearance of a form of thinking that is guided by what are sometimes called 'sacred values' – principles that are not necessarily religious, but which transcend immediate best socio-economic interests and are neither negotiable, nor measureable with ordinary economic metrics. The life of my child is one such value – I will die rather than trade. It is not negotiable and offering me more money brings a more angry reaction rather than a further response of bargaining (Atran, 2016). Nor does the passage of time bring a diminution of the strength of feeling involved. The emotions of Palestinians about their 'right of return' to the homes they were forced to leave in 1948 in the Nakba or 'catastrophe', is just as strong in later generations that never lived in Israel.

At different points, the Irish conflict showed both the phenomena of victory/defeat and of stalemate. Repeatedly over the centuries, Irish rebellions were put down, but, because the people survived as a people, defeat did not mean the extinguishing of the ideal or the will.

It was most notably expressed by Padraig Pearse at the funeral of the veteran republican Jeremiah O'Donovan Rossa in 1915: '... the fools, the fools, the fools! – they have left us our Fenian dead; and while Ireland holds these graves, Ireland unfree shall never be at peace' (Pearse, 2015). Defeated the following year, but not destroyed, Irish Republicanism arose again and within five years had driven the British out of most of the island. Later the Irish Republican Army (IRA) re-emerged in the North, which had remained British, and, after a number of desultory campaigns, embarked, in the late 1960s, on what was to be 30 years of terrorism. In this case, there was neither defeat, as in the 1916 Easter Rising, nor victory, as in the Anglo-Irish War of Independence of 1919 to 1921. Instead, both sides – the British military and political establishment and the leadership of the IRA and the Republican movement – concluded that neither could win but neither would be defeated. What is so interesting about that particular intractable conflict is that it then moved into a different form of engagement with a Peace Process that addressed the passions and relationships between the peoples of the island and ultimately brought the intractable violent struggle to an end, though political disagreement remains over the ultimate vision for the political future of the territory.

This takes us to the second of my four questions.

How and Why Can Some Intractable Conflicts Subsequently Find Resolution?

Faced with an ongoing violent conflict or terrorist campaign, the natural reaction is to regard it as breach of criminal law and to look to security responses. Sometimes this is successful, but the essence of intractable conflicts is that, despite all such interventions, the conflict continues.

One of the reasons that some conflicts prove so refractory is that they are vicarious conflicts, maintained not alone by the stubborn refusal of the partisans to either negotiate or accept defeat, but because there are external stakeholders who maintain the conflict. Indeed, where conflicts have major external stakeholders – such as India and Pakistan in the case of Kashmir, Greece and Turkey in the case of Cyprus, Britain and Ireland in the case of Northern Ireland and the USA and the Soviet Union in the case of the old apartheid South Africa – no resolution is possible without the cooperation of these external stakeholders.

In the case of Northern Ireland, a peace process became possible because of the radical change in the historic relationship between Britain and Ireland when they both joined the European Union on 1 January 1973. For Jean Monnet, Robert Schuman and Konrad Adenauer, the French and German architects of the European Union, the driving force was not primarily the development of economic liberalism in a supranational market, but a reaction to the horrors and unprecedented destruction of two world wars that began in Europe. These wars had demonstrated that the traditional rivalries of nationalism and imperialism were now just too dangerous, and scientific advance had created the prospect of even more catastrophic wars in the future. The freedom for people to trade (goods, services and capital) and travel were not the purpose of the European project but the instruments through which intractable conflicts in Europe could be moved away from violence and war and channelled into economic and social cooperation.

People in Northern Ireland had been much affected by the two world wars and to see the French and Germans cooperating despite the history of centuries of bloody conflicts provided both a model of possible cross-border cooperation and an inspirational vision of how relationships between former enemies could be transformed. In the early 1990s, the indications (at the time) of progress in the Middle East Peace Process between Israelis and Palestinians and the successful and largely peaceful transition to democracy in South Africa added to the sense that even some of the most intractable conflicts could be resolved.

In addition to inspirational models elsewhere, and practical demonstrations of how cross-border structures were working between Britain and Ireland in the European context, there was a transformational recognition that these conflicts, however intractable, were ultimately all about disturbed historic relationships between communities of people.

What are the Challenges of Completing Such a Peace Process?

Even when exhaustion has sapped the belief that physical force can bring about victory and the external stakeholders have concluded that a peace deal is in their interests, the two (or more) sides in the internal conflict and the significant external stakeholders have some distance to go to construct a peace process.

Contrary to popular belief, trust is not a prerequisite for, but rather an outcome of, fruitful negotiations. However, initial and often risky engagement, by interlocutors, is almost always necessary in putting together the preliminary agreements about how to engage – 'Talks about Talks'. Since this usually takes place in advance of a cessation of violence, it is often laden with personal and political danger, so all participants must be extremely cautious, initially backing off at any sign of threat or perfidy. However, at every stage the process is, as Vamik Volkan says, more like playing an accordion than riding a bicycle (Volkan, 2004). It is not a question of creating sufficient momentum to ram through obstructions, but an acceptance that every step forward will produce anxiety and will be followed by some degree of retrenchment before the next step can be taken.

External powers can make or break such a process. If they provide a constant and relatively reliable containment and encouragement for progress, the prospects for resolution are good. On the other hand, if they continue to use the conflict to conduct the rivalries in their own troubled relationship, they can scupper any prospects for progress. Lebanese politicians often complained to me that their country was a playground for the power games of external powers that frustrated domestic attempts to work together.

One of the most important understandings to emerge from the Irish Peace Process was the appreciation that the structure of negotiation should be based on and involve the people who represented the various strands of the historic disturbed relationships that contributed to the conflict. Strand 1 addressed relationships between Protestant Unionist Loyalist communities and Catholic Nationalist Republican communities, and was facilitated by the British Government. Strand 2 addressed the relationships between the communities in Ireland, north and south, and the Strand 1 parties were therefore joined by the Irish Government. Strand 3 addressed the historic disturbed relationship between Britain and Ireland and only involved the two governments. When this structure was observed, progress could be made. On those occasions when parties chose to go outside the structure, it almost inevitably caused problems in the process.

The degree of painstaking administrative and procedural discussion necessary in the pre-negotiation period should also be noted. This requires commitment and devotion by small teams of civil servants and party officials behind the scenes, setting up arrangements, smoothing the way and keeping records, notes and contacts in place. This work is necessary to hold a process together and to facilitate the involvement of people in all the communities through their own representatives, without which little progress can be made. People do not feel a sense of confidence in, or ownership of, a process or its outcome unless their own representatives are involved, but creating the structure and the political context in which that can happen is painstaking and frustrating work.

The wider international community is important not only in giving moral support but also in providing economic assistance, encouragement, expertise and mediation, and visits to other parts of the world to see conflict resolution at work can be very helpful. Expatriate communities also need to be engaged. If left outside, they can be destructive, but, if engaged, they can, for example, provide financial aid to small businesses and community groups that are trying to build a more entrepreneurial post-conflict economy. Just as the political task in Ireland was to enable the divided community to take shared responsibility for its own governance, so the economic emphasis has to be to help people build their own wealth, take control of their own affairs and increase their engagement in commerce and trade with the outside world.

However, the conduct of any multi-party talks is critical. Listening patiently and carefully for a very long time to all the different parties to the problem, excluding no-one and creating a process in which the parties bring their proposals forward, as far as possible in the presence of each other, may not achieve agreement, but it can build the trust that makes possible an informed intervention from the chair of the talks. This work of building a process, rather than conjuring up a solution, is the heart of conflict resolution. It requires skill and stamina and, like the preparatory phase, may take years. There are many aspects to this negotiation: the careful use of deadlines, gradual building of respectful behaviour (even in the absence of feelings of respect), devices to break through when there is deadlock and the imaginative use of different formats for the talks are just a few of the skills needed in this key phase of the process.

All these components – a significant preparatory period of pre-negotiation, the critical part played by influential international relationships, the sustained political commitment over a long period of time whatever government is in power, the difficult but necessary inclusion (in so far as is at all possible) of the representatives of all parties, the creation of sustainable economic development and cross-border trade, the deployment of patient, imaginative and skilful mediation through a long-term talks process, an element of institutional creativity, and the embedding of international instruments of human rights protection – are all vital aspects of conflict resolution, but they are not themselves sufficient for success. There are some others.

Rebuilding the rule of law is critical. Demilitarisation, decommissioning illegal weapons and reform of policing and the criminal justice system are usually some of the most difficult and contentious issues, and DDR (Disarmament, Demobilisation and Re-integration) for the fighters is crucial.

Rights, responsibilities and respect for minorities are difficult issues, but they cannot be avoided for they are at the core of many conflicts. The classic liberal commitment to freedom under the rule of law creates an environment for the protection of minorities, but even international legal norms and structures are rarely a sufficient guarantor for the partisans in a conflict and usually particular political protections are required for, at least, a transitional period.

There must also be a spirit of generosity and respect. Without them, the process and the new structures cannot flourish, and unless there are changes in attitudes as well as in the political institutions, the administration of justice and shared socio-economic benefit, the conflict is never truly put to the past. Rules and rights can provide the context for a conflict to be stopped, but only a new culture of mutual respect can prevent it returning.

What is the Role of Leadership in Achieving a Positive Outcome?

James MacGregor Burns, the recently deceased doyen of leadership studies in the USA, has pointed out that the direction in which a community moves depends as much on followership as on what is usually called leadership (MacGregor Burns, 1978). In this way, he helped to move the focus of leadership studies away from an almost total concentration on the personalities and behaviour of great people to the interaction and relationships between leaders and the communities on and through which they try to exercise influence. This is especially important in understanding the causes and modalities of terrorism, which are largely informed by large group psychology.

However, the personalities of political leaders are still important not only because they can provide inspiring role models in moving things forward, but they are also representative of some key elements of the psychology of the groups they lead. Some stay in place for a very long time, because the conflict freezes development of the group and the same leader is still an 'appropriate' representation of the 'personality' of the group. Studies of the psychology of particular leaders can shed an interesting light on their cause and their followers because, in their very personality, they tell us something about the group (Falk, 2004).

This is not only the case for the formal, established leaders that would be widely recognised, but also for those who are chosen by young people as models to admire and emulate. Some of the people with whom they identify are sporting celebrities, but others are mates in their football teams and urban gangs. The person who most deserves the appellation 'leader' is the one who can not only represent his or her community but also find a way of taking that community beyond its current position, improve its context and hand leadership over to the next generation with the community in better order.

Such transformational leaders, who may have made their names in the violent struggle, may, with courage and imagination, be able to use that credibility to persuade their people to grasp the opportunities for a political negotiating process as an alternative to continued violence. However, peace, progress and an end to violence only come through strong, persistent, persuasive and courageous leadership of a high order.

Practical political leadership often requires an undue confidence in one's own abilities, perspectives and principles and a certitude that 'my people' are in the right. One may wish that leaders could allow for more doubts, but most leaders will feel that this is liberal, wishful thinking and not something in which practical politicians can indulge. Any consideration of the role of leadership in bringing terrorist campaigns to an end must appreciate the really difficult challenge for the leader of a terrorist organisation who believes it is time to end the campaign. What are the key elements?

When a campaign of politically motivated violence is firmly entrenched, removal of the primary 'causes' will not bring a campaign to a close: just as removing a patient from a toxic environment does not necessarily cure them of a resultant disorder that has taken hold. Leadership is not only crucial for getting to the table and negotiating a settlement, but it is vital right on through the implementation phase. Closing down a substantial community-based terrorist operation is not easy if one is going to avoid damaging splits between those who want to change and those who want to continue, and splits in a terrorist organisation almost inevitably involve internecine violence and murder. The first criterion for leadership in such circumstances is physical and moral courage.

However, the context must be conducive if leaders are to be successful. I have referred to how leaders come to prominence because, through their personalities, they represent something of the 'personality' of the community they represent. The leader of a community is not necessarily the most intelligent, ambitious or talented candidate, but the one who fits best the community's way-of-being-in-the-world at that time – angry communities are likely to choose truculent leaders.

Good fortune is also a key requirement. Some leaders do seem to be blessed with more regular breaks than others. However shrewd, strategic and tactically adept a leader may be, unless he or she is presented with some opportunity for movement, it may be impossible to change. It is doubtful that even the extraordinarily charismatic leadership of Nelson Mandela would have led to the end of apartheid in South Africa had not the end of the Cold War changed external attitudes. Leaders can take active steps, but they need the context. If key groups still believe that they can have things their own way through the exercise of sufficient force, good leaders may fail because the key internal and external forces are not in positive alignment. It needs to be said that it is also essential to have courageous, imaginative leadership on the official side.

While some of these remarks may seem very obvious it is only since 9/11 that the challenge of ending terrorism has become the subject of wider study than just mitigation through robust security measures. Two very thoughtful books on the genesis of terrorist campaigns from Louise Richardson (*What Terrorists Want*; Richardson, 2007) and their ending by Audrey Kurth Cronin (*How Terrorism Ends*; Kurth Cronin, 2011), address issues of leadership.

In-fighting, a loss of momentum or relevance, state repression or decapitation of their organisation through killing or imprisoning the leadership can all play a role. Generally, imprisonment is more effective in destroying the myth of the leader's power, while assassination can produce martyrs. In the minority of cases in which there was some success, negotiations tend to reduce the death and damage caused and may lead into democratic politics, or into the alternative of organised crime. In all six overlapping outcomes identified by Kurth Cronin – decapitation, negotiation, success, failure, repression and reorientation – leadership plays a role in success or failure, since negotiation is a role of the leaders, and reorientation requires reframing the group narrative in a new direction.

The most important development in recent years, however, is the widespread destabilisation of states from Afghanistan right across the wider Middle East and much of North Africa, and the chaos left in the wake of this phenomenon. In the late nineteenth and early twentieth centuries, anarchist terrorism contributed to the end of empires in the outcome of World War I. After World War II, the USA and USSR channelled their rivalries into support for terrorist groups and the end of the Cold War between them brought to a close some long-standing terrorist campaigns. I fear that the current wave of terrorism and destabilisation has ushered in the third global conflict. The failure of weak states to sustain themselves is not just a crisis of certain regions, but of leadership in liberal democracy, reminding us again of the requirements for leadership on the 'official' political side and in non-governmental 'civil society'.

Leadership by elements in both the civil service and in civil society is very important. Business organisations and trade unions as well as religious leaders and non-governmental organisations that are established for peace-building can help overcome the barriers of de facto segregation. The press can play a positive role if so minded, but this does involve some challenge to their own community as well as merely appealing for a beneficent attitude to peace-building.

When a leader has decided that, for the good of his or her people, things have to change and is courageous enough to move, he or she should work to frame the people's understanding of their dilemmas. The term 'narrative' is often used to connote the way a group construes its place in history. Volkan has identified how chosen traumas and chosen victories fulfil a powerful role in determining how a group feels about itself and reacts to others (Volkan, 2004). Such seminal historic incidents as well as the language and understanding a leader conveys to his people are crucial.

In the Irish context, the Northern Nationalist leader and Nobel Laureate, John Hume, developed a new political language, based on relationships. 'The problem is not that that the island is divided', he would often say, 'but that the people are divided about how they should share the island' (Drower, 1995). The implication of this reframing was that the political task was no longer to maintain control of territory or wrest it from the other side, but to resolve the disagreement about how to share the territory – the problem of disturbed historic relationships on the island.

When he engaged with the IRA leadership, his question was whether the method (terrorism) was more sacred than the cause (Irish unity). The answer – that it was the cause – gave him the opportunity to ask whether violence could be abandoned if there was a better alternative. When Republicans replied in the affirmative, Hume's challenge to the British Governments created an opportunity for Irish Republicans to abandon the argument of physical force and espouse the force of democratic argument.

This development of a shared 'peace process language' is very important. Terrorists do not need to speak of abandoning a failed struggle, but can characterise their efforts as 'courageously taking risks for peace'. Their opponents in government do not have to speak about defeating the terrorist enemy but can say, as did the Unionist Nobel Laureate, David Trimble, 'We have never said that the fact that someone has a certain past means that they cannot have a future. We have always acknowledged that it is possible for people to change' (Trimble, 1998).

Communication through action is at least as important as that of words and much of the process of peace or war involves political choreography and drama. When political enemies start to share a programme in a broadcasting studio, or meet or shake hands, it can convey progress in an exquisitely delicate process. These are necessary, but not sufficient, achievements of leadership in the resolution of intractable conflict. Real change must be seen if it is to be believed. If the community has been torn apart and lives destroyed, the weapons of war and the organisations that used them must be transformed and that part of the process must be independently verified. The same is true of agreed changes to the police, courts and security apparatus.

In addition to all the qualities I have described here – courage, context and timing, commitment, creativity in developing new narratives and communicating them persuasively, and the value of external monitors – there is at least one other element.

Concluding Thoughts

When people get involved in terrorism, their groups develop a different way of thinking. Stable societies expect people to act rationally in their own best social and economic self-interest. However, terrorists are not rational actors in that sense; they are devoted actors who will defend sacred values at enormous personal cost. The flag of a country may be a sacred value that you defend to the death even though you can't eat a flag or even stay warm wrapped in it. This kind of thinking is characteristic of groups living in situations of existential threat.

As combatants transition to civil society and take responsibility for the day-to-day decisions of government, the transformation from 'devoted actors' operating on 'sacred values' to 'rational actors' functioning on 'socio-economic best interest' is a daily challenge for political leaders who try to take their people into a new dispensation. Going beyond into exploring how these changes of attitude and culture can be facilitated in historic conflicts is the key challenge at the outer edge of our understanding of how to bring intractable conflict to a close.

References

Atran, S. (2016). The devoted actor: Unconditional commitment and intractable conflict across cultures. Current Anthropology, 57: 13.

Drower, G. (1995). John Hume, Peacemaker. London: Victor Gollancz.

Falk, A. (2004) Fratricide in the Holy Land: A Psychoanalytic View of the Arab–Israeli Conflict. Madison, WI: University of Wisconsin Press.

Kurth Cronin, A. (2011). How Terrorism Ends: Understanding the Decline and Demise of Terrorist Campaigns. Princeton, NJ: Princeton University Press.

MacGregor Burns, J. (1978). Leadership. New York, NY: Harper & Row.

Pearse, P. (1915). Manuscript of speech, Pearse Museum, Rathfarnham, Dublin.

Richardson, L. (2007). What Terrorists Want: Understanding the Terrorist Threat. London: John Murray.

Trimble, D. (1998) Hansard of the Northern Ireland Assembly, volume 1, p. 17.

Volkan, V. (2004) Blind Trust. Charlottesville, VA: Pitchstone Press.

Chapter 22

Agency as a Source of Recovery and Creativity

John Drury, Tim Healing, Richard Williams, Catherine Haslam and Verity Kemp

Introduction

This chapter draws together a selection of the key themes that recur in Section 3 of this book. One of the features of this section is that the authors focus on occurrences that are, statistically, uncommon. In terms of risk, these events are relatively moderate to low in probability but high in psychosocial impact. Thus, each of the serious events and types of incident covered in this section of the book pose threats to people, their families and communities, and to whole societies.

Perhaps, then, it might appear odd that the editors have selected these matters for inclusion in this book. Commentaries on them, which range from disasters through sectarian division and bloodshed to extremism, radicalisation and terrorism, are included in our quest for learning and inspiration in general terms as much as finding solutions to these and other circumstances that affect people. Put another way, does our understanding of social connectedness explain how people cope with extreme events and also throw light on how people are drawn to commit antisocial and deadly acts?

We note that even the most extreme events throw up important human experiences, altruistic acts and aspects of their relationships that allow people to cope with these events more effectively than they might, without people around them. Indeed the extremity of these events, and the simplification of life and focussing of activities that can accompany them, can have a permanent effect on people, altering the course of their lives. As well as long-term suffering and the pain of memory, they may even also leave some people with a permanent nostalgia for a period in their lives that was extremely fulfilling, an experience that can affect their lives and relationships. It is these matters that we seek to identify in Section 3.

Here, we draw together the common themes and the positive learning from these, all-too-often, horrible events in order to contribute lessons that might be built on in Section 4, or at least to substantiate that the importance of social connectedness is as, if not more, important in tough scenarios as they are in more ordinary circumstances.

We begin by summarising what we see as the foci of each of the chapters and then draw out our perception of recurrent themes that emerge from the, apparently, disparate subject matter.

A Commentary on the Themes in Section 3

Chapter 15 introduces basic principles of crowd psychology. In the past, psychology and cognate disciplines have characterised crowds as psychologically inferior to individual persons. In these accounts, not only are crowds supposedly more emotional, but they are also less intelligent and less rational than a lone person. This perspective on crowds has long existed in both popular culture and scholarly accounts (see, for example, Carey, 1992). However, its persistence in some domains today is of more than academic interest because these constructions of collective life serve as justifications and rationales for institutional practices (Drury et al., 2013; Stott & Reicher, 1998).

Speaking to this problem, Chapter 15 suggests an alternative way of thinking about the psychology of being part of a crowd, drawing upon the social identity approach in social psychology. A key point is that the transformations entailed provide the basis for cooperation. In short, far from inhibiting meaningful action, crowds enable such action; and sharing identity in a crowd enables people to act together. These points about the basic psychology of crowds are in fact relevant far beyond crowds, since they apply to group and collective contexts more generally, as other chapters in the book have shown.

Chapter 16 suggests that disasters can rob people of all six dimensions of the human condition that are identified in Chapter 2, or at least alter people's experience of them (i.e. embodiment, finiteness, sociability, cognition, evaluation and agency). Displacement is a major factor in damage to physical and mental health after disasters, and an important component of this impact on people who are affected is that it disempowers them. We have observed this in diverse cases, including those in which people were moved from their homes following the floods in York (UK), in 2015–2016, and in people who were dispersed to emergency accommodation and separated from each other, following the Grenfell Tower fire, London, UK of 2017.

While psychological and psychiatric responses have often focused on the experiences of individual persons, using a medical model, the approach that is known as psychological first aid emphasises the way in which simple, practical measures can serve to restore a level of self-efficacy. Thus, professional responders to disasters should consider the need to maintain people in their homes, if possible, thereby allowing them a chance to retain not just agency, but also self-continuity in a period of major change and uncertainty. If displacement is essential or inevitable, then families and other social groups should be kept together as far as possible, to allow people to maintain their relationships and their identities. This means that, for example:

(1) Schools should be re-opened as soon as possible: they promise hope for the future, an orientation to recovery, and places for chance meetings between people to re-establish relationships, and for more organised events.
(2) One-stop-shops for all services are required: the premises and responders who are preferred by those people affected by events should be readily available to people who are affected by events.
(3) On arrival at a reception centre or displaced persons' camp, groups should be kept together if possible. Otherwise, displacement can break up social groups, remove agency and cause considerable social tension. As soon as possible after arrival in a camp, people should be given roles and activities that allow them to maintain a feeling of agency.
(4) If displaced persons are to be housed in communities, families should be kept together, and social groups housed close together, if possible. But care must be taken with these activities. There is a risk that host families may feel a loss of agency due to the presence of strangers and the need to alter routine behaviours and activities to accommodate them. Also, they may experience loss of privacy and risks to family cohesion. There is also a risk to communities by introducing displaced families or social groups, or by establishing

a displaced persons facility, especially if the resources of the community are limited and become overstretched by the addition of extra people. Indeed, great care must be taken to ensure that communities are not disadvantaged by the presence of displaced persons or by siting a place or camp for displaced persons in the immediate area. Resentments can grow if the assistance given to displaced people by aid agencies is perceived as being better than that available to the host community.

Chapter 17 brings together certain topics that recur in the previous two chapters. It shows that ad hoc crowds of people with few previous connections can act as regulators of behaviour in emergencies and disasters. During events such as these, an individual person in a crowd can be at risk when everyone else also acts individually; for example, if they compete for a limited exit. Shared social identity in a crowd can enhance the likelihood of survival, by motivating people in the crowd to cooperate and by providing shared cognitions and expectations that make cooperation practically possible.

These psychological features of crowds allow people to achieve agency, or at least greater agency than they would if the crowd were divided, in a situation that would, otherwise, be beyond their control. Put differently, while it is true that disasters often undermine or reduce access to the resources that allow people to act as a community, including, for example, community locations, they can also provide opportunities to *create* a sense of community. This emergent community identity is the basis of the cooperation and mutual aid that has commonly been observed across all phases of disasters. In addition, some of the same processes (common fate, shared social identity, social support) that have been shown to operate in crowds in disasters, to produce resilient behaviours, have also been found to take place for refugees of war in developing countries; in this case, shared social identity reduces some of the negative effects of secondary stressors.

Chapter 18 describes how survivors of serious trauma, such as torture and imprisonment, lose agency and lose trust. Focusing on displaced persons seeking asylum, it shows how they may be separated from families, friends and support networks. Moreover, the trauma experienced by some asylum seekers is complex and repeated; they suffer not only the torture or trafficking itself, but also disempowering management by the authorities in the 'sanctuary' country, which includes detention and uncertainty. Further, through the process of displacement, the loss of skills and inability to work cause a serious lack of self-esteem, even if people are with their families or own social groups. Failing to meet their needs and to value them as contributors to society makes things worse for asylum seekers. Their experiences of loss, including loss of valued relationships, skills and activities, undermine their identity and hence their agency. This is because identity, which is the basis of agency, is grounded in social relations and practices with others. Thus, if we have no self, how can we act in a meaningful way? Solutions include a coordinated, multidimensional, multi-agency approach to integrated care, thereby addressing multiple needs and human dimensions.

Chapter 19 focuses on the experiences of military groups, which are tight-knit and closed to outsiders, with defined cultures that may have slightly different norms compared to those of other parts of society. These peer groups can provide essential support to their members when living and fighting in extreme and dangerous situations. When members of armed forces leave combat, the military culture and its shared experience act as support mechanisms, helping members to adjust to the changed situation.

Sometimes, this comes at a cost because members of armed forces who leave the service may have difficulties integrating into society outside, due to loss of this tight-knit group and the identity it provides. Similarly, reservists who return to their usual roles and relationships lack this continued support, and they face mental health problems more frequently. The chapter shows empirically that the 'resilience' of military personnel in a military context is best explained in terms of social support within groups; actual deployment measures are far less predictive of resilient outcomes. This has been found to be the case across a range of mental health indicators. However, the process is less clear with veterans, who may not have these supportive relations, despite veterans' associations, such as the British Legion, having an important role to play. Again, this highlights the role of being a member of a psychological group. The concept of agency is less apparent; but here too we can see its importance, since mental disorders such as depression and other conditions that affect ex-military personnel are associated with low self-efficacy. In summary, studies of military personnel show that the risk of developing mental health problems is mitigated by unit cohesion and morale, elements which diminish when they leave the service.

The authors of Chapter 20 suggest that so-called radicalisation is a poorly understood process. However, from what we know from research, it seems that radical groups may provide the same support and reinforcement of social identity for their members that groups do, in general, in society. This is in line with more recent conceptualisations of the 'lone wolf' phenomenon, for example. Individual persons may strike alone, but they are more often aligned psychologically with ideological motivations of extremist groups, which inspire and influence their thoughts, beliefs and actions. As this suggests, the identity that radical groups may provide is a valued one, and their practices serve to construct alternative worlds, based on radical values to which individual radical people can aspire. The research shows that common factors across radicalised persons all relate to psychological group membership. They act as if they are group members and share the same 'sacred values', which Alderdice describes in Chapter 21, even in events in which they act alone. Across different continents and at different times, common factors include the benefit from belonging and being part of a powerful group, and, therefore, love of the group and the need to be loved by it. In addition, the persons involved come to this through a process of socialisation. This involves influence from parents, teachers, wider society, clubs and religious and social institutions, on the precise attitudes and behaviours that are considered normative, i.e., appropriate and valued.

Therefore, this chapter suggests that radicalised groups operate like movements in general: they form and re-form around new aspirations, political ideologies and manifesto pledges, to persuade new followers; and, often, there is significant conflict and competition between these groups. These groups provide their members with social capital, more resources, networks, and trust in those resources. Research (see Chapters 3, 4 and 20) has found that social capital is often associated with better health outcomes; people who are better connected feel secure themselves and are, therefore, in a good position to develop further movements. The social identity approach adds to this by suggesting that these network connections are based on social categorisation and that the trust in the 'bank' can be an effect as well as a cause of social connectedness (see also Chapter 15).

Chapter 21, on intractable conflicts, suggests that resolution of conflicts between groups, with different cultures that their members perceive as inimical to each other, can be very difficult. Alderdice identifies a core triad of factors that create this kind of circumstance, which include groups of people experiencing shared feelings of humiliation, a sense of deep unfairness and an inability to resolve the causes of these feelings through democratic development. In his opinion, these group experiences provide the vulnerability for a violent explosion. Alderdice also identifies a number of other factors that contribute to making conflict intractable. Sometimes, a conflict may be reinforced or maintained by external stakeholders, and its resolution requires that these persons and/or groups and/or nations be brought onside, which may prove more difficult than achieving resolution between combative groups that are becoming war weary. Conflict resolution requires changing the thinking of the members of the groups or even removing them from those groups. Group leaders have a major part to play in the structure of groups and the collective thinking of each in guiding the group towards resolution.

As we have noted, Chapter 21 also points to the role of sacred values in our understanding of extreme or terrorist groups. Psychologically, this concept is useful in allowing us to transcend the false rational–irrational dichotomy in understanding collective behaviour and intergroup conflict. It is in line with the notion that all meaningful action is identity-based because values reflect identities. The chapter also reinforces the important point that trust can be an outcome and not, just, a condition of social relations. Alderdice argues that, contrary to popular belief, trust is not a prerequisite for, but rather a result of, fruitful negotiations. However, initial, and often risky, engagement by interlocutors is almost always necessary in putting together the preliminary agreements about how to engage: 'talks about talks' may be necessary before the 'real' negotiation takes place. The chapter also refers to the role of followership in leadership and the concept of transformative leadership. The concept of followership helps to move the focus of leadership studies away from an almost total concentration on the personalities and behaviour of great people to the interaction and relationships between leaders and the communities on and through which they try to exercise influence.

As Chapter 21 argues, however, social context matters; it must be conducive if leaders are to be successful, and that social context consists of groups and their relations with each other. As we see in Section 4, resolution of conflict and intervening, in almost all circumstances, requires that the people affected are involved in the manner of coproduction and that interveners build a process.

Overarching General Themes

It is clear from our commentary that there are a number of themes that recur within and across the chapters that comprise Section 3. An overarching general theme that recurs in a variety of forms in most of the chapters, either directly or by implication, is that of *agency* generated, or enhanced, through people's membership of groups, whether temporary or longer-lasting. In ordinary discourse, the concept of agency is usually associated only with individual persons. The chapters in this book have argued that groups are a source of *collective* agency. In both groups and single people, there are the same psychological conditions for agency. The core requirement is an identity; for, without a sense of who we are, there cannot be purposes, aims and goals. The main difference between the agency of the lone person and that of the group is in terms of power. When people share identity, they share beliefs about the world and expectations about each other's behaviour. This enables coordination and hence plans to be put into action that could not be achieved by lone persons, though, as we have learned, it may also contribute to intractability.

Groups are sometimes accused of pathology, because they are associated with extremes of behaviour. A different way to look at the extremes of behaviour that take place in groups is to suggest that groups enable ideologies to be lived out and enacted. They enable people, particularly those who lack power, to act out values and beliefs in a way that they cannot do when acting alone – they provide agency. In this analysis, it is the ideology of, for example, terror or racism, that is detrimental to society, not the fact of groupness.

It is also understandable that in different contexts, such as disasters, change (e.g. leaving military service), trauma, imprisonment and humiliating treatment of asylum seekers, distress and mental disorders are linked to lack of shared identity and lack of agency. The corollary of this, therefore, is that restoring group membership contributes strongly to restoring agency and wellbeing. Otherwise, people may well seek other forms of identity and agency when what is currently on offer doesn't meet their needs or if they feel rejected by their current group. These notions are clearly recognisable in the construct of horizontal epidemiology that is raised by Chapter 7.

We recognise that humans, human systems and the circumstances in which humans are placed or find themselves are messy. Some are potentially and actually injurious and destructive. But from these analyses, there is also evidence that human relationships work especially well when people close to the frontline of services are empowered with the intention that the environments in which they work, create social connections and help people to solve problems locally. Tim Harford's book (2016) identifies that, often, creativity arises from events and circumstances that are not well-ordered, and it is clear that we have much to learn about societies and top-down policies for caring from studying situations that imperil people. A corollary is the risk of our thinking that we have created order by defining and labelling responses to people's needs when that process fails to recognise the expectations of the spectrum of people who use and deliver services of all kinds.

Other General Lessons

The chapters in Section 3 provide important information about how crowds and other social groups regulate the behaviour of people within them despite there being no formal methods of communication. Many of the chapters show that groups can provide strong social bonds, maintain resilience and assist people to exceed expectations. Furthermore, as we have identified earlier, people seek a group to belong to but the price of admission may be large especially if it involves deviance from societal norms.

We have also learned about the importance of the legitimacy of people who respond to the needs of people who are affected by disasters. As an illustration, this appears to us to have been most strongly shown by our prima facie examination of the Grenfell Tower fire in London in 2017, when the legitimacy of local and national government in the eyes of the people who were affected was, and remains, very low. By contrast, the firefighters and volunteers who provide social support are, apparently, seen as much more legitimate by the people who were directly affected.

Conclusions

There are three important conclusions from our overview of Section 3. The first is that we should continue to be mindful, in all we plan for persons, families, communities and society, of trying to look at circumstances and events through the eyes of the people affected. Bottom-up perspectives are often instructive in defining what best to do from the top down. We must endeavour to balance between top-down planning with bottom-up perspectives by ensuring we are in tune with people's needs as *they* see them. This is an mportant lesson that resonates with learning that emerged in our scoping in Section 2, ncluding Chapter 7 on horizontal epidemiology and Chapter 8 on parity of esteem.

Second, we must be continually aware of the importance to people of their agency as effective persons in their recovery from ill health and how important this is to people remaining healthy. Because there are different loci of agency, we must consider the agency that people gain through some group memberships, as well as the usual notion of individual or personal control.

Third, health is not solely about embodiment and finiteness but also the other four dimensions of being that Smith describes in Chapter 2. This means that it is important, in finding solutions to problems, that we recognise, accommodate and absorb wider preexisting conceptions and misconceptions into our health promotion and healthcare responses if we are to reduce the stressors that accompany people's embodiment, in the range of circumstances depicted by these chapters. In other words, there is a socially connected dimension to planning and delivering all services.

References

Carey, J. (1992). The Intellectuals and the Masses: Pride and Prejudice Among the Literary Intelligentsia, 1880–1939. London: Faber and Faber.

Drury, J., Novelli, D. & Stott, C. (2013). Psychological disaster myths in the perception and management of mass emergencies. Journal of Applied Social Psychology, **43**: 2259–2270.

Harford, T. M. (2016). Messy: The Power of Disorder to Transform Our Lives. New York, NY: Riverhead Books.

Stott, C. & Reicher, S. (1998). Crowd action as intergroup process: Introducing the police perspective. European Journal of Social Psychology, **28**: 509–529.

Section 4 Scaffolding

Chapter 23 Making Connectedness Count: From Theory to Practising a Social Identity Model of Health

Stephen Reicher

Introduction

The purpose of this chapter is to serve as a bridge between the chapters in the previous three sections and those in this fourth section. Thus far, we have sought to analyse the social bases of mental and physical wellbeing. Now, we turn to the question of how the fruits of these analyses can be applied in practice. That is, we have been reporting and interpreting the way the world impacts individual people for long enough; it is time to consider how we might change the world in order to improve our wellbeing.

Interrogating Connectedness

Let us start by considering what has been learnt thus far. Cath and Alex Haslam start Chapter 3 with a strikingly bold assertion, 'Social relationships affect health. Of that we are certain'. If anyone was sceptical on reading this, hopefully they will by now have been converted. The ensuing pages contain a litany of ways in which our connectedness to others not only protects us from physical and mental health problems and helps us to recover from them, but also enables us to flourish more generally and realise our human potential, even in the face of the most extreme stressors, including war, terrorism and natural disasters.

The case is indeed compelling enough to make professionally sceptical researchers experience certainty. But the case is not new. As long ago as 1623, John Donne famously wrote in his Meditation 17, 'No man is an island, entire of itself; every man is a piece of the continent, a part of the main' (Donne, 2018). We are implicated in others, and they in us. We are completed by others, and incomplete without them.

It might be argued that Donne's views soon became outdated with the advent of the Enlightenment, with its stress on individual reason and enquiry in contrast to the received collective wisdom that was handed down by the ancients, by bishops or by absolute monarchs. But that would be a misunderstanding. Writing from St. Andrews, in Scotland, it is perhaps appropriate that I illustrate my point through reference to the Scottish enlightenment. Broadie explains (Broadie, 2007, p. 20).

> It is one thing to think *for* yourself, another to think *by* yourself, and the enlightened ones were not much given to thinking by themselves. On the contrary, thinking was regarded as essentially a social activity. People thought with each other, that is, they *shared* their thoughts.

These are points I shall expand upon presently. For now, my argument is simply that the editors of this book are far from unique in insisting that human flourishing, from its most mundane to its most spectacular manifestations, depends less on what happens *within* people than on what happens *between* people.

More seriously still, to assert a link between connectedness and mental and physical wellbeing is not simply derivative but largely useless. Because, however positive our connections to others can be in certain circumstances, they can be equally negative in others. Mick Billig advises us that, whenever we come across someone extolling one proposition to the extent that it seems self-evident, connectedness is good for you, think of the opposite proposition, connectedness is bad for you, and run as hard as you can with that (Billig 1987). Do others confirm your views? Yes, but they also contradict you. Do others support you? Yes, but they also impede you. Do you feel lonely and bereft without others? Yes, but you feel suffocated with them. Which of us has not, at one point or another, cried 'give me space!', even, perhaps especially, from those people to whom we are most connected. As we once put it in a review of some of the relevant literatures, and echoing Sartre, others can be heaven. But they can also be hell (Haslam et al., 2012).

So, without being able to specify when our connections to others impact positively and when they impact negatively, we really cannot say anything of much use at all. This is a major limitation of models of social capital which, for all their power and eloquence in warning of the collapse of social ties in contemporary society tend to treat all the connections in one's social network as more or less equivalent and supportive (Putnam, 2001). Robert Putnam, for instance, defines social capital as, 'connections among individuals – social networks and the norms of reciprocity and trustworthiness that arise from them' (Putnam, 2001, p. 19). Pierre Bourdieu, who popularised the term, sees it as, 'the aggregate of the actual or potential resources which are linked to possession of a durable network of more or less institutionalised relationships of mutual acquaintance and recognition' (Bourdieu, 1986).

To be more precise, there are three issues with these sorts of conceptions of social ties and of the way in which they constitute a key resource for people. The first is that they are *over*-extensive: it is implied that everyone with whom one has some acquaintance is of equal value or, at least, even if of varying degrees, they are all of positive value. As we have argued, this is plainly not the case.

Second, these conceptions are simultaneously *under*-extensive. They limit the benefits of connectedness to those we already know and who form part of pre-existing social networks. Yet, as John Drury and Khalifah Alfadhli show in Chapter 17, sometimes it is the support of strangers that is critical to our wellbeing or our very survival. Moreover, as a number of writers show us, in both fictional and non-fictional accounts, it is the aggregation of small signs of civility, for example whether others make eye contact or not as they pass in the street, whether or not they angle their bodies to give you space as you pass, whether they treat you as visible or invisible, which constitute our social experience and impact our mental wellbeing (Ellison, 1952; Souief, 2012). Many of us will remember the tragic case of Damilola Taylor, a young black man who bled to death on a London street because no-one intervened to help him, and of the, then, Home Secretary, Jack Straw, bemoaning our 'walk on by society'. That may be an extreme example of the unkindness of strangers, but it does need to be addressed, and social capital, as traditionally construed, is of little help to us in doing so.

The third issue concerning the relationship between social ties and social capital is that it is overly static. This has implications both at an explanatory and at a practical level. Thus, while networks, self-evidently, change over time, they do so rather slowly and by small increments through, for example, a new colleague, a couple of people who meet at a party or whatever. This fails to address the fact that the same people may or may not be supportive at different times and in different places, or the ways in which whole communities can suddenly cohere in, say, a conflict, or when snowed in by a severe winter, even after a great sporting success. Along with a group of colleagues, for instance, I am currently working on data showing that, in New Zealand, the day after the All Blacks won the 2015 Rugby World Cup, the quality of interactions, even with complete strangers at a bus stop or in a local shop (people one might have seen every day for years but never previously spoken to) became much more intimate and people felt far better for it.

If one could understand how this variability came about, if one could then harness it in order to create cohesive communities in which not only families, friends and acquaintances but also strangers come to constitute social capital, then one would not only have an explanation of the social bases of wellbeing, one would have a practical tool of inestimable worth to mental and physical wellbeing in society.

Conversely, it is arguable that our inability to understand when those people in our existing networks fail to sustain us, and when those outside do so, underlies the relative decline in social models of health over recent years and hence the urgent need to reinvigorate the field. We might have known for centuries that there is something that sometimes makes others sustain and complete us. That knowledge may have been massively reinvigorated by the work of Putnam and others, showing us that contemporary society, for all its technological advances (perhaps because of them), is in danger of destroying that precious something for all time. But still, there is very little one can do with this knowledge unless one can be precise about what that something is, and when it is effective. And if there is one thing worse than our models being wrong, it is for our models to be useless.

From Connectedness to Shared Social Identity

What is novel, and also useful, about the work presented in this book is not the stress on connectedness, but rather a model of what makes our connections into a valuable resource and hence when they are likely to support and sustain us. This model is rooted in the social identity approach to social psychology, which starts from the premise that the self is not single but multiple and not static but variable (Reicher et al., 2010b, Tajfel & Turner, 1986).

That is, if you ask anyone, 'Who are you'?, they are likely to respond with characteristics that render them individually distinctive (I am friendly, I have brown hair, etc.). But, they are also likely to respond with group memberships that render them collectively distinctive (I am a woman, I am British, etc.). The former, what makes 'I' distinct from 'you', is termed personal identity. The latter, what makes 'us' different from 'them', is termed social identity and we have many social identities deriving from the various categories to which we see ourselves as belonging.

What is more, these different elements of the self-system are more or less salient in different contexts. One may be walking down the road, psychologically separate from others, one's personal identity to the fore, then one sees a newspaper stand with yet more headlines about sexual harassment and one's gender identity comes to the fore, and soon after one passes a television store, showing images of Britain winning a medal at the Olympic Games, and gender gives way to national identity.

This leads to a simple but radical claim. The reason why the connection between self and other changes is rooted in the variability of selfhood. As an individual, I am disconnected from others in the street. In terms of gender identity, my self now encompasses other men and connects me to them. And, when I shift to national identity, I now feel connected to anyone, man or woman, supporting the national team; but disconnected from others, women as well as men, who cheer for another team.

Let me illustrate this with a very simple study that we conducted a number of years ago (Levine et al., 2005; Chapter 3 in this book). Manchester United football fans are brought into the laboratory, and we stress their Manchester United identity. We tell them that they need to go to another building and, as they walk there, they see someone running along, falling and clutching their knee in apparent agony. This person is wearing a Manchester United shirt, a Liverpool shirt or a plain red t-shirt. Do the fans provide help? Or do they walk on by? The results were clear. The participants help the person wearing a Manchester United shirt. They do not help the person wearing a Liverpool or plain red t-shirt. To generalise, they help the ingroup member to whom they are connected by a shared social identity.

What makes the study more interesting, though, is that we repeat it. Again, we use Manchester United fans who walk to another building and see someone wearing a Manchester United shirt, a Liverpool shirt or a red t-shirt fall and hurt themselves. This time, however, we have stressed their identity as football fans, not as Manchester United fans. The results are very different at a surface level. Now they help the person wearing a Manchester United or a Liverpool shirt, but not the person wearing a red t-shirt. But, the results are the same at an underlying process level. They help the ingroup member. But now the ingroup is more extended. As football fans, they now include the previously excluded Liverpool fans in their shared identity and that connection shapes their action.

Lest this study seems somewhat contrived, let me complement it with a personal anecdote. Many years ago, in 1996, I went to see England play Germany in the semi-finals of the European football championships. England lost on penalties, of course, and I missed my last train back to Exeter (where I then worked). I had to sleep the night on Paddington station – not a pleasant experience, especially when I saw various dubious-looking characters begin to prowl the concourse. But then, I noticed others on the station with football programmes in their pockets. And though they were people I might ordinarily run a mile from (no neck, no hair, but a lot of tattoos), now I felt a bond. As fellow England fans, I knew I could call on their help should anything happen. Any tension disappeared. The night passed well.

So, shared social identity creates connections, and transforms our social experience. As Hinemoa Elder puts it, in Chapter 10, referring to a very different context, it is through group processes that social capital is mobilised. Or rather, to be more precise, it is through group processes that social connections are created and made to constitute social capital.

Shared Identity and Human Flourishing

We have already begun to illustrate how shared social identity in groups not only creates functional connections, but also has transformative consequences for group members. Now let us build on the arguments of John Drury and colleagues in Chapter 15 by considering more systematically the transformations that come about when people see each other as belonging to the same social group and hence sharing the same social identity. As we shall see, these transformations are intimately connected to various basic features of the human condition as identified by Steven Smith in Chapter 2.

Cognitive Transformations

Early work in the social identity tradition, and especially work on *self-categorization* processes (Turner et al., 1987) focused on the cognitive consequences of group membership. These take two broad forms. On the one hand, there is a transformation in terms of content. Instead of acting on individual values, beliefs and interests, we act on the basis of collective values, beliefs and interests (Reicher, 1985). We see the world through the prism of collective representations of reality; our goals are framed by what is important to the group. Our interests are connected to the fate of the group rather than our own fate. As a consequence, people can be prepared to sacrifice their own benefit, at the extreme that they may even sacrifice their own lives, so that the group can thrive. In many ways, this is the most profound implication of the social identity approach. Rational actor theories presume that people act in order to maximise self-interest. Social identity theorists interject, 'Yes, but that doesn't get us very far unless we interrogate the self of self-interest'.

On the other hand, there is an ontological transformation. The glory of being human is that our relationship to reality is mediated through representations. That allows us to model the world, to plan ways of transforming it, and thereby have the potential to construct new worlds. The downside is that our grasp on reality is necessarily contingent and, critically, we are aware of this (Reicher, 2017). We know our perceptions and memories; our values and beliefs are contested and might be wrong. But through shared identity, we are able to reach consensus about the world (Haslam et al., 1997). This consensus is critical. It validates our positions. It removes our doubts. It transforms *individual opinions* into *social facts*. And such ontological security then provides a firm foundation for action.

Relational Transformations

In recent years, social identity research has increasingly addressed the ways in which shared identity affects relations between people. The helping experiments that I summarise above are one example of this, but they are but one example of a plethora of studies that show, among other things, that shared identity increases trust, respect and cooperation between people; it leads to enhanced social support and solidarity; it even leads to people preferring greater physical proximity and losing disgust at the smell of others (for reviews, see Haslam et al., 2011; Reicher & Haslam, 2010).

These last two findings are especially relevant in the light of Smith's comments on embodiment. When it comes to human relations, psychology tends to concentrate on what we think of each other. But this misses the fact that we are smelly, slimy creatures of blood, sweat and body odour. Being together or being apart depends as much on our ability to tolerate the embodied presence of others as on what we think of them. Disgust, in particular, is the great social ordering emotion: I might be able to stay in the same room as someone I despise, but proximity to someone whose sight and smell physically disgusts me is far more difficult. The point, then, is that shared social identity helps us to overcome disgust (Reicher et al., 2016).

This capacity for shared identity to produce relational transformations is critical. It allows people to come together, coordinate their actions and, thereby, become both individually and collectively empowered. Shared identity, in other words, gives people a sense of mastery over their world (Drury & Reicher, 2009).

The health implications of this came to us, or at least to me, almost by serendipity. Alex Haslam and I were involved in research that revisited Philip Zimbardo's famous Stanford

Prison Study. We created an environment in which Guards had multiple privileges, such as good food, leisure facilities and control over their environment, while Prisoners had to endure harsh conditions: basic rations, demeaning uniforms and being locked up in hot, cramped cells (Reicher & Haslam, 2006). To our surprise, though, it was the Guards, not the Prisoners, who were feeling stressed. It was the Guards, not the Prisoners, who were becoming burnt out.

When we looked closely, it became clear why. The Prisoners quickly formed a sense of shared identity. They worked together to undermine the Guards. And while, physically, they had much to endure, they had a strong sense of accomplishment in achieving their goals. Conversely, the Guards never cohered as a group. And though, individually, they worked just as hard as the Prisoners, they never aligned their efforts, serving instead to undermine each other and to cancel out each other's efforts. The harder they tried separately, the less they achieved together and the less they had a sense of being in control, or of coping. Whereas bonds of shared identity allowed the prisoners to flourish, the lack of them left the Guards broken and burnt out (Haslam & Reicher, 2006).

More recently, we have found equally striking phenomena in a real-life event. The Magh Mela at Allahabad, North India, is, arguably, the greatest collective phenomenon on Earth. It is a month-long Hindu festival that occurs each year, but which operates on a 12-year cycle. Every year, millions of pilgrims assemble for the month-long event. Every six years, tens of millions come, and it is claimed that, on the twelfth year, the Kumbh Mela, up to 100 million people come over the month, to bathe at the sacred confluence of the Ganges and Yamuna rivers.

Now, by every tenet of received wisdom, this event should be extremely bad for one's wellbeing and health. It is so densely crowded that it should create high levels of stress. It is so loud, that, according to World Health Organization (WHO) guidelines, 45 minutes of exposure should start to cause harm; and yet the noise continues for 24 hours a day, for the whole month. It is deeply unsanitary, with a basic sewage system and people relieving themselves all around the Mela site. Yet despite all this, people describe themselves as being serene. They find the noises soothing. The word they typically use to characterise their experience is 'anand' (bliss). And indeed, data from longitudinal matched samples show that their mental and physical wellbeing improves because of their participation. The same data explain why shared identity leads to people expecting social support from others and this, in turn, leads people to feel they can cope with the challenges of everyday life. The outcome is lowered stress along with enhanced wellbeing (Khan et al., 2015; Shankar et al., 2013; Tewari et al., 2012).

Here, we see clearly the way in which shared identity transforms other people from an impediment into an asset. John Bowlby's notion of a secure base refers to the way parenting gives a child confidence to go out and explore the world (Bowlby, 2008). Adapting from attachment theory, we can speak here of the way in which shared social identity constitutes *a socially secure base* whereby people can go out into the world with confidence, knowing that, if they encounter difficulties, others will help them in overcoming their challenges.

Emotional Transformations

Here again, shared identity produces two types of transformation. Thus, to start with, emotions are experienced in relation to what happens to the group rather than what happens to myself as an individual person. I can feel exhilarated at the accomplishments of a fellow group member (a Nobel prize, an Olympic gold, a winning goal) even if I had nothing to do with them at all. Equally I can feel shame and guilt at what my group has done to others (slavery, genocide) even if I had nothing to do with these acts and, indeed, even if they happened long before I was born (Branscombe & Doosje, 2004).

More interesting, however, given present concerns, is a second type of transformation. This has to do with that sense of excitement and exhilaration which, for many people, is the defining characteristic of group and, particularly, crowd, participation. Emile Durkheim captures the bubbling character of this feeling in the term effervescence (Durkheim, 1912).

Classically, psychology tends to see such strong emotions as a sign of a loss of identity and a loss of rationality in crowds: see, for instance, Gustave Le Bon's classic text, *The Crowd* (Le Bon, 1947; originally published in 1895). Emotions, then, substitute for the lack of ideas in the crowd. But, as should now be clear, social identity theorists argue that identity is not lost in a crowd but, rather, *shifts*. We start to act in terms of social, not individual or personal identity. What is more, as we have just been discussing, shared social identity allows people to converge on a common world view, it enables them to work together to advance that world view. These ontological and relational convergences empower people to achieve their goals; that is, to transform social-identity-based values and beliefs into lived reality. We refer to this as *collective self-realisation* (CSR; Khan et al., 2015).

Another way of looking at collective self-realisation is in terms of agency. It denotes the fact that people are creating their own social worlds rather than living in a world made by other people. That idea, and the understanding that agency, of this nature, is a collective accomplishment, is beautifully expressed by the great French historian Georges Lefebvre in his essay on crowds in the French revolution (Lefebvre, 1934). Perhaps it is only in the crowd, argues Lefebvre, that people lose their petty day-to-day concerns and become the subjects of history.

The subjects of history. The term is worth underlining and retaining. It is a rare and fleeting experience for most of us to be a subject of history. But it is truly exhilarating when that happens. I caught a glimpse of this long ago, back in 2005. Each year, I teach a crowd seminar to my students. And I tell them that they should experience the phenomenon before they study it. I tell them to attend a crowd event, any crowd event, before we start delving into the academic literature. In 2005, the students came back to the class and, when they explained their experiences, they had tears of joy in their eyes. They had attended a 'Make Poverty History' demonstration, which was a huge event in Edinburgh that coincided with the G8 summit that occurred in Scotland that year. I asked why they were so excited, so effervescent, one might say. They replied, 'for most of our lives, governments tell us what to do, but for once we were telling governments what to do'.

Of course, anecdotes are hardly definitive data. So, I return to the Magh Mela as the focus. My colleagues and I collected survey data during the event that showed a clear path from shared identity, to a sense of collective self-realisation, to extreme positive emotions (Hopkins et al., 2016). The joy of the crowd, then, is the joy of self-determining agency.

At one level, this accords with those liberal philosophies, which see this as the fullest expression of human potential and hence the highest expression of human flourishing (see Steven Smith on agency in Chapter 2). At another level it marks a decisive break with these philosophies by making it clear that certain accomplishments can only be achieved together through shared identity, rather than in isolation.

If we return to Broadie's account of the Scottish enlightenment with which I began, we can see that independence of thought meant challenging the power of traditional authority.

It was something impossible to do alone, either in terms of formulating alternatives or expressing them. Collectivity gave people the confidence to think differently. It gave them the power to talk openly without being crushed. The enlightenment worthies were able to think for themselves precisely because they thought, and talked, together.

Once more, a social identity analysis gives rise to a foundational argument: collectivity and individuality are not counterposed. Rather, they are interdependent. In a world where we are so often constrained by the power of others, it is only with collective support that we can act on our own terms and create social realities that reflect our own values.

Harnessing the Power of Groups: A Simple but Subversive Idea

The argument, thus far, can be summarised in a sentence: shared identity in social groups has the potential to improve our wellbeing and to allow us to flourish fully as human beings. The practical question becomes how to realise that potential. Such a message has both the benefits and the problems of simplicity. If it were really that straightforward, then why hasn't it been thought of before and implemented before? The answer is twofold. First, the notion that group psychology might be our most valuable asset goes against a culturally ingrained common sense, summarised by Rupert Brown as the idea that groups are bad for you (Brown, 1999; Spears, 2010). Second, it is the case that successful implementation of group-based strategies only works if one observes a series of key caveats. I deal with the former issue in this section and the latter in the next.

The notion that groups are bad for you is omnipresent in many different forms. Groups, we are told, diminish your intellect, destroy your judgement, blunt your morality and either lead you to do appalling things or else impede you from doing good things (Manning et al., 2007). In terms of health, we are told that groups, especially peer pressure in groups, leads you to take drugs, smoke and drink alcohol, to eat unhealthily and to take unwarranted risks (Hopkins, 1994).

Thus, for instance, we have described how events such as the Magh Mela can impact positively on health and wellbeing. We have published these findings in special issues of journals devoted to the new WHO specialism of mass gatherings medicine (Hopkins & Reicher, 2016). But our positive evidence goes very much against the grain of a specialism that was founded out of the fear that mass gatherings, such as the Hajj, would be the place where people from many countries come together, pass on infections, then go home to spark the global pandemic (see, for instance, the special collection of articles published online by *The Lancet* (2014)).

The roots of this negativity run very deep. Psychology, and social psychology in particular, emerged in the nineteenth century as a response to the growth of an industrialised mass society and the question of social order which it posed (Giner, 1976). The overwhelming fear was that the masses would reject the status quo and combine in order to overthrow it, and the crowd, the mass in action, constituted the sum of all these fears (Barrows, 1981). The power of crowds and the way they allow people to make their own history was not something to be celebrated but something either to be repressed or else channelled into safer passions such as nationalism. That was the project that motivated crowd scholars such as Gustave Le Bon, whose work we have already encountered.

But elite fear is not the only root of anti-collectivism. There is also the need for authorities to justify their own existence. The standard Hobbesian justification of government is that, left to themselves in a state of nature, people will not be able to create any functional society but will tear themselves apart. Therefore, it is worth their while to cede a little bit of their freedom and autonomy to a government that will then ensure the peace and order within which they can then live safely and thrive. The fundamental notion is that people are fragile and, especially in states of emergency, cannot look after themselves. They need the state and its agencies to look after them.

Not surprisingly, this ideology is at its clearest during emergencies (Tierney, 2003). There is concern about giving information about dangers to the public since they may not be able to cope with it and it could lead to panic. The overwhelming priority is to get emergency services, including first responders, to the situation as quickly as possible, in order to stablise the situation. And yet, as the work of John Drury and his colleagues has shown (see Chapter 17), it is lack of information which is the biggest cause of loss of life in emergencies. Moreover, as we have already seen, when emergencies do happen, it is normally the public themselves who act as first responders in supporting and sustaining each other. The emergency services, which are often taken aback by this self-organisation, can even disrupt and undermine it on the grounds that they alone are in a position to deliver succour. For all their remarkable heroism during 9/11, it is arguable that the firefighters who ran into the twin towers did more to get in the way than to help those people who were already self-organising their escape (Solnit, 2009).

My argument, and the argument of this book, is that the State and its services (including health services) should not ignore mutual support among ordinary people, but, instead, create the conditions under which it should thrive. In a slogan, policy and practice must orient to the need for scaffolding and not become a substitute for public self-help.

Thanks to the work of many authors of this book, this understanding is starting to gain traction among policymakers and practitioners. But there is still much further to go. And in seeking progress, we must be aware of multiple possible misunderstandings and resistances that derive from the profound extent to which the notion of 'scaffolding' reworks our understanding of state–society relations, demands a shift from paternalism to partnership and requires elites to trust the people.

Applying the Power of Groups: Six Conditions for Success

If the notion of scaffolding is to have impact, it is critical that we are precise about when and how groups improve health. There are many potential pitfalls in applying group psychology to benefit wellbeing, and many conditions for successful application. Here are some of the most important among them.

1. Maintain Conceptual Precision

It is essential to be clear about what we mean by a group. As we have stressed, our perspective is that a group is not simply a set of people who have historical links of kinship, friendship or acquaintance. It is a set of people who have a sense of shared identity, and it is this identity which not only creates bonds even with erstwhile strangers, but which unlocks the positive potential of these links. Shared identity creates the secure base that makes the world a more manageable place.

Accordingly, both in my own and my colleagues' studies and in our applications, we must be very careful not to over-extend the use of the term 'group' beyond this specific usage and, say, re-describe networks as groups. This would be an over-extension that dilutes the usefulness of our concepts. It undermines understanding of the processes that produce benefits. It is an act of hubris, and hubris destroys all empires, be they intellectual or geographical.

2. Interrogate Group Boundaries

If the benefits of group membership are a function of shared identity, it follows that they are unlikely to extend to people who are beyond the group boundary. This makes critical the definition of group boundaries. We have already seen, for instance, that when Manchester United fans define themselves in terms of support for the club rather than the sport, they ignore the plight of Liverpool fans. More relevantly, perhaps, we also find that, when Scots define their nationhood in ethnic terms, they do not come to the help of a young woman of Chinese descent though, when Scottishness is defined in civic terms, help is forthcoming (Wakefield et al., 2011).

Inclusiveness, then, is not only a matter of how we define 'them', and our stereotypes and prejudices about the other. It also, perhaps even more critically, depends upon how we define 'us'. And if we want communities in which all members gain from the many benefits of shared identity that are described in this book, it is critical to interrogate this definition carefully.

This is not just a matter of explicit pronouncements but also practices and policies that lead certain people to feel that they don't belong. They are often trivial (e.g. the timing of a meeting, the refreshments at a social event, the naming of a street or building) and the effects are unintentional, but that makes them, nonetheless, powerful in their exclusionary effects (Reicher et al., 2010a).

3. Interrogate Identity Content

In this chapter, I have been careful to stress the potential benefits of shared identity rather than suggest that shared identity always benefits our wellbeing. In the face of such strong messages in our culture (and also in the academic world) that groups are bad for you, it is easy to retort that, no, groups are good for you. But it is plainly not the case that this is always true. Indeed, it is easy to think of many occasions on which groups behave in appalling ways, from lynchings to Nuremburg rallies. But as John Drury et al. put it so well in Chapter 22, the problem here is not one of groupness per se but rather of the specific ideologies of specific groups. This means that, in order to understand the impact of any given group on wellbeing, we need to interrogate the content of an identity as closely as its boundaries.

Let me elaborate, because this point is pivotal. After the Kosovo conflict of 1998–1999, Blerina Kellezi and I examined the psychological effects of Kosovan war experiences. On the one hand, we found that group processes could buffer against extreme events such as losing a limb or losing a loved one. If the loss was sustained in a way that affirmed identity, notably in fighting the Serbian enemy, then it could be talked about, celebrated and commemorated with the support of others. But if the loss was sustained in a way that did not affirm identity, say in fleeing the enemy, then no such support and no such buffering occurred.

Still worse, if the loss was sustained in a way that undermines identity, most notably in the case of rape which sullied both the women themselves and the men who let it happen, then the victim was shamed, spurned and often excluded from the community. Here, the group process invoked a second insult, which compounded the effects of the original injury (Kellezi et al., 2009; Kellezi & Reicher, 2014).

Identity content, then, doesn't just shape the general norms that guide our behaviour. It shapes our interpretations and reactions to specific events, serving either to mitigate or accentuate their psychological impact as a function of relations of consonance or dissonance between the meaning of the event and the definition of identity.

4. Analyse Social Context

The more general point to be derived from the previous discussion in this chapter is that one cannot apply social identity processes to real-world settings, or determine their health effects, without considering the specific groups, specific identities and specific contexts involved. This is not true solely when it comes to the way that groups impact the content of our values, beliefs and interests. It is also true of all the psychological transformations that occur in the group. And, as in the case of content, the impact on wellbeing can be negative as well as positive.

Nick Hopkins and I have spelt this out, drawing on evidence from a range of mass gatherings (Hopkins & Reicher, 2017). Thus, when it comes to cognitive transformations, it is normative to eat a simple healthy diet at the Magh Mela, but it is normative to consume alcohol and drugs to excess at certain other gatherings, such as large music festivals. Relational transformations at the Hajj can lead to people helping each other in a gruelling climate, but, elsewhere, it may lead to unsafe sexual practices. And when it comes to affective transformations, this can enhance one's sense of mastery but, equally, can lead people to ignore ominous symptoms until it is too late.

All-in-all, social identity interventions can never take a one-size-fits-all approach. They require us to look closely at the social world and to take account of the key parameters that moderate the operation of psychological processes (for examples, see Haslam et al., 2018). Consequently, effective practitioners should be culturally as well as theoretically aware

5. Consistent Application

It is critical to align process and content if social identity interventions are to be effective. Often, though, this is not the case and, consequently, interventions are doomed before they even start. I offer an example. An attempt to foster green norms among staff at my own institution began with 'please switch off the light' stickers appearing in all our offices. This act felt like a violation of our own space by managers and led to the initiative being seen as an outgroup imposition rather than an expression of ingroup norms. This led to resistance even among those who were not averse to the content of the message.

In the same way, any group-based initiative must evolve from the ground up (one of the attractions of the scaffold metaphor is that scaffolding can never be built from the top down). Any attempts at producing change must pay heed to principles of influence and leadership that are aligned to, and informed by, knowledge of social identity theory (see Chapter 4). That is, the leader should preferably be seen to be of the group and must always be seen to be acting and achieving results for the group (Haslam et al., 2011).

But, consistency of application has another dimension. It is not just about what you do, but to whom you do it. Indeed, as Adrian Neal, Verity Kemp and Richard Williams suggest in Chapter 28, one won't get very far in providing care if one doesn't care for the carers, whether they are relatives, volunteers or professional practitioners. Still worse, if enhanced care for the general public places additional burdens on healthcare workers, imposes conditions of service that atomise them, stress them and undervalue them, they are unlikely to invest in these initiatives and the potential for abuse is likely to be increased.

The very same principles that have been discussed throughout this book, the need to: trust and respect people; support them; help them come together; and help each other must all be applied to healthcare staff. Sadly, the managerialist, target-driven ethos of the National Health Services in the UK, like that of other healthcare systems around the world, does not bode well in this respect.

6. Provide Adequate Funding

A few years ago, I was invited to participate in a joint workshop of the Economic and Social Research Council (ESRC) and Scottish Government on community resilience. When I got there, I realised that the clear context of the meeting was 'we are going to have to cut spending on local communities, so we want to know how you can be made to look after yourself'. The notion of building the self-organisation of communities went hand in glove with reducing public spending.

So, it is important to be absolutely clear, creating communities of shared identity is the *effective* option, but it will not be possible if it is seen as the *cheap* option. The concept of scaffolding is about redirecting, not reducing, spending. It is about providing the means for people to form their own groups, not leaving them alone. And that costs money. Small, but nonetheless significant, examples include people needing spaces in which they can come together. Inclusivity requires those spaces to be accessible, and heating, lighting and audio aids are necessary. Childcare support should be made available. People's different dietary requirements must be catered for. The list goes on. Moreover, the merest suspicion that scaffolding means cuts will ensure that it is seen as an attack on the community rather than community facilitation. All the good work in the world will be lost.

Conclusion

A couple of days ago, a colleague mentioned that he had seen an online video entitled 'Prof Steve Reicher explains social identity in just a minute (available at https://vimeo.com/224205888 if anyone is interested). He was very kind about it, but he did point out that it is 2 minutes 26 seconds long. Equally, I was asked to write this chapter in less than 6,000 words and I am already at 7,000. So, I apologise. Brevity is not my strong point. But I had better be brief in bringing this chapter to a close. Thankfully, though, that is easy, and I can summarise my argument in three points:

(1) Shared social identity in groups creates bonds between people and converts those bonds into social capital.

(2) The key to a new social model of mental and physical health lies in understanding how to support people in building and consolidating their own social groups.

(3) Projects with these objectives can only be successful if they integrate a knowledge of psychological principles with a cultural understanding of the social, institutional and political contexts in which they are to be applied.

If we address these three points, then we have a tool of immense power to improve wellbeing and enable people to realise their full potential. The remaining question is whether there is the will to do so.

References

Barrows, S. (1981). Distorting Mirrors. Newhaven, CT: Yale University Press.

Billig, M. (1987). Arguing and Thinking. Cambridge: Cambridge University Press.

Bourdieu P. (1986). The forms of capital. In Richardson, J. F., editor, Handbook of Theory of Research for the Sociology of Education. Santa Barbara, CA: Greenword Press, pp. 241–258.

Bowlby, J. (2008). A Secure Base: Parent–Child Attachment and Healthy Human Development. New York, NY: Basic Books.

Branscombe, N. R. & Doosje, B. (2004). Collective Guilt: International Perspectives. Cambridge: Cambridge University Press.

Broadie, A. (2007). The Scottish Enlightenment. Edinburgh: Birlinn.

Brown, R. (1999). Group Processes. Oxford: Blackwell.

Donne, J. (2018). Meditation XVII. See www.online-literature.com/donne/409/, accessed on 29 May 2018.

Drury, J. & Reicher, S. D. (2009). Collective psychological empowerment as a model of social change: Researching crowds and power. Journal of Social Issues, **65**: 707–725.

Durkheim, E. (1912). The Elementary Forms of Religious Life. Oxford: Oxford University Press (Oxford World Classics, 1988, Cladi, M. S., editor; translated by Cosman, C.).

Ellison, R. (1952). Invisible Man. New York, NY: Random House.

Giner, S. (1976). Mass Society. London: Martin Robertson.

Haslam, C., Jetten, J., Cruwys, T., Dingle, G. A. & Haslam, S. A. (2018). The New Psychology of Health: Unlocking the Social Cure. London: Routledge.

Haslam, S. A. & Reicher, S. D. (2006). Stressing the group: Social identity and the unfolding dynamics of responses to stress. Journal of Applied Psychology, **91**: 1037–1052.

Haslam, S. A., Reicher, S. D. & Levine, M. (2012). When other people are heaven, when other people are hell: How social identity determines the nature and impact of social support. In Jetten, J. Haslam, C. & Haslam, S. A., editors, The Social Cure: Identity, Health and Well-Being. Hove: Psychology Press, pp. 157–174.

Haslam, S. A, Reicher, S. D. & Platow, M. J. (2011). The New Psychology of Leadership. Hove: Psychology Press.

Haslam, S. A., Turner, J. C., Oakes, P. J., McGarty, C. & Reynolds, K. J. (1997). The group as a basis for emergent stereotype consensus. European Review of Social Psychology, **8**: 203–239.

Hopkins, N. P. (1994). Peer group processes and adolescent health-related behaviour: More than 'peer group pressure'? Journal of Community and Applied Social Psychology, **4**: 329–345.

Hopkins, N. P. & Reicher, S. D. (2016). Adding a psychological dimension to mass gatherings medicine. International Journal of Infectious Diseases, **47**: 112–116.

Hopkins, N. P. & Reicher, S. D. (2017). Social identity and health at mass gatherings. European Journal of Social Psychology, **47**: 867–877.

Hopkins, N. P., Reicher, S. D., Khan, S. S. et al. (2016). Explaining effervescence: Investigating the relationship between shared social identity and positive experience in crowds. Cognition and Emotion, **30**: 20–32.

Kellezi, B. & Reicher, S. D. (2014). The double insult: Explaining gender differences in the psychological consequences of war. Peace and Conflict: Journal of Peace Psychology, **20**: 491–504.

Kellezi, B., Reicher, S. D. & Cassidy, C. (2009). Surviving the Kosovo conflict: A study of social identity, appraisal of extreme events, and mental well-being. Applied Psychology, **58**: 59–83.

Khan, S. S., Hopkins, N. P., Reicher, S. D. et al. (2015). Shared identity predicts enhanced health at a mass gathering. Group Processes & Intergroup Relations, **18**: 504–522.

Le Bon, G. (1947). The Crowd: A Study of the Popular Mind. London: Ernest Benn (originally published in 1895).

Lefebvre, G. (1934). Foules revolutionnaires. Annales historiques de la revolution Francaise, **61**: 1–26.

Levine, M., Prosser, A., Evans, D. & Reicher, S. D. (2005). Identity and emergency intervention: How social group membership and inclusiveness of group boundaries shape helping behavior. Personality and Social Psychology Bulletin, **31**: 443–453.

Manning, R., Levine, M. & Collins, A. (2007). The Kitty Genovese murder and the social psychology of helping: The parable of the 38 witnesses. American Psychologist, **62**: 555–562.

Putnam, R. (2001). Bowling Alone: The Collapse and Revival of American Community. New York, NY: Simon and Schuster.

Reicher, S. D. (1985). The St. Pauls' riot: An explanation of the limits of crowd action in terms of a social identity model. European Journal of Social Psychology, **14**: 1–21.

Reicher, S. D. (2017). Biology as destiny or as freedom? On reflexivity, collectivity, and the realization of human potential. In Dovidio, J. & van Zomeren, M., editors, The Oxford Handbook of the Human Essence. Oxford: Oxford University Press, pp. 173–184.

Reicher, S. D. & Haslam, S. A. (2006). Rethinking the psychology of tyranny: The BBC prison study. British Journal of Social Psychology, **45**: 1–40.

Reicher, S. D. & Haslam, S. A. (2010). Beyond help. The psychology of prosocial behavior: Group processes, intergroup relations, and helping. In Sturmer, S. & Snyder, M. editors, The Psychology of Prosocial Behavior. Chichester: John Wiley & Sons, pp. 289–310.

Reicher, S. D., McCrone, D. & Hopkins, N. P. (2010a). A Strong, Fair and Inclusive National Identity: A Viewpoint on the Scottish Government's Outcome 13. Manchester: The Equality and Human Rights Commission.

Reicher, S. D., Spears, R. & Haslam, S. A. (2010b). The social identity approach in social psychology. In Wetherell, M. & Mohanty C., editors, Sage Identities Handbook. London: Sage, pp. 45–62.

Reicher, S. D., Templeton, A., Neville, F., Ferrari, L. & Drury, J. (2016). Core disgust is attenuated by ingroup relations. Proceedings of the National Academy of Sciences, **113**: 2631–2635.

Shankar, S., Stevenson, C., Pandey, K. et al. (2013). A calming cacophony: Social identity can shape the experience of loud noise. Journal of Environmental Psychology, **36**: 87–95.

Solnit, R. (2009). A Paradise Built in Hell: The Extraordinary Communities That Arise in Disaster. New York, NY: Viking.

Souief, A. (2012). Cairo: My City, Our Revolution. London: Bloomsbury.

Spears, R. (2010). Group rationale, collective sense: Beyond intergroup bias. British Journal of Social Psychology, **49**: 1–20.

Tajfel, H. & Turner, J. C. (1986). The social identity theory of intergroup behavior. In Worchel, S. & Austin, W. G., editors, Psychology of Intergroup Relations, Chicago: Nelson-Hall, pp. 7–24.

Tewari, S., Khan, S. S., Hopkins, N. P., Srinivasan, N. & Reicher, S. D. (2012). Participation in mass gatherings can benefit well-being: Longitudinal and control data from a North Indian Hindu pilgrimage event. PLoS One, **7**: e47291.

The Lancet (2014). Mass gatherings medicine. The Lancet, 21 May. See www.thelancet.com/series/mass-gatherings-medicine).

Tierney, K. (2003). Disaster beliefs and institutional interests: Recycling disaster myths in the aftermath of 9–11. In Clark, L., editor, Terrorism and Disaster: New Threats, New Ideas. Bingley: Emerald Group Publishing Limited, pp. 33–51.

Turner, J. C., Hogg, M. A., Oakes, P. J., Reicher, S. D. & Wetherell, M. (1987). Rediscovering the Social Group. Oxford: Blackwell.

Wakefield, J. R., Hopkins, N. P., Cockburn, C. et al. (2011). The impact of adopting ethnic or civic conceptions of national belonging for others' treatment. Personality and Social Psychology Bulletin, **37**: 1599–1610.

Chapter 24

Public Health Values and Evidence-Based Practice

Jonathan Montgomery and Richard Williams

The Public Nature of Health

The foci of this book are on the social determinants of health, and the importance to our health of our social connectedness and social support that turn on shared social identities. In Chapter 23, Reicher surveys these matters and makes three important concluding points. First, shared social identity in groups creates bonds between people and converts those bonds into social capital. Second, he asserts that the key to a new social model of mental and physical health lies in understanding how to support people in building and consolidating their own social groups. But, importantly, he also points out that social identity can work for good outcomes but also for those that are seen as less positive. Thus, his third concluding point is that projects with the objectives of supporting people to achieve positive outcomes can only be successful if they integrate a knowledge of psychological principles with a cultural understanding of the social, institutional and political contexts in which they are to be applied.

In Chapter 12 in Section 2, one of us (JM) considers values in relation to tolerance of different ideas. But, Reicher's third conclusion about effectively applying the important constructs that run through this book raises the importance of our revisiting values, but with a societal focus this time. So, we turn here to consider the resources that can be drawn from public health ethics and practice in understanding how health can be sustained, and also recovered, in the face of shocks and challenges to wellbeing at community level. Public health ethics is a complex area, and a social focus has recently emerged, bringing to the fore 'concepts of group, community, population, public goods, common goods, solidarity, reciprocity, welfare, well-being and justice', which provide a 'substantive' approach that transcends the modified liberal approaches that have been dominant (Dawson, 2011).

As in Chapters 15, 17, 22 and 23, there is a substantial focus throughout this book in reframing or challenging, as appropriate, frequently repeated myths about the power and risks of groups. Therefore, we begin this chapter by comparing what is implied by the oft-misunderstood terms, *common good* and *collective good*. In this respect, we take up the challenge identified by Steve Reicher. He identifies that scaffolding has to be bottom-up. By implication, the conception of social scaffolding, which this book crystallises in Chapter 25, sets out to enable and support people who wish to work in coproductive relationships with members of the public to improve services for them. So, in endeavouring to bring culture and values into conjunction with social connectedness and social support and provide a solid base for social scaffolding, we explore, albeit briefly, matters of public trust in experts and public decision-making. We identify the values and three key issues that are explicit and, more often, implied in creating a framework for public health ethics. We think such a framework must accompany our application of the lessons for health and social care that flow through this book from people's potent shared identities with the many groups of which they are members. Then, we illustrate these matters in action by describing how a group created a framework for the UK of public health ethics for pandemic influenza with a view to influencing and supporting policymakers. It has been tested in action.

Common Good or Collective Good?

The essence of the core question for public health ethics can be captured in understanding how concepts of the common good relate to those of the collective good.

The common good captures those elements of our interests that we all share. Defining such goods precisely is challenging. Coggon offers discussion of various approaches to giving definition to this idea (Coggon, 2012, pp. 170–183). However, the basic idea is easily grasped. We all share, for example, an interest in basic securities in relation to food, shelter and safety. It follows that we have an equal interest in participating in those goods and that society should be organised in a way that secures these common goods for all. This is not easy, and may require hard choices to be made. However, there is a mutuality about the common good that gives citizens an equal stake in making those decisions.

The idea of the common good is not to be confused with the way in which the concept of 'public good' is used by economists to describe goods that everyone can enjoy in common, because their use does not reduce the possibility of others enjoying them too (for example, breathing air). Technically, they are described as 'non-rivalrous' goods because people are not in competition for them. This terminology is used to distinguish public from private goods, which are goods that individual persons benefit from using, to the exclusion of others. In this usage, while food security is something for which we all have a common need, food itself is a rivalrous good because it must be consumed by some persons, and, therefore, not by others, if the common need for nutrition is to be satisfied. Food security requires a distribution system that provides it to people for their personal use. The element of commonality is that everyone has the same claim to the provision of food security because all require food to live, not that they are all entitled to the same meal. It is, therefore, doubtful that public health interventions are properly described as concerned with 'public goods' in this technical sense (O'Neill, 2011). Rather, they raise questions about the appropriate allocation of resources.

It is also important to distinguish the commonality of the interests that we share from the idea that society's collective health and wealth can be increased through the way in which it is organised and governed. We all benefit from stability in the social, economic and political institutions of our community. However, the interests that we have in common can sometimes be overtaken by the good of society as a whole. This is because the collective good can sometimes be pursued in ways that sacrifice individual interests in order to secure or maximise these wider benefits.

This is, in part, an issue about aggregation – the way in which assessing net benefits does not properly take into account the fairness of distribution. This is one of the common criticisms of utilitarian theory – the pursuit of the greatest good for the greatest number. However, we should also remember that even the poorest people in society might be better off if the society in which they live is more productive and functions better than a state of anarchy. John Rawls captures this idea within liberal political philosophy in his argument that we should aim to improve the position of the least advantaged members of society and that inequality could be justified if it delivered such improvements (Rawls, 1971). If this were achieved, then even resource-poor people might have reasons to accept their position in an unequal society because they would be better off in absolute terms. An example of this was the claimed 'trickle down' effect of neoliberal economics, which has not shown in practice the effect that was claimed for it in relation to poor people (Stiglitz, 2012, pp. 6–7). It is unreasonable to expect people to trust the institutions that oversee these kinds of choice and accept the outcomes of their decisions when they do not appear to be in the public's immediate interests, unless everyone has a stake in those decisions about resource allocation.

We should aim to secure fundamental common interests for everyone and to ensure equal participation in them. Pursuing the collective good beyond this may be politically and ethically attractive, but should not be at the cost of these basic interests. This approach can be explored through the idea of the human right to health. However, it should be noted that, in a holistic assessment of people's needs, we must mitigate against the risks of inappropriate medicalisation that might occur if we give automatic priority to a narrow conception of people's health needs over other aspects of human life. This point resonates with the points made by Smith in Chapter 2.

Achieving the Common Good

Rather, achieving the common good for people's health is understood by the World Health Organization (WHO) to require three types of state responsibility. The first is to *respect* people's health rights by refraining from interfering with their opportunities to enjoy good health. The second is to *protect* people's health from being compromised by the actions of others, including organisations. Most important for our concerns is the third category of responsibility, which is to *fulfil* the right to health by taking positive steps to ensure that it is realized (WHO, 2008). Concerns that ambiguous definitions of health can undermine this realisation have been addressed by considering state obligations as requiring the *progressive realisation* of the right to health (General Comment 14, adopted at the Twenty-second Session of the Committee on Economic, Social and Cultural Rights, 11 August 2000 – see Wolff, 2012, especially chapter 2) Thus, states are held to account in human rights law for their efforts towards continuous improvement in fulfilling their citizens' health rights.

The idea of the human right to health roots our concerns in the value of public health to individual persons, not merely aggregated groups. However, the idea of the collective good is superficially attractive when considered from a public health perspective, and is intrinsic in working to maximise the efficient use of resources through health technology assessments, such as that undertaken in the UK by the National Institute for Health and Care Excellence (NICE) to determine whether interventions are clinically and cost effective. Here, the interests of the community are taken as a whole. One objective might be to secure the maximum net aggregated benefit for the members of the community. In the classic utilitarian tradition, this is formulated as to promote the greatest good for the greatest number. Such an approach pays little attention to the way in which those benefits are distributed to individual persons and struggles to take into account the problems created by inequality. This approach seems committed to two unsatisfactory positions.

The first is that an unequal distribution of goods is actually desirable if the aggregate welfare is increased and that this principle holds even if some people are sacrificed to achieve a net gain. This seems incompatible with our idea of human rights (Hart, 1983). The demands of *respect* and *protection* of human beings' rights to health provide side constraints which preclude the pursuit of collective gains that infringe people's health rights. Thus, a core entitlement to a basic standard of health must be protected against being traded off for collective benefit (Tasioulas, 2017a, b).

The second unsatisfactory position that utilitarian aggregation adopts is that we cannot rationally choose between different patterns of distribution that have the same net effect. However, there is, as this book shows, compelling evidence now that inequality is itself associated with poor health and other costs to society (Stiglitz, 2012, Wilkinson & Pickett, 2009). It turns out that interventions that seek to reduce inequality benefit all members of society, even those who are comparatively advantaged and, in that sense, distributive justice is something in which we have a common interest.

We have also seen how important social identity is in securing sustainable good health, including mental health. We should consider how we secure the participation of everyone in the good society and not merely enhance net outcomes, and thereby reduce the alienation that comes from individuals feeling that they have no stake in governance. Pursuing the aggregate collective good without regard for these constraints provides little reason for those people who feel disadvantaged to accept the value of public health action. An inclusive society is, thus, more likely to be a resilient one.

There are other important strands of thinking about the collective good that should not be abandoned because of our concerns about unconstrained utilitarianism. One emphasises the need for collective action to achieve individual or common goods (for example, pollution control, and security of access to water, food and energy). Here, our interests are necessarily public in nature because they require collective action (Dawson, 2011). Another focuses on the importance of the institutions of society in conserving the public good, including over time. We have already explored some elements of this in the discussion of tolerance in Chapter 12. In this chapter, we are more concerned with the resilience of such institutions in the face of challenges to public health rather than communal values.

We have in mind a range of such challenges. Some could be considered as 'shocks': public health emergencies such as disease outbreaks, including pandemics, and terrorist attacks using biological and chemical agents. Here, the collective good may require not just the unequal distribution of benefits, but also the unequal allocation of burdens to promote the collective needs of society. This requires us to explain how differential responsibilities relate to our common interests in a resilient and well-ordered society when the longer-term perspective is adopted. Such 'shocks' also tend to exacerbate pre-existing vulnerabilities (Buccieri & Gaetz, 2013; Kaposy & Bandrauk, 2012; Lee et al., 2008), and sound public policy would need to mitigate the risks of cumulative injustices.

We can also learn from public health ethics about how we should best make anticipatory decisions about interventions that are aimed at promoting more resilient societies and conditions in which good health, including mental health, can more easily be sustained. Typically, decisions such as these are taken in conditions of considerable uncertainty. Yet, they may create significant 'path dependencies', which may lock societies onto a direction of travel that then excludes potential alternatives (Nuffield Council on Bioethics, 2012). When evidence is uncertain, the scope is increased for decision-making to be adversely affected by heuristic biases (Gluckman, 2016), and good processes are essential to reduce the risks of poor decisions that have far-reaching consequences.

Questions of Trust

Evidence-Based and Expert Decision-Making

A particular anxiety has arisen in contemporary societies that are technologically developed about trusting evidence-based and expert decision-making. Both individual persons and professional practitioners are liable to privilege experience from those known to them over scientific evidence, and to suspect that evidence to be compromised by conflicts of interest (Academy of Medical Sciences, 2017). Public health ethics has been required to address problems of trust, of various forms. One is distrust of the reliability of expert evidence, such as was observed in the face of bovine spongiform encephalopathy (BSE) and Creutzfeldt–Jakob disease (CJD) (Phillips, 2000), the anti-MMR (measles, mumps and rubella) campaign, as well as, more generally, the anti-VAXX movement. Another is distrust of public institutions to be competent (linked with, but not limited to, the expertise problem), non-discriminatory and focused on the public interest rather than corrupt or self-serving activity.

Stewardship of Health Data

Particular issues are arising currently in relation to the stewardship of health data. Anxieties about personal privacy and commercial exploitation are in tension with the public interest in using data to support sound epidemiology, rational resource allocation and maximising the opportunities of 'big data' techniques in planning and research. Public health practice is experienced at seeking to reconcile these competing interests to accommodate legitimate concerns without failing in the obligation of progressive realisation of health rights.

Social Licence and Legitimacy

Trust can be understood as a socio-psychological phenomenon. It can easily be lost, as in the case of the UK when a poorly managed programme for bringing health data together forfeited the 'social licence' required for it to be accepted (Carter et al., 2015). Rebuilding trust in such a sense requires a form of social contract in which all can see the benefits that they will gain from collaboration (Academy of Medical Sciences, 2015; Lucassen et al., 2017). However, rebuilding trust is not, in itself, an appropriate objective because it may be no more than a form of deceit.

Just as importantly, trust is a matter of legitimacy. It would be inappropriate to invite people to trust in institutions that are not, in fact, trustworthy. Public health practice has needed to develop ways of demonstrating the legitimacy of decision-making in the face of commercial hostility (e.g. the experience of NICE) and unsympathetic political ideology (HIV/AIDS). The key elements of trustworthiness in public decision-making have been articulated by Onora O'Neill in terms of competence, reliability and honesty (O'Neill, 2002). Institutions that are responsible for public decision-making should acquire these virtues and also demonstrate that they have them so that other people and organisations can place their trust in the decisions that are made.

Recognising the importance of trustworthiness is important, but it remains at a formal rather than substantive level. As Onora O'Neill has pointed out, it is irrational to consider whether to place trust in a person or institution without regard to the particular tasks that they are undertaking. Although we sometimes talk about whether we trust, or not, people in the abstract, this is a dangerous tendency that undermines sound decision-making. It is rational to trust a Hollywood star to turn in a good acting performance, but it is not rational to place trust in her as a scientific expert. We must, therefore, elaborate a sense of the task that is in issue before questions of trust can properly be considered. Where the task is thought to require promotion of the common good, then we also need to explore the values that are involved in that pursuit.

Values in Public Health Ethics

These problems of legitimacy are particular examples of the challenges of promoting the public good through collective and individual action. As it was put by the Nuffield Council on Bioethics (2007) in its report, *Public Health Ethics* (paragraph 1.21)

> the collective efforts of all parts of society, including individuals, healthcare professionals, industries, urban planners, health policy and other policy makers and politicians, should contribute to generating and supporting measures that improve the health of all.

Sometimes, as, for example, in relation to vaccinations, we ask individual people to accept a personal burden in the interests of the community as a whole. Sometimes, individual persons or groups are particularly well-placed to carry out work in the wider interests of communities; perhaps, because they undertake essential activities (such as securing energy supplies or clean water) or because they have skills that are particularly vital in the face of specific threats (such as health professionals in a disease outbreak). People may be called upon to work in ways that may be in tension with their own self-interest in order to promote public health.

In a resilient society, people tend to perceive little tension between the collective good and their common benefits from community membership. There will, then, be good reasons for people to accept particular burdens because they believe they will be engaged in promoting the common good from which they all ultimately gain. This requires widespread trust that collective actions are orientated to promote the common good, that everyone's interests are duly taken into account and that differential treatment is not a mark of people being less valued.

The problems that occur when this trust breaks down can be illustrated by experiences in the USA when faced by terrorist attacks (Anthrax in 2001) and infectious diseases (Ebola in 2014–16). In each case, suspicion and stigma led to victimisation of those people who were perceived to be associated; with reports that physicians refused to treat, employers prevented employees from working, schools turned away children (Kayman et al., 2009; Malecki, 2001; US Presidential Commission for the Study of Bioethical Issues, 2015). The risks run by health practitioners who deployed in the Ebola crisis is a good example. A number of healthcare staff reported being shunned rather than being supported by colleagues, because of people's fears, after they returned home from the deployment. This increased the burden on people who put themselves at risk altruistically. There was a report of two Senegalese–American children being beaten up by their peers (US Presidential Commission for the Study of Bioethical Issues, 2015, p. 11).

Three Key Issues

The Role of the State: Beyond Libertarianism

The dominant principlist tradition of medical ethics has been highly individualised and the suggestion of community obligations has been seen as an intrusion into patients' rights. This reluctance to entertain collective action for the common good is amplified by well-recognised cognitive biases and widespread scepticism about expertise. Thus, the immediate loss of freedom that comes from pressure to vaccinate is more keenly felt than the nebulous gain that will come from a society becoming free from an infectious disease. Actions in the collective good are seen, from this perspective, as infringements of individual freedom, which require strong justifications. This may reflect the origins of this approach in the USA, where government is regarded with more suspicion than in mainland European traditions.

The UK has found itself between these positions, and, in relation to public health ethics, this has been articulated as a modified liberalism under the banner of the 'stewardship state' (Nuffield Council on Bioethics, 2007). In this model, states are held to have obligations to look after people's important health needs, both individually and collectively, by providing the conditions for good health and taking measures to reduce health inequalities. However, they should not coerce people into living healthy lives, they should seek mandates (individual or community consents) and they should avoid unduly intrusive interventions. 'The stewardship-guided state recognises that a primary asset of a nation is its health: higher levels of health are associated with greater overall well-being and productivity' (Nuffield Council on Bioethics, 2007, p. xvii).

An infrastructure for public health is, thus, a common good from which we all stand to benefit. It is consistent with the obligation to fulfil the right to health. Well implemented, it can prove trustworthy, but this requires consideration of what it sets out to do (i.e. those interventions it seeks to make) and how it goes about selecting them.

The Ethics of Interventions

We have seen how the importance of public health cannot justify interventions merely because they are likely to improve net outcomes. The protection of individual liberty is important and many theorists promote the idea that the least restrictive or intrusive interventions should be adopted. In this vein, the Nuffield Council on Bioethics offered a heuristic of an 'intervention ladder' in which less intrusive interventions were preferred to more intrusive ones (Nuffield Council on Bioethics, 2007, paragraphs 3.37–3.38). However, as Dawson (2016) has pointed out, this tool only operates along the dimension of liberty and does not assist with balancing concerns about liberty against the other values that public health ethics introduce.

Other proper concerns of public health ethics, such as reducing inequality or protecting those people who are at particular risk and/or unable to protect themselves, may require more intrusive interventions and the metaphor of the ladder does not assist decisions that involve trading liberty off against these other values (Dawson, 2016). Faust and Upshur (2009, p. 274) add a principle of proportionality as a way of ensuring that the benefits outweigh any 'moral infringement', as broadly understood, that they involve, which is less rigid as a tool for evaluation.

There are a number of other values that are important in public health ethics. They include questions of evidence, such as that on the effectiveness of interventions. This can be challenging during public health emergencies not only because of the limitations of the available evidence, but also because of difficulties in making decisions when we are faced with uncertainty. Decisions in these circumstances are likely to be acutely affected by cognitive biases; such as aversion against loss, familiarity and confirmation bias, and the tendency to maintain the status quo (Gluckman, 2016, Part 2, chapter 2). They also bring to the fore tensions between public and expert decision-making. Thus, technically similar risks may appear outrageous to members of the public when they involve features such as lack of control over exposure, unfair distribution, human-made rather than 'natural', unfamiliarity, dread (i.e. anticipatory fear of future harm), or when hazards are concentrated into time and specially limited events (Sandman, 1989).

Of particular importance to this conversation is the notion of 'solidarity' or 'fraternity'. The Nuffield Council preferred to formulate this as a value of 'community', which it defines as 'the value of belonging to a society in which each person's welfare, and that of the whole community, matters to everyone' (Nuffield Council on Bioethics, 2007, paragraph 2.34).

Dawson and Verweu (2012) have argued that solidarity can take two forms. 'Rational solidarity' offers citizens reasons to 'stand together' in order to address a common threat or to secure a collective benefit. 'Constitutive solidarity' is different: 'a social concept: a function of shared values, meaning and identify' (Dawson and Verweu, 2012, p. 2). It can be seen that choosing public health interventions on the basis of rational solidarity can easily focus on the collective good, with inadequate recognition of distributive values. The philosophical idea of the common good can be linked with the development of a constitutative solidarity, and societies that can address shocks from such a foundation are likely to prove more resilient. Therefore, in pursuing collective or community resilience, the ethics of interventions need to be connected to the sense of community. This is best achieved by creating decision-making processes so as to ensure that the values that underpin choices are broadly accepted by the relevant society.

Good Decision-Making

The most discussed framework for public health decision-making is probably Norman Daniels' 'accountability for reasonableness' (Daniels, 2000, 2008). This requires decisions to be accountable, inclusive, open and transparent, reasoned and responsive (Daniels, 2000). Faust and Upshur draw attention to the importance of public justification and transparency in ensuring that there is public deliberation on the principles and policies before they are enshrined in legislation, and that there is public articulation of reasons for infringements, to show that they are consistent with the values that have emerged from those deliberative processes (Faust & Upshur, 2009, p. 275). This requires a blend of process and substantive values.

The aspiration to good decision-making can be operationalised in two main ways. First, by focusing on actions that are being contemplated and exploring the basis for choosing between them. Grill and Dawson (2015) advocate such a model, based on five steps:

(1) Identifying relevant options;
(2) Distinguishing the relevant empirical differences between the options;
(3) Ranking the options from best to worst;
(4) Evaluating explicitly the senses in which some are better than others; and
(5) Submitting a documented assessment to a designated oversight institution.

This approach assumes that some values have been established to guide decision-making, but it is not, in itself, committed to a particular set. Rather, it describes a process that is designed to ensure that decision-making is both values-based and evidence-based. It provides a practical approach to integrating both substantive and procedural values with the careful consideration of evidence in the light of available options. It also allows for that fact that values are necessarily rooted in particular communities, that they are not arbitrary but can, and should, be subjected to critical scrutiny. Grill and Dawson's final step draws attention to the importance of sponsorship from a legitimate authority (Grill & Dawson, 2015), and this point is also made by Thompson et al. (2006).

The second approach is to begin with an actual or anticipated challenge and to reflect on the values that might be at stake. This can be done in a way that generates a statement of those values that can then, in turn, be used as a measure against which to assess planning decisions. Such an approach recognises that new social shocks may require new thinking about values as well as merely extrapolating from existing statements. But it also recognises the importance of solidarity around a values-based social identify. You might say, it is a mechanism for enabling communities to remain true to the 'better selves' of members (the community that they would like to be, having reflected on what they stand for) in the face of threats which might lead them to abandon the very values that they share and which constitute them. We now turn to a practical example of engagement with these key problems and, thereby, to operationalise public health ethics in preparation for anticipated flu pandemics. This concerns our experience of being part of the group charged with creating and implementing an ethical framework for the UK's preparations for pandemic flu.

Operationalising the Principles: The CEAPI Ethical Framework for Responding to Pandemic Influenza

Ethical Governance

Operationalising good public health practice depends, in part, of the nature of the challenge. Coggan et al. (2017) identify a number of dimensions of ethical governance. This chapter has already explored one of them, the focus on *ethical justification*, which is, 'a generalised account of what kinds of institutions, policies, or actions are ethical' (Coggan et al., 2017, p. 30). We now turn to consider how this might be operationalised in a more specific context and we use to illustrate this the ethical framework for pandemic planning that the UK developed in 2007 and with which we were both involved.

Coggon et al. also draw attention to the differences between possible aims in operationalising ethics (Coggan et al., 2017, pp. 30–31). One is to *increase ethical awareness*, so that actors can be prompted to overcome their cognitive and affective biases. A second is *ethical action guidance*, for which the objective is to prescribe behaviours that have been identified to lead to the desired objectives. The third is an approach that is intended to promote *ethical deliberation*, by education or codifying values that should be brought to bear.

The UK's Committee on Ethical Aspects of Pandemic Influenza

These distinctions are helpful to make sense of the work of the UK's Committee on Ethical Aspects of Pandemic Influenza (CEAPI), which we use to illustrate how public health values can be integrated with scientific knowledge to support evidence-based practice and, thereby, also support resilience and sustainable good health in the face of socially disruptive challenges.

The need for anticipatory governance in this field was identified in many countries (Thompson et al., 2006), and the UK's experience provides a useful case study in its operation. The work was aimed at elaborating a set of public health ethics principles and 'hard-wiring' them into institutional decision-making. An invited group of 'experts' was convened by the Department of Health in England, in response to a request from the Cabinet Office in the UK, in order to draw up an ethical framework to guide the planning processes that were being established to help the UK prepare for an anticipated pandemic. Some members of that group held expertise in ethics and law, but the majority were drawn from those experienced in the services that might be engaged in responding to a pandemic, including from the public and private care sectors and from trades unions. There were also members who were involved with healthcare ethics as lay representatives.

Three Dimensions of CEAPI's Work

The work of the Committee proceeded through three broad dimensions, overlapping in terms of time. First, there was deliberation within the group to develop a draft ethical framework. This required the creation of a 'public' rather than private ethical position, through a collegiate exploration of the anticipated challenges and the articulation of what was at stake and how it might be adequately protected. Individual members had to accept some degree of compromise in order to reach a consensus on how best to guide public decision-making (Montgomery, 2013). The aim was to produce a framework that reflected international learning, but was also sensitive to the cultural and institutional context in which decisions would be taken for the UK. In the process of doing so, the Committee established a common set of values and became a 'group' that shared an identity in the sense described by Reicher in Chapter 23.

The second dimension, validation of that framework through consultation with public and professional groups, involved the Committee in working through case-study scenarios, to elaborate and improve the principles. This ensured that the principles resonated with a wider group of stakeholders and also served to increase their ethical awareness. This work provoked some healthy and, sometimes, robust debate, especially about prioritisation in relation to intensive care facilities, and over the relevance of age in that process. It also exposed an important issue about the role of ethical action guidance. A number of professional groups felt critical that the ethical framework was insufficiently precise to guide their actions. These critics wanted ethical action guidance to determine decisions and to absolve the decision-makers from the need to exercise their own judgement. The Committee deliberately resisted this objective as it believed that resilience in a pandemic required thinking to be flexible and adaptive. In its view, the purpose of the framework was to support ethical thinking. If action guidance became rigid and determinative, it would replace the exercise of judgement with a regime of compliance with rules.

Rather than determining outcomes, the framework was intended to provide a measure against which policies and decisions could be considered. This constituted the third dimension of its work: applying the framework to emerging policy documents. These policies were considered by the Committee in draft form, with a view to ensuring that the planning framework was consistent with the ethical principles that had been adopted. It was a matter of some satisfaction to members of the Committee when commentators made a favourable comparison between the, positively received, prescription of the policy documents and the vagueness of the ethical framework, which was disliked. In the view of the Committee, the former was achieved because of the latter. Later, the wisdom and experience of the Committee members was made available to support Ministerial and Departmental decision-makers during the pandemic of 2009–2010. This did not remove their democratic responsibility, but was a resource that was available to confirm consistency with the ethical framework (Department of Health, 2010, paragraph 33). The Hine Review into the handling of the 2009–2010 pandemic highlighted the importance of the CEAPI approach and concluded that 'it would have been very difficult to reach a consensus over the ethical issues concerned in the heat of a pandemic response' (Hine, 2010, paragraph 6.62). In effect, this third dimension ensured the integration of the three functions that Coggon et al. identified (Coggan et al., 2017).

These process elements of public health ethics in operation are possibly as important as the substance of the principles that were set out in the CEAPI framework (Department of Health, 2007). However, we have also found that those principles have proved themselves adaptable to a number of policy contexts and conclude that they have merit beyond the specific pandemic context.

The Fundamental Principle

The fundamental principle that underpinned the planning framework was *equal concern and respect*. This principle aimed to recognise that social solidarity would be forfeit if any members of society felt that their interests were being disregarded. But, provided they were confident that they were not being excluded from proper consideration, then it was anticipated that citizens would accept that differential treatment would be necessary to promote the collective good. The CEAPI framework explained the meaning of this principle in the following terms:

- Everyone matters.
- Everyone matters equally – but this does not mean that everyone is treated the same.
- The interests of each person are the concern of us all, and of society.
- The harm that might be suffered by every person matters, and so minimising the harm that a pandemic might cause is a central concern.

This formulation aims to ensure that the common and collective goods are held together, and not permitted to come into conflict, by ensuring that an individual person's interests cannot be sacrificed to the collective good. Differential treatment at a particular time might be acceptable if a longer time perspective shows how it does not constitute a devaluing of individual persons' value. However, it is only reasonable to expect people to accept this if they have reasons to be confident that their interests are being respected, and that the response to shocks is based on solidarity rather than separation.

Honouring the Fundamental Principle

The CEAPI framework sought to flesh out what would be required to ensure that this fundamental principle was honoured by elaborating eight further principles, which, if kept in mind, would help to ensure that planning was ethically defensible. Five of these principles could be described as ethical orientations, the substantive aims that would need to be pursued, and the remaining three as concerning the process values that should underpin ethical planning.

Ethical Orientations

Respect

Respect means recognising people's agency; keeping them informed, enabling them to express views, respecting choices as far as possible while recognising and being open about the fact that it might not be possible to provide all the treatments that they might like or which might benefit them during a pandemic, and recognising the full range of their interests if they cannot make decisions for themselves.

Harm Minimisation

Harm minimisation recognises that harm (broadly understood, so as to include adverse physical, social and economic effects) is inevitable, but that the impact of a pandemic can be reduced. The framework illustrated steps that might be taken in order to pursue this principle in terms of global actions to: prevent spread in and from other countries; reduce contagion, reduce the impact and complications of infection (e.g. through the use of antiviral medication); and minimise social disruption, which may be as harmful as the disease itself.

Fairness

Fairness generally requires that people who have an equal chance of benefiting from health or social care resources should have an equal chance of receiving them. Some approaches to harm minimisation might be unfair if they do not reflect the fact that everyone matters equally. Where some people are treated differently to others, the reasons for doing so should be explained so that it can be seen that the differences are fair.

Reciprocity

Reciprocity might provide one example of such a reason. The Committee used this term to capture the mutuality of obligations between members of society, and, in particular, the fact that it would be wrong to ask some members of that society to take on greater risk or burdens without accepting a responsibility in planning to minimise them, so far as is practicable.

Proportionality

Proportionality requires that actions that affect people's lives, such as 'social distancing' strategies that limit people's freedoms in order to reduce transmission risks, should ensure that the risks are proportionate to the anticipated benefits.

Process Values

Elements of the principle of proportionality also address process values. Communications, both by officials and the media, should aim to neither exaggerate nor minimise the situation so as to be as accurate as possible. The CEAPI framework recognises that this can be challenging, because much was likely to remain unknown about the situation. It identifies a number of other process values that recognise this without compromising the other principles. They are the following.

Flexibility

Flexibility requires plans to be adaptable, and to provide as much chance as possible to take into account concerns or disagreement from the people who are affected (linking here with the principle of respect).

Good Decision-Making

Good decision-making was elaborated for the purposes of the CEAPI framework in terms of openness and transparency, inclusiveness, accountability and reasonableness. The explanations of these concepts are broadly consistent with their discussion in the wider literature on public health ethics, but a few specific points are worth noting. In the framework's explanation, *openness* includes being consultative and transparent about what decisions are being considered as well as explaining the reasons. *Inclusiveness* is also relevant, both to process and to impact. It requires active steps to involve people, including those who may find it difficult to express views. It also requires decision-makers to take into account any disproportionality in the way their conclusion might impact on particular groups of people. *Reasonableness* is used to describe decisions that are rational, not arbitrary, based on appropriate evidence, taken after an appropriate process, bearing in mind the urgency and circumstances, and which have a reasonable chance of working.

Working Together

The final principle is *working together*, which sets out a vision of social solidarity. It asserts that all persons have a role in responding to a pandemic by: helping families and friends; and keeping the community going by continuing day-to-day activities, including work, unless there is a particular reason not to do so (such as when infectious). It also sets out an expectation of cooperation between public agencies and civil society, recognising that this would require national, regional and local coordination. The precise implications of such an approach depend on societal dynamics. As an illustration and for a Canadian perspective, see Faust et al. (2009) on the SARS crisis in Toronto and the role of faith-based organisations.

Conclusions: The Importance of Public Health Values in Social Scaffolding and Healthcare

This chapter focuses on the way in which the UK's CEAPI framework for developing policy, strategy and practice was developed and used. Our intention is to illustrate how the matters concerning the common good and collective good, public health values and ethics that we explore in the first half of the chapter can be used to develop a framework for action.

The breadth of contributions in this book show that matters relating to the social determinants of health are important. They explore the power and effects of people's social identification with the groups of which they are members. This places demands on us to consider values and ethics from a standpoint that recognises the properties of groups and group processes if we are to exploit them appropriately, sensitively and effectively.

We observe that many frameworks of ethics are based on considering the people to whom they apply as being separate persons. This is done with the intention of assisting them, and the people who make decisions with or for them, to make choices that are good for them as individuals. While this disciplined approach is enormously helpful, although also demanding, it might also be seen as incomplete in settings in which we recognise people's interdependency and the importance of their relationships. In this regard, we refer readers to the commentary in Chapter 14. Put another way, there may be tensions between decisions made appropriately, ideally jointly by practitioners and individual persons, and similar decisions that recognise the implications of taking into account the collective good and common good that groups raise. Thus, values-based practice should not be seen as reflecting solely the approaches that focus on single persons, and then grossing them up by a process of multiplication. Neither is values-based practice context-free. We think that the public health and values-based approach, which was taken when creating the CEAPI framework, has much to offer widely.

Extending the Principles in the CEAPI Framework

One of the tensions includes the finite nature of resources, in human and financial terms, and this was introduced in Chapter 1. Making a perfectly acceptable decision to allocate resources for one person may threaten to deprive others of use of that resource. Thus, collective values and ethics abound in healthcare. This has become apparent to us in the context of commissioning healthcare, in which strategic considerations are given to allocating scarce resources to different populations of people, who have differing needs. Making these decisions demands similar considerations as does developing policy and practice for pandemics. Thus, we have applied the fundamental principle, and similar notions of the ethical orientations and process values, to a number of other circumstances.

These matters were articulated when constructing the, then, Welsh Assembly Government's ethical framework for commissioning health services to achieve the healthcare standards for Wales in 2007 (Welsh Assembly Government, 2007). More recently, commissioning by separate health service bodies has been discontinued in Wales and the responsibilities integrated into organisations that are responsible for both commissioning and providing healthcare. However, our stance is that these considerations remain highly pertinent despite the structures having been changed by the Welsh Government. Changing the structure of the decision-making bodies does not remove the challenge to public health ethics that allocating scarce resources raises!

Another arena into which the principles explicated in the CEAPI framework have been extended concerns how we apply values and ethics to applying restraint to some highly disordered young people who are in public care, education and detention in the criminal justice system, as a consequence of their behaviour and needs. A moment's thought shows that there are huge demands in balancing competing interests in this field. Thus, when the Restraint Advisory Board (RAB), appointed by the Ministry of Justice for England and Wales, reported on the acceptability of a new system of restraint in 2011, the Board included in its report an approach to working with the values involved that takes in the considerations and approach created by CEAPI (Restraint Advisory Board, 2011). Similarly, the RAB's successor body, the Independent Restraint Advisory Panel to the Ministry of Justice (IRAP) included these considerations in the approach it recommended to the ministries, agencies and authorities that were and are responsible for implementing the new restraint programme in secure training centres and young offender institutions, and in education services (IRAP, 2014a, b).

Reflexive Practice: Learning As We Go Rather Than Just Reacting

Generally, we see systems of public ethics as essential to using the lessons that flow from the well-researched material in this book. They should underpin systems of reflective, but also reflexive practice, in order to assure the quality of new responses to people's needs in which bottom-up and top-down approaches are better balanced within systems of co-design and coproduction.

One of the clear advantages of the CEAPI framework is that it focuses attention on the matter of ethics in emergencies as well as in other challenging circumstances. It has *increased ethical awareness*, so that actors can be prompted to overcome their cognitive and affective biases. It has offered *ethical action guidance*, in which the objective was to prescribe behaviours for those planning responses that have been identified as more likely to lead to the desired objectives. It has promoted *ethical deliberation* through education and codifying values that should be brought to bear. We commend these objectives when applying the lessons that flow from this book and when choosing between the preferences of different groups of people. Therefore, active awareness of, reflection on, and engagement with values and ethics must be a core component part of the process of social scaffolding.

References

Academy of Medical Sciences (2015). Exploring a new social contract for medical innovation. See https://acmedsci.ac.uk/file-download/38377-5673dcc2f036b.pdf.

Academy of Medical Sciences (2017). Enhancing the use of scientific evidence to judge the potential benefits and harms of medicines. See https://acmedsci.ac.uk/file-download/44970096.

Buccieri, K. & Gaetz, S (2013). Ethical vaccine distribution planning for pandemic influenza: Prioritizing homeless and hard-to-reach populations. Public Health Ethics, 6: 185–196.

Carter, P., Laurie, G. T. & Dixon-Woods, M. (2015). The social licence for research: Why care.data ran into trouble. Journal of Medical Ethics, 41: 404–409; doi: 10.1136/medethics-2014-102374.

Coggon, J. (2012). What Makes Health Public? Cambridge: Cambridge University Press.

Coggon, J., Syrett, K. & Viens, A. M. (2017). Public Health Law: Ethics, Governance and Regulation. New York, NY: Routledge.

Daniels, N. (2000). Accountability for reasonableness. British Medical Journal, 321: 1300–1301.

Daniels, N. (2008). Just Health: Meeting Health Needs Fairly. Cambridge: Cambridge University Press.

Dawson, A. (2011). Resetting the parameters public health as the foundation for public health ethics. In Dawson, A., editor, Public Health Ethics: Key Concepts and Issues in Policy and Practice. Cambridge: Cambridge University Press, pp. 1–19.

Dawson, A. (2016). Snakes and ladders: State interventions and the place of liberty in public health policy. Journal of Medical Ethics, 42: 510–513.

Dawson, A. & Verweu, M. (2012). Solidarity: A Moral Concept in Need of Clarification. Public Health Ethics, 5: 1–5.

Department of Health (2007). Cabinet Office and Department of Health Responding to Pandemic Influenza: The Ethical Framework for Policy and Planning. London: Department of Health.

Department of Health (2010). Independent review of the swine flu response: Memorandum by the Department of Health. See www.gov.uk/government/uploads/system/uploads/attachment_data/file/61261/doh.pdf.

Faust, H., Bensimon, C. & Upshur, R. (2009). The role of faith-based organisations in the ethical aspects of pandemic flu planning: Lessons learned from the Toronto SARS experience. Public Health Ethics, 2: 105–112.

Faust, H. S. & Upshur, R. (2009). Public health ethics. In Singer, P. & Viens, A. M., editors, Cambridge Textbook on Bioethics. Cambridge: Cambridge University Press, pp. 274–280.

Gluckman, P. (2016). Making Decisions in the Face of Uncertainty: Understanding Risk. Auckland: Office of the Prime Minister's Chief Scientific Advisor.

Grill, K. & Dawson, A. (2015). Ethical frameworks in public health decision-making:

Defending a value-based and pluralist approach. Health Care Analysis, 25: 291–307.

Hart, H. L. A. (1983). Between utility and rights. In Hart, H. L. A., editor, Essays in Jurisprudence and Philosophy. Oxford: Oxford University Press, pp. 198–222.

Hine, D. (2010). The 2009 Influenza Pandemic: An Independent Review of the UK Response to the 2009 Influenza Pandemic. London: Cabinet Office.

IRAP (2014a). Report of the Independent Restraint Advisory Panel to the Ministry of Justice. Implementation of the Minimising and Managing Physical Restraint System in Secure Training Centres and Young Offender Institutions. London: Independent Restraint Advisory Panel.

IRAP (2014b). Report of the Independent Restraint Advisory Panel to the Ministry for Education. A Review of Restraint Systems Commissioned for Use with Children Who are Resident in Secure Children's Homes. London: Independent Restraint Advisory Panel.

Kaposy, C. & Bandrauk, N. (2012). Prioritizing vaccine access for vulnerable but stigmatized groups. Public Health Ethics, 5: 283–295.

Kayman, H., Radest, H. & Webb, S. (2009). Emergency and disaster scenarios. In Singer, P. & Viens, A. M., editors, Cambridge Textbook on Bioethics. Cambridge: Cambridge University Press, pp. 281–288.

Lee, C., Rogers, W. A. & Braunack-Mayer, A. (2008). Social justice and pandemic influenza planning: The role of communication strategies. Public Health Ethics, 1: 223–224.

Lucassen, A., Montgomery, J. & Parker, M. (2017). Ethics and the social contract for genomics in the NHS. In Davies, S. C., editor, Annual Report of the Chief Medical Officer 2016, Generation Genome. London: Department of Health, ch. 16.

Malecki, J. (2001). Letters Laced with Anthrax. Palm Beach, FL: Health Commission.

Montgomery, J. (2013). Reflections on the nature of public ethics. Cambridge Quarterly of Healthcare Ethics, 22: 9–21.

Nuffield Council on Bioethics (2007). Public Health Ethics. London: Nuffield Council on Bioethics.

Nuffield Council on Bioethics (2012). Emerging Biotechnologies: Technology, Choice and the Public Good. London: Nuffield Council on Bioethics.

O'Neill, O. (2002). A Question of Trust: The BBC Reith Lectures. Cambridge: Cambridge University Press.

O'Neill, O. (2011). Broadening bioethics: Clinical ethics, public health and global health. Nuffield Council on Bioethics Lecture. See http://nuffieldbioethics.org/wp-content/uploads/Broadening_bioethics_clinical_ethics_public_health_global_health.pdf.

Phillips, N. (2000). Report of the Inquiry into BSE and Variant CJD in the United Kingdom. London: Stationery Office. See https://webarchive.nationalarchives.gov.uk/20060525120000/http://www.bseinquiry.gov.uk/report/index.htm.

Rawls, A. (1971). Theory of Justice. Cambridge, MA: Harvard University Press.

Restraint Advisory Board (2011). Report of the Restraint Advisory Board to the Ministry of Justice. Assessment of Behaviour Recognition & Physical Restraint (BRPR) for Children in the Secure Estate. London: Restraint Advisory Board.

Sandman, P. M. (1989). Hazard versus outrage in the public perception of risk. In Covello, V. T., McCallum, D. B. & Pavlova, M.T., editors, Effective Risk Communication: The Role and Responsibility of Government and Nongovernmental Organizations. New York, NY: Plenum Press, pp. 45–49.

Stiglitz, J. (2012). The Price of Inequality. London: Allen Lane.

Tasioulas, J. (2017a). Minimum Core Obligations: Human Rights in the Here and Now. Washington, DC: World Bank.

Tasioulas, J. (2017b). The Minimum Core of the Human Right to Health. Washington, DC: World Bank.

Thompson, A. K., Faith, K., Gibson, J. L. & Upshar, R. E. G. (2006). Pandemic preparedness:

An ethical framework to guide decision-making. BMC Medical Ethics, 7: 12.

US Presidential Commission for the Study of Bioethical Issues (2015). Ethics and Ebola: Public health planning and response. See https://bioethicsarchive.georgetown.edu/pcsbi/sites/default/files/Ethics-and-Ebola_PCSBI_508.pdf.

Welsh Assembly Government (2007). An Ethical Framework for Commissioning Health Services to Achieve the Healthcare Standards for Wales: WHC (2007) 076. Cardiff: The Welsh Assembly Government.

World Health Organization (2008). The right to health: Factsheet 31. See www.ohchr.org/Documents/Publications/Factsheet31.pdf.

Wilkinson, R. & Pickett, K. (2009). The Spirit Level: Why More Equal Societies Almost Always Do Better. London: Allen Lane.

Wolff, J. (2012). The Human Right to Health. New York, NY: W. W. Norton.

Chapter 25

Social Scaffolding: Supporting the Development of Positive Social Identities and Agency in Communities

Catherine Haslam, S. Alexander Haslam and Tegan Cruwys

Masons, when they start upon a building,
Are careful to test out the scaffolding;

Make sure that planks won't slip at busy points,
Secure all ladders, tighten bolted joints.

And yet all this comes down when the job's done,
Showing off walls of sure and solid stone.

So if, my dear, there sometimes seems to be
Old bridges breaking between you and me,

Never fear. We may let the scaffolds fall
Confident that we have built our wall.

Seamus Heaney, 1966

Introduction

This poem, by the Irish poet and Nobel Laureate, Seamus Heaney, is as applicable to sustaining healthy communities as it is to sustaining marital harmony, which is the purpose for which it was originally written. As the scaffolding provided the foundational structure from which Heaney and his wife built the walls of their marriage, so too we can develop communities through our own collective efforts, drawing on support from health and social care practitioners of various persuasions where and when required. Once it is established, we can gain confidence from the fact that we can use what we have built together to help our communities to endure and thrive when they, too, are threatened by adversity.

It is in this spirit that we consider in this chapter practical approaches to the ongoing and ever-present challenge of helping communities to build the physical and psychological structures that are likely to sustain them. Key to achieving this outcome, and a central theme of this volume, is the importance of agency. Here we focus on developing a framework to help people to realise that agency through harnessing the power of social groups.

We must understand five things to deliver this agenda:

(1) What is meant by social scaffolding;

(2) Why social identities are critical both for successful scaffolding and good health;

(3) How identity-based social scaffolding works (i.e. its mechanisms of action);
(4) How such scaffolding can be constructed in partnership with various parties, invested in the health of communities (with community members as active agents in the process); and
(5) What can be done to ensure that the community endures after scaffolding has been dismantled.

In responding to these questions, we hope to elaborate on a common theme in the conclusions drawn in preceding chapters about how to engage people in doing the work on social identity that is needed to help communities to thrive.

1. What Is Social Scaffolding?

The field of education introduced the notion of scaffolding as a psychological concept and developed it as a metaphor for the process of resourcing and nurturing learners in ways that enhance their potential and allow them to achieve more than they might otherwise do on their own (Bruner, 1975; Wood et al., 1976). In this use of the term, support is gradually withdrawn until the students can manage independently; this is similar to the ways in which psychotherapy sessions are scaled down when clients have learned how to control negative thoughts. This notion of *tapered support* is vital, as it ultimately empowers learners to achieve autonomous performance while also allowing for prudent husbandry of finite resources. As Vygotsky (1978) stressed, social interaction plays a crucial role in this process because it provides an essential testing ground for dynamic processes of learning and development. In essence, then, scaffolding bridges the gap between students' current states and their optimal ones through appropriate investment in collaborative resources, guidance and support.

Some key elements of this original educational conceptualisation of scaffolding are certainly relevant to health and social care. In particular, we stress the importance of supported learning through social interaction that facilitates autonomous functioning. However, in the light of the social identity framework that is introduced in Chapter 4, we also highlight two significant differences between the domains of education and health. First, in the educational field, scaffolding was originally conceived in the context of a learning paradigm. While this process can be generalised to activities in diverse contexts and populations (Pea, 2004), we note that good health is not just a matter of knowledge and skill acquisition. Clearly, such knowledge can be helpful (e.g. see Hammond, 2002; Feinstein & Hammond, 2004), but, alone, it is insufficient to change entrenched attitudes, beliefs and behaviour (see Chapters 16, 19, 20 and 21 on managing disasters, veteran health, radicalisation and conflict). Second, in education, the social relationship emphasised is the one-on-one interaction between a teacher and pupil. The effect of this relationship on students' outcomes is often understood in individualistic terms, in much the same way that we understand other interpersonal relationships (e.g. between a couple, or two friends). However, we argue that, in most health contexts, the dominant form of interaction and development typically centres on *group memberships*; whether as a member of a particular practitioner group or as a representative of a particular population of clients or patients; usually those who are at greater risk.

The example of depression allows us to consider how these principles apply in the mental health context. Most people who live with the realities of depression are acutely aware that physical and psychological symptoms are not the only challenges associated with this condition. It also impacts on families, employment, finances, physical health and social relationships. Viewing depression through this lens allows us to see how easily the condition can become embedded in communities, and particularly among those who are at greater risk because, for example, their members face financial hardship, disability or discrimination. In this context, individualised education and treatment are likely to fall short in addressing the origins of illness; notably, the broader social and economic factors that have contributed to its escalation. Stigma associated with depression is high, and limited access to professional services leads many people to seek help from family and friends. This is an ideal context in which professional practitioners can work collaboratively with communities to understand their realities and use this as a basis to develop meaningful social interventions. Not only may they help communities to manage the presenting mental illness, but this collaboration may act as a scaffold from which continued support can be drawn to better manage problems in other life domains.

Drawing on this reasoning, we conceptualise social scaffolding as *the process through which practitioners work to promote health and wellbeing with community groups through structured activities that enable them to develop a positive shared social (community) identity from which to harness ongoing support*. The community groups we refer to here can comprise any meaningful collection of people who share common experiences, attitudes or characteristics, which range from communities of people living in supported accommodation, to those taking part in a psychotherapy group, or those who represent an ethnic minority in a particular neighbourhood. This framing resonates with that of social prescribing, highlighted by Maughan and Williams in Chapter 26, but extends this to recognise that building a shared sense of identification (i.e. not just prescribing *any* group) lies at the heart of successful scaffolding.

As we will see, the value of social scaffolding lies largely in cultivating meaningful and sustainable forms of group activity. Facilitation can be helpful in the process, and particularly so if experiences of loneliness and disconnection make it difficult to know where to start. However, these groups must ultimately be identified and developed *from the ground up*; by the people who engage in those activities (along the lines highlighted in Chapter 23 on making connectedness count). Facilitated, collaborative activity serves three goals. First, in itself, this activity is directly beneficial to participants' health and wellbeing to the extent that it promotes a sense of positive social identity. Second, it helps to generate workable solutions to practical health-related problems, because it is based on the knowledge and experience of the community in question. And third, this activity increases ownership of those solutions (e.g. Wegge & Haslam, 2003).

Going further, our definition also recognises that people are more open to, and hence more likely to benefit from, the support that others offer when their sense of group membership is shared, whether as practitioners, clients or participants, in some form of therapeutic alliance. This is largely because shared social identity is the basis for a sense of mutual connectedness and trust (Haslam et al., 2009, 2012). We argue, too, that in the absence of shared identification, attempts at scaffolding are liable to fail or at least prove suboptimal. After all, why would we trust those people who are perceived as not sharing our perspective or interests to build the supports on which our lives depend?

2. Why are Social Identities Central to Both Scaffolding and Health?

There is now abundant evidence that interventions that help to develop a sense of shared social identity within a given community (a sense of 'us') provide the members of that community with a powerful basis for scaffolding social connections to enhance health. Our own research with older adults residing in care shows that building a sense of identification with others offers a platform for improvements in both their cognitive and their mental health. This has been found in a series of intervention studies in which shared identity was developed through collective activity as members of: (a) design teams, responsible for redecorating communal spaces in care homes (Haslam et al., 2014a; Knight et al., 2010); (b) reminiscence groups, sharing past memories together (Haslam et al., 2010, 2014b); (c) water clubs, formed to tackle the issue of dehydration (Gleibs et al., 2011a); and (d) men's clubs to combat isolation in a group, which tends to be the minority in care (Gleibs et al., 2011b).

The value of promoting shared identity appears even more pronounced in the case of depression, because social disconnection is a defining feature of the condition (Cruwys et al., 2014b, 2014c). Indeed, some of our work with large representative samples in the UK has shown that, if older adults with depression belong to no social groups but join one, then their risk of relapse is reduced by 24 per cent (Cruwys et al., 2014c). If they join three, the risk of relapse is reduced by 63 per cent. Importantly though, research has shown that it is not merely showing up for group activities that delivers benefits (Sani et al., 2012). Rather, it is the sense of social identification with these groups – feeling that you belong, and that the groups are an important part of who you are – that is critical.

This point was confirmed in research that sought to create connections for adults who were considered to be at greater risk by inviting them to take part in activity- and arts-based groups with others who shared similar interests (e.g. in yoga, art or soccer). The impact of the intervention was negligible for those people who did not identify with their groups (in other words, people who were below the sample median for social identification), and they still had a 52 per cent chance of meeting the diagnostic cut-off for depression at the study's conclusion. However, the intervention proved very successful for those who *did* identify (whose social identification was above the sample median). Among this group, fewer than 30 per cent met the cut-off for depression at the study's end (Cruwys et al., 2014a).

Moreover, these findings were replicated in a follow-up study that sought to understand the contribution of social identification in a therapy context. Here, 92 adults presenting with depression and/or anxiety received group cognitive behaviour therapy. And again, identification with the therapy group was the driver of treatment outcome, irrespective of primary diagnosis. Specifically, 50 per cent of clients below the median in therapy group identification remained depressed on completion of treatment, but this reduced to just a third among those with higher identification. These studies show that identification is at least as important as, and some would argue more important than, therapy content. Accordingly, the more people identify with their therapy group, the greater their improvement in response to treatment (Cruwys et al., 2014a).

Similar findings have been observed in other studies in which members of disadvantaged groups (e.g. groups of people who were experiencing mental, intellectual or physical disability) have been helped to join a community choir (Dingle et al., 2012). The choir increased participants' sense of connectedness to others and helped members to develop a collective voice, both physically and symbolically, which, in turn, delivered dramatic improvements to health and wellbeing; most notably, in resolving negative emotional states and problems with pain. Moreover, it is notable that these benefits emerged in the face of the various forms of stress, anxiety and fatigue that such activity might otherwise be expected to induce among those people for whom public performance is anything but normative.

Another study that has explored these processes even more directly was conducted with a sample of homeless people who were living in temporary supported accommodation, offered by a charitable organisation, the Salvation Army. The nature of support that participants received varied as a function of the particular service from which they received support. Some received only food and a bed, while others were assigned a dedicated case-worker and had opportunities to take part in recreational and community activities with other service users. The people who reported having a positive social experience and a sense of social identification with the homelessness service had better outcomes at three-month follow-up. This was characterised by a reduced sense of social isolation and greater openness to becoming involved with and joining other groups in the community. Indeed, a positive experience with the Salvation Army proved to be an important turning point in participants' lives, acting as a scaffold to develop the social and personal resources that they needed to break the cycle of homelessness (Cruwys et al., 2014b).

In their different ways, then, each of these studies provides insights into the power of various forms of identity-based social scaffolding to deliver profound benefits for health and wellbeing. However, before we can build the active ingredients of these interventions into relevant programmes, we first need to understand what those ingredients are.

3. What are the Mechanisms Through Which Social Scaffolding Works?

There are multiple ways through which social scaffolding achieves its positive effects. As demonstrated by the studies to which we refer earlier in this chapter, the most pertinent is creating *positive social bonds*. They are developed through meeting and engaging with other people who are in the process of building new social identities (e.g. as a member of a choir, an arts group, a soccer team). All these studies showed that the identity-based ties were developed through positive group experiences and had the effect of increasing participants' appetite for more constructive group engagement. Indeed, the evidence suggests that one positive experience can be sufficient to kick-start future social engagement, even among the people who were at greater risk and whose negative experiences were considerable. Here, then, positive group experiences can set in train a virtuous cycle in which the group they join acts as a scaffold which supports further positive experiences in other groups.

Nevertheless, and as noted in previous chapters (e.g. Chapters 20 and 23), it is also the case that not all group experiences are beneficial for health. In some circumstances, groups can have deleterious effects, both emotionally and physically. This may be the case, for example, if the group encourages and promotes normative behaviours or activities that are destructive (e.g. substance misuse, self-harm, etc.). Where there is the possibility for harm, practitioners are professionally bound to facilitate their clients or patients breaking away from these groups. However, breaking away from groups such as these also proves easier, and is more sustainable, when there are opportunities for positive identity gain to mitigate the costs of identity loss. This is illustrated in work by Dingle and colleagues (Dingle et al.,

2015) that examined the processes through which people recover from substance abuse. That research identified two ways in which social identity was critical to people's journeys of recovery. On the one hand, the path to recovery involved breaking ties with substance-using groups that promoted drug and alcohol use. On the other hand, this substance-user identity had to be replaced by an alternative identity that promoted more positive forms of group-related behaviour, by promoting a recovery identity. In effect, then, the role of those who help people through this difficult transition centres on the dual process of dismantling a harmful social identity and replacing it with one that is more constructive and which can scaffold longer-term health.

Importantly, this discussion points to the importance of understanding *identity content*, that is, what a group stands for and does, when facilitating development of new social connections. As Dingle et al.'s (2015) study illustrates, this is a critical factor in health behaviour. But awareness of social identity content is also important to ensure that, when helping people to forge new group ties, we facilitate identities that are likely to be subjectively meaningful. Indeed, insensitivity to this is a barrier to constructive identification (Haslam, 2014). This is because a person's subjective experience of their fit with a particular group, which is highlighted as key to the long-term survival of groups in Chapter 27, is a major determinant of their strength of identification, and this explains why social scaffolds cannot be successfully instigated in a top-down fashion. Our care home studies showed that few benefits accrue to atheists or agnostic people if all we try to do is help them join a religious group (Ysseldyk et al., 2013).

It is through understanding of the processes we outline in this chapter, and working with them in practice, that practitioners can play a vital role in defining the structures that are likely to best facilitate constructive forms of social identification. Working as *social scaffolders* in partnership with communities requires practitioners to understand, and to provide access to meaningful and constructive community-based social identities (e.g. familial, recreational, cultural, religious). How, then, might this be achieved? As one concrete framework for this kind of activity, in the next section, we draw upon previous work informed by the Actualizing Social and Personal Identity Resources (ASPIRe) framework (Haslam et al., 2003; Peters et al., 2014). ASPIRe gives an example of how practitioners might derive an understanding of the identities at play in a given community, and work with them to promote collective health.

4. How Can We Help to Construct Social Scaffolds?

The ASIPRe framework was originally developed in a work environment to provide organisational psychologists with a model for developing and harnessing the power of shared organisational identity in the context of diverse subgroup identities. It outlines a four-phase process of *social identity management* and recognises that effective teamwork hinges upon the cultivation of a collective sense of us to which everyone in an organisation, or community, contributes. A key observation here, as Reicher observes in Chapter 23, is that this sense of organic social identity needs to be forged through a bottom-up participatory process, rather than imposed from the top down (e.g. Eggins et al., 2002).

The importance of this agenda in organisational contexts is illustrated by the growing costs of low organisational identification that may be manifested not only in low productivity but also in compromised employee health (see, for example, Haslam, 2004). This is demonstrated most vividly in research that links low organisational identification both to reduced job and life satisfaction, and to high levels of stress and burnout (Haslam & Reicher, 2006; Steffens et al., 2014a, b; van Dick & Haslam, 2012). It is worth noting, though, that this call for bottom-up participatory processes can meet with resistance. In particular, this is because interventions such as these can be resource-intensive and challenge the managerial prerogative, the manager's perceived right to manage (after Taylor, 1911). Much the same is true in the context of healthcare for people who are perceived as vulnerable. Here, what we might term the practitioner prerogative can equally mitigate against participatory forms of identity building and health promotion; even if the underlying motivations are benevolent.

Nevertheless, the need for participatory solutions to problems of health is as apparent in the health domain as it is in the organisational. Indeed, the spiralling costs of healthcare throughout the world (e.g. Orszag & Ellis, 2007) alone make efforts to involve communities more actively in their own health seem prudent. This is also the basis of horizontal epidemiology (see Chapter 7) and is especially true in the case of communities whose members are at great risk because they lack access to treatments and in whom governments may be unwilling to invest (Haslam et al., 2017a). In this context, the importance of an ASPIRe-like process is that it specifies activities that can be adapted to a range of domains to help practitioners work with communities in order to develop a shared sense of identification and to scaffold their resources and potential. In what follows, we summarise the key elements of this process in a community context, but also refer interested readers to relevant papers in the organisational domain for a more detailed description of the approach and for evidence of its utility (e.g. Haslam, 2014; Haslam et al., 2003; Peters et al., 2013).

The first two phases of the ASPIRe process involve activities that develop an understanding of the social identities that exist within a community. The first of these is Ascertaining Identity Resources (*AIRing*). This involves efforts to understand the group memberships that are potentially important for members of a given community and which are, therefore, an actual or potential basis for their sense of social identity. This centres on a process of *social identity mapping* that attempts to establish the groups that are part of people's lives, their importance and their interrelationships (e.g. Cruwys et al., 2016). Indeed, mapping has been found to raise awareness of a person's social group world and, through this, of where best to seek support in the context of responding to adversity (Jetten et al., 2009). This is the reason why it is a tool that has proved to have significant value as a core component of both health interventions (notably Groups 4 Health; Haslam et al., 2016) and leadership programmes (notably 5R; Haslam et al., 2017b) that aim to build upon and harness social identity. Within a community health context, we can use this same mapping process to identify the main cultural, religious, social and recreational groups in which people come together. On the back of this, we can also ask a range of important secondary questions. What are the events that bring those groups to life? Where do they take place? And, critically, who participates, and who does not?

Following this, a Subgroup Caucusing (*SubCasing*) phase is undertaken with the various groups that have been identified through AIRing, bringing their members together to discuss and raise awareness of their particular group's goals and aspirations, and also any barriers to these being achieved in the community. How would particular cultural or recreational groups, for example, like to develop and grow? What is stopping this from happening? What would sustain the group to allow it to survive in the long term?

The third phase, of Superordinate Consensualising (*Super-Casing*), brings the different subgroups in the community together to share the outcomes of the previous discussions. What this process promotes is the idea of working with the multiple and diverse groups in a community for the collective good. Doing so clearly requires some careful management to ensure that all groups are recognised positively. To this end, people are encouraged to discuss differences in their experiences and aspirations as well as commonalities, and also to identify barriers to their achieving their different goals. Essentially, this allows the different groups in a community to specify the goals that are important to them (e.g. more communal play and social areas, increased housing support, greater access to mental health support groups) and the goals they have in common (i.e. building and strengthening community infrastructure). Research suggests that it is only through this process of alignment, accompanied by an appreciation and recognition of meaningful forms of group differences, that a sense of community identity is able to emerge (e.g. Eggins et al., 2002).

The final phase in the ASPIRe process, Organic Goal Setting (*ORGanizing*), seeks to develop and formalise a strategic plan that addresses the goals identified in previous phases. This might focus on what is required, for example, to ensure that new initiatives, such as developing a recreational club, can thrive by identifying activities that members can collectively pursue, identifying and designating a safe accessible space for these activities, and considering any barriers to participation, such as timing and transport. This plan should centre on strategies that are Realistic, Implementable, Timely and Engaging (RITE) if it is to provide a framework to guide future activity that is oriented towards realising the community's other goals and aspirations.

The ultimate value of a process such as ASPIRe for health practitioners is that it serves to construct a meaningful and workable social scaffold. There are at least five particular ways in which this process feeds into health-related benefits. The first is by aligning existing social identities with an overarching community identity in ways that ensure diverse identities and groups work with, rather than against, each other. This means that forming a new and broader community identity does not necessarily involve forgoing older ones. Second, the process raises people's awareness of their own and others' multiple social identities. This is important in the light of evidence that these identities provide social psychological capital that proves to be a vital health-promoting resource under conditions of adversity and challenge (Jetten et al., 2012, 2014). Third, working with existing identities means that practitioners do not continually have to reinvent the wheel, because the scaffold they create is constructed out of existing resources and capabilities. Indeed, a key benefit of the ASPIRe process is that, in itself, it serves to define and consolidate potentially valuable community identities. Fourth, recognising that these resources are actually within one's control also increases confidence within a community that it can achieve the ultimate goal of self-management. In the realm of health, this has been shown to be immensely important, especially for marginalised and disadvantaged communities (see, for example, Chandler & Lalonde, 1998). Fifth and finally, ASPIRe is an organic process in which emergent community identity is constructed from the realities of the people living in it. Thus, by generating their own community identity, people come to see this as an extension of themselves and are more likely to take ownership of the process and its products in ways that allow the community and its members to thrive.

Yet as we have already noted, for all its benefits, it is clear that the ASPIRe process, or any other intervention that works to develop and harness a sense of shared community identity, requires considerable investment. Identity building requires investment on the part of activists and practitioners to engage with, facilitate and oversee the process. It also requires investment on the part of community members to ensure that: (a) the process articulates with meaningful identities and with groups' psychological and material circumstances; and (b) they are translated into actions that move groups forward. Our sense is that if people are committed to the business of identity building, such investment is unavoidable. While it is true that communities can be quickly destroyed, the process of building them up generally proves to be far more demanding. Neither Rome, nor any other successful society, was built in a day.

5. How Can We Embed Newly Developed Social Identities?

So once forged, how can we ensure that newly developed, or newly invigorated, social groups, and the identities that underpin them, are sustained and endure? For a social identity to endure, the emergent abstract sense of 'us' that ASPIRe (or any similar process) helps to create, must be a lived reality of the people in those groups. This requires that identities be embedded (see Steffens et al., 2014a, b) in ways that help community members coordinate their joint activities. This, we argue, is achieved primarily through interrelated processes of *shared cognition* and *shared practice*.

Shared cognition in any community resides, to a large extent, in its members' *transactive memory*, which is their shared, communal, knowledge-base (Wegner et al., 1985). This is partly comprised of the shared language that members of the community group use to describe and understand the world in which they live as seen, for example, through the language of sport for a football club, or of recovery for a therapy group. However, it also incorporates multiple forms of local knowledge (e.g. about various activities in the community and where they take place) as well as expertise about, for example, how to access resources and services for health, employment, finance and housing, and not least knowledge about the people and places in which this knowledge resides.

Shared social identity provides a platform for transactive memory of this form. In part, that is because it creates the motivation to: invest in this knowledge; accrue it over time; draw on it when needed; and give back to it when possible. Encouraging community groups to explore and develop shared language through social interaction offers a vehicle for members to develop a common understanding of the various issues they might face, such as experiences of racial conflict or the stigma of mental illness. Group-focused interventions that help to build this understanding are also more likely to be effective in dealing with the origins of the social barriers that challenge particular groups (e.g. discrimination, poverty) than those that are targeted only at individual persons. They also help communities develop confidence in their shared knowledge and this is something that is furthered by opportunities to put that knowledge to the test by attempting to solve the specific problems that groups confront (Liang et al., 1995).

Similarly, shared practices that are informed by social identities offer another means for those identities to be lived out. These practices can range from those that are exalted and special (e.g. ceremonial events and festivals), to those that are seemingly banal and mundane, such as, for example, attending a football match, going to the local pub or writing a local newsletter. Where community identities are newly formed, there may clearly be a need for these practices to be actively promoted and facilitated in order to increase both awareness and participation. At the same time, their success also hinges on their being seen to map onto goals and aspirations that the community group recognises (e.g. as part of the ORGanizing process in ASPIRe).

In the end, though, the success of this entire enterprise can be measured by the extent to which social scaffolding has served its purpose and, ultimately, becomes unnecessary. This would be evident in the formation of highly identified community groups (e.g. a local soccer club) that embrace norms and practices (i.e. attending social functions, playing weekly matches) and where members benefit from sustained engagement in coordinated activities that increase their sense of belonging and commitment to the community.

Concluding Comments

The main goal of this chapter has been to develop the argument that much is to be gained by investing in efforts to help communities to develop and live out constructive shared identities through providing social scaffolding. Largely, we have made this case by drawing on the theoretical framework that is provided by the social identity approach, and on practical models, in particular the ASPIRe model, and activities such as social identity mapping that derive from this.

Yet there would, of course, be little requirement for health and social care professionals to invest in social scaffolding were it the case that communities could do this for themselves, without their help. Sadly, though, it is often the case that those people who are most in need of social scaffolding are least able to source it, due largely to a lack of various forms of capital. Indeed, one of the greatest advantages one can have in contemporary society, and one of the key advantages conferred by education, wealth and social standing, is the ability to construct and access a social scaffold as and when it is required.

It is plainly the case, then, that social scaffolding is neither universally nor uniformly available. Furthermore, the communities in which social scaffolds are most needed tend to be the places where the services of both healthcare professionals are often hardest to access (Saxena et al., 2007). In these contexts, risk factors and disadvantage can make it difficult for members of a community to build scaffolds on their own. Accordingly, a core professional priority should be to empower communities to break negative social spirals and promote positive social experiences. In this context, empowerment recognises that ordinary people are as important as the experts in finding solutions to what appear to be insurmountable problems. Indeed, in order to be effective, intervention should engage with groups and their identities, rather than impose identities and associated cognitions and structures from above.

As powerful as Heaney's scaffolding metaphor is, perhaps equally important in this context is his injunction to "never fear" and to be prepared to stand back once our scaffolding has done its job. Indeed, like scaffolding for a building, the scaffolding that practitioners (e.g. physicians, social care workers, psychologists, psychiatrists) provide is, by necessity, often short-lived and temporary. Yet, if it is properly constructed and positioned, its benefits will be felt long after it has been delivered. Indeed, at the risk of pushing the metaphor a little further, we can go so far as to suggest that the best forms of scaffolding are precisely those that go on to become unnecessary, and where the only long-term evidence of their value is the quality of the more permanent structures that the social processes make possible.

References

Bruner, J. S. (1975). From communication to language: A psychological perspective. Cognition, **3**: 255–287.

Chandler, M. J. & Lalonde, C. (1998). Cultural continuity as a hedge against suicide in Canada's First Nations. Transcultural Psychiatry, **35**: 191–219.

Cruwys, T., Dingle, G. A., Hornsey, M. J. et al. (2014a). Social isolation schema responds to positive social experiences: Longitudinal evidence from vulnerable populations. British Journal of Clinical Psychology, **53**: 265–280.

Cruwys, T., Haslam, S. A., Dingle, G. A. et al. (2014b). Feeling connected again: Interventions that increase social identification reduce depression symptoms in community and clinical settings. Journal of Affective Disorders, **159**: 139–146.

Cruwys, T., Haslam, S. A., Dingle, G. A., Haslam, C. & Jetten, J. (2014c). Depression and social identity: An integrative review. Personality and Social Psychology Review, **18**: 215–238.

Cruwys, T., Steffens, N. K., Haslam, S. A. et al. (2016). Social identity mapping: A procedure for visual representation and assessment of subjective multiple group memberships. British Journal of Social Psychology, **55**: 613–642; http://doi.org/10.1111/bjso.12155.

Dingle, G. A., Brander, C., Ballantyne, J. & Baker, F. A. (2012). 'To be heard': The social and mental health benefits of choir singing for disadvantaged adults. Psychology of Music, **41**: 401–421.

Dingle, G. A., Cruwys, T. & Frings, D. (2015). Social identities as pathways into and out of addiction. Frontiers in Psychology, **6**; doi: 10.3389/fpsyg.2015.01795.

Eggins, R. A., Haslam, S. A. & Reynolds, K. J. (2002). Social identity and negotiation: Subgroup representation and superordinate consensus. Personality and Social Psychology Bulletin, **28**: 887–899; doi: 10.1177/01461672020280070З.

Feinstein, L. & Hammond, C. (2004). The contribution of adult learning to health and social capital. Oxford Review of Education, **30**: 199–221.

Gleibs, I., Haslam, C., Haslam, S. A. & Jones, J. (2011a). Water clubs in residential care: Is it the water or the club that enhances health and well-being? Psychology and Health, **26**, 1361–1378.

Gleibs, I., Haslam, C., Jones, J. et al. (2011b). No country for old men? The role of a Gentlemen's Club in promoting social engagement and psychological well-being in residential care. Aging and Mental Health, **15**: 456–466.

Hammond, C. (2002). Learning to be Healthy. London: Institute of Education, University of London.

Haslam, C., Cruwys, T., Haslam, S. A., Dingle, G. & Chang, M. X.-L. (2016). Groups 4 Health: Evidence that a social-identity intervention that builds and strengthens social group membership improves mental health. Journal of Affective Disorders, **194**: 188–195.

Haslam, C., Haslam, S. A., Jetten, J. et al. (2010). The social treatment: Benefits of group reminiscence and group activity for the cognitive performance and well-being of older adults in residential care. Psychology and Aging, **25**: 157–167.

Haslam, C., Haslam, S. A., Knight, C. et al. (2014a). We can work it out: Group decision-making builds social identity and enhances the cognitive performance of care home residents. British Journal of Psychology: **105**, 17–34.

Haslam, C., Haslam, S. A., Ysseldyk, R. et al. (2014b). Social identification moderates cognitive health and well-being following story- and song-based reminiscence. Aging and Mental Health, **18**: 425–434.

Haslam, S. A. (2004). Psychology in Organizations: The Social Identity Approach, 2nd edition. London: Sage.

Haslam, S. A. (2014). Making good theory practical: Five lessons for an Applied Social Identity Approach to challenges of organizational, health, and clinical psychology. British Journal of Social Psychology, **53**: 1–20; doi: 10.1111/bjso.12061.

Haslam, S. A. & Reicher, S. D. (2006). Stressing the group: Social identity and the unfolding dynamics of responses to stress. Journal of

Applied Psychology, **91**: 1037–1052; doi: 10.1037/0021-9010.91.5.1037.

Haslam, S. A., Eggins, R. A. & Reynolds, K. J. (2003). The ASPIRe model: Actualizing Social and Personal Identity Resources to enhance organizational outcomes. Journal of Occupational and Organizational Psychology, **76**: 83–113.

Haslam, S. A., Jetten, J., Postmes, T. & Haslam, C. (2009). Social identity, health and well-being: An emerging agenda for applied psychology. Applied Psychology: An International Review, **58**: 1–23.

Haslam, S. A., McMahon, C., Cruwys, T. et al. (2017a). Social cure, what social cure? Exploring the propensity to underestimate the importance of social factors for health. Social Science and Medicine, **198**: 14–21.

Haslam, S. A., Reicher, S. D. & Levine, M. (2012). When other people are heaven, when other people are hell: How social identity determines the nature and impact of social support. In Jetten, J., Haslam, C. & Haslam, S. A., editors, The Social Cure: Identity, Health and Well-Being. Hove: Psychology Press, pp. 157–174.

Haslam, S. A., Steffens, N. K., Peters, K. et al. (2017b). A social identity approach to leadership development: The 5R program. Journal of Personnel Psychology, **16**, 113–124.

Jetten, J., Haslam, C. & Haslam, S. A., editors (2012). The Social Cure: Identity, Health and Well-Being. Hove: Psychology Press.

Jetten, J., Haslam, C., Haslam, S. A., Dingle, G. & Jones, J. J. (2014). How groups affect our health and well-being: The path from theory to policy. Social Issues and Policy Review, **8**: 103–130.

Jetten, J., Haslam, S. A., Iyer, A. & Haslam, C. (2009). Turning to others in times of change: Social identity and coping with stress. In Stürmer, S. & Snyder, M., editors, The Psychology of Prosocial Behavior: Group Processes, Intergroup Relations, and Helping. Oxford: Blackwell, pp. 139–156.

Knight, C., Haslam, S.A. & Haslam, C. (2010). In home or at home? Evidence that collective decision making enhances older adults' social identification, well-being and use of communal space when moving to a new care facility. Aging and Society, **30**, 1393–1418.

Liang, D. W., Moreland, R. & Argote, L. (1995). Group versus individual training and group performance: The mediating role of transactive memory. Personality and Social Psychology Bulletin, **21**: 384–393.

Orszag, P. R. & Ellis, P. (2007). The challenge of rising health care costs: A view from the Congressional Budget Office. New England Journal of Medicine, **357**: 1793.

Pea, R. D. (2004). The social and technological dimensions of scaffolding and related theoretical concepts for learning, education, and human activity. The Journal of Learning Sciences, **13**: 423–451

Peters, K., Haslam, S. A., Ryan, M. K. & Fonseca, M. (2013). Working with sub-group identities to build organizational identication and support for organizational strategy: A test of the ASPIRe model. Group and Organization Management, **38**: 128–144.

Peters, K. O., Haslam, S. A., Ryan, M. & Steffens, N. (2014). To lead, ASPIRe: Managing diversity and building social capital by empowering subgroups and embedding organic organizational identity. In Otten, S., van der Zee, K. & Brewer, M., editors, Towards Inclusive Organizations: Determinants of Successful Diversity Management at Work. Hove: Psychology Press, pp. 87–107.

Sani, F. (2012). Group identification, social relationships, and health. In Jetten, J., Haslam, C. & Haslam, S. A., editors, The Social Cure: Identity, Health and Well-Being. Hove: Psychology Press, pp. 21–37.

Saxena, S., Thornicroft, G., Knapp, M. & Whiteford, H. (2007). Resources for mental health: Scarcity, inequity, and inefficiency. The Lancet, **370**: 878–889.

Steffens, N. K., Haslam, S. A., Jetten, J., Schuh, S. C. & van Dick, R. (2014b). The contribution of social identifications in organizations to employee health: A meta-analysis. Unpublished manuscript, University of Queensland.

Steffens, N. K., Haslam, S. A., Kerschreiter, R., Schuh, S. C. & van Dick, R. (2014a). Leaders enhance group members' work engagement and reduce their burnout by crafting social identity. German Journal of Research in Human Resource Management, **28**: 183–204.

Taylor, F. W. (1911). The Principles of Scientific Management. New York, NY: Harper and Brothers Publishers.

van Dick, R. & Haslam, S. A. (2012). Stress and well-being in the workplace: Support for key propositions from the social identity approach. In Jetten, J., Haslam, C. & Haslam, S. A., editors, The Social Cure: Identity, Health and Well-Being. Hove: Psychology Press, pp. 175–194.

Vygotsky, L. S. (1978). Mind in Society: The Development of Higher Psychological Processes. Cambridge, MA: Harvard University Press.

Wegge, J. & Haslam, S. A. (2003). Group goal-setting, social identity and self-categorization: Engaging the collective self to enhance group performance and organizational outcomes. In Haslam, S. A.,van Knippenberg, D., Platow, M. J. & Ellemers, N., editors, Social Identity at Work: Developing Theory for Organizational Practice. Philadelphia, PA: Taylor & Francis, pp. 43–59.

Wegner, D. M., Giuliano, T. & Hertel, P. (1985). Cognitive interdependence in close relationships. In Ickes, W. J., editor, Compatible and Incompatible Relationships. New York, NY: Springer-Verlag, pp. 253–276.

Wood, D., Bruner, J. S. & Ross, G. (1976). The role of tutoring in problem solving. Journal of Child Psychology and Psychiatry and Allied Disciplines, 17: 89–100.

Ysseldyk, R., Haslam, S. A. & Haslam, C. (2013). Abide with me: Religious group identification amongst older adults promotes health and well-being by maintaining multiple group memberships. Aging and Mental Health, 17, 869–879; doi: 10.1080/13607863.2013.799120.

Chapter 26

Synthesising Social Science into Healthcare

Daniel Maughan and Richard Williams

Introduction

This book presents a compelling weight of evidence about how belonging to social groups confers advantages that help people to achieve and sustain good physical and mental health. A huge volume of work has been done to take the evidence-base to where it currently stands. But, arguably, the work required to embed these psychosocial understandings and, importantly, their implications for healthcare, is a larger and more challenging task. The contents of Chapters 23, 24 and 25 should be real assets in so doing.

One of the intentions of this book is to identify effective methods that can be applied to improving healthcare outcomes and delivery. However, linking people's social relationships with their health, their social groupings, their communities and, within them, health and social care service functioning is undeniably complex involving far more than changing or adding a service. It requires rethinking how we design, deliver and provide care in order to capitalise on the substantial health benefits derived from people's social connectivity and shared identities. Thus, evidence-based healthcare at the scale of communities requires a path that leads to the skills for redesign that were identified between the 1980s and the present (e.g. Warner & Williams, 2005; Williams & Kerfoot, 2005). This is clear from the contents of Chapters 23 and 25. But Chapter 24 identifies that decision-making in these domains raises matters of value for groups, communities and nations, and the practical matter of how we allocate scarce resources in ways that are fair in response to the competing preferences of different groups.

This chapter reviews the current context of healthcare, relating specifically to the challenges inherent in developing services that straddle both health and social care. It defines the stakeholder groups that are involved in making the changes to services that are necessary. It proceeds to address potential barriers to implementation. This chapter resonates with a number of the themes introduced in Chapter 1. It concludes with a review of the practical steps that are needed to broaden the focus of health and social care; to move beyond interventions for individual persons towards building dynamic social capacity, through enhancing the ways in which we communicate, form groups, develop relationships and spend our leisure time.

The Current Context of Healthcare Development

Healthcare is always changing, but the pace of change has accelerated throughout the twentieth and twenty-first centuries. Changes in the last 70 to 100 years reflect developments in five broad areas:

- Growth in evidence-based public health (health promotion, illness prevention and rehabilitation) and healthcare interventions;

- Improved understanding of the organic causes of, and treatments for, diseases;
- The rapid rise of technology;
- Funding of public health and healthcare services; and
- The ways in which governance of health and healthcare services has been implemented.

These developments have provided the foundation for substantial improvements in public health and care of patients. Evidence-based healthcare, with its three components of obtaining core evidence, reviewing and synthesising the evidence, and applying the evidence (Croft et al., 2011) has allowed healthcare systems to prioritise the most appropriate interventions to the right people at reasonable cost. Improved understanding of the organic causes of health conditions has transformed patients' outcomes and is going to continue to have a profound impact on the nature and the ways in which healthcare is delivered in the future. Over the past four decades, advances in technology have provided a revolution in designing and delivering healthcare. They range from surgical procedures to online healthcare records and, now, developing wearables that enable people to track their own physiological markers.

The three factors that comprise the evidence-based approach are the main drivers of constant change in healthcare systems. Consequentially, they evoke two other drivers, funding and strategy. Advances in improving human health have influenced the direction of developments and funding in healthcare. They also call forth national, community, family and personal choices in a resource-limited world. Arguably, however, this trajectory towards more interventionist and technical assessments, care and treatments has been interpreted by some people as requiring strategic and managerial approaches that are contrary to some of the social interventions suggested in this book. Thus, the notions that arise from the social cure, horizontal epidemiology and coproduction, for example, raise another driver; that of recognising the contribution of each of these constructs to rising pressure for a better balance between bottom-up and top-down processes in designing, developing, delivering and governing healthcare services and practice. Chapter 24 provides an overview of the issues of principle and public ethics that are involved in making choices together with a framework for drawing public health ethics into the decisions that are required, when balancing the needs of different groups against finite budgets.

Evidence-Based Public Health and Healthcare

Evidence-based healthcare has led to our tendency to rely on certain types of evidence; notably, randomised controlled trials (RCTs) that are able to demonstrate differences in clinical outcomes with statistical clarity in controlled conditions (Croft et al., 2011). But, as Tudor Hart (2001) has pointed out, these controlled circumstances and carefully selected patients are not necessarily common in day-to-day clinical practice. Emphasis on RCTs as the gold standard for questions related to the effectiveness of preventive or therapeutic interventions favours the more simple interventions or those with binary outcomes, which can be adequately controlled (Grimshaw et al., 2011). More complex interventions, such as certain of the social and public health interventions that are suggested in this book, are often not easily amenable to these types of trials. This level of evidence is hard to attain due to the sheer complexity of these types of interventions, the wide range of possible effects and the difficulty inherent in randomisation for larger-scale group-based interventions (Croft et al., 2011). While drawing on RCT evidence is largely a good thing, limitations in the suitability of this methodology for examining the efficacy of complex interventions lead us to conclude that such a gold standard cannot be set as an absolute. The downside of reliance on RCT evidence to inform funding is that interventions that are not amenable to such methodology are not supported, despite other forms of evidence being readily available, such as longitudinal or case–control studies.

Improved Understanding of the Organic Causes of, and Treatments for, Diseases

Advances in scientific knowledge of the organic causes of, and interventions to relieve, many health conditions has created a tide of public interest in personalised medicine and magic-bullet interventions, based on each person's genetic make-up (Hedgecoe, 2004). However, investment in neuroscience and in genetic research that targets these organic causes has been to the detriment of investment in social interventions (Priebe et al., 2013). This is, perhaps, another way of putting into words the matter raised by Alex Haslam and colleagues in Chapter 14. It is how we are to understand and practise personalised care and reap the important contribution of the social sciences without running the risks of over-individualising care and failing to adequately recognise the huge importance of people's social relationships and needs.

Contributing to this is the intense pressure on academics and practitioners to publish in high-impact-factor journals and to be cited by other researchers, which risks a narrowing focus on what is mainstream. The consequence has been that research is conducted in 'areas that will generate funding and impact-factor points' (Priebe et al., 2013), which has been and appears to remain with the hard sciences rather than health services research or public health interventions. In making this argument, we do not deny the significant developments that have been, and will continue to be, made in the organic aspects of health and healthcare. But we also call for greater balance in investment in the wider, social aspects of science that have a demonstrable impact on people's health and their care. The topic of horizontal epidemiology, which is focused on in Chapter 7, provides an example; it shows that people's experiences of their ill health and their needs fall into the social science arena.

The Rapid Rise of Technology

Technology has changed the face of healthcare worldwide (Chaudhry et al., 2006). However, often, the focus of these technological developments in mental healthcare has been on providing personalised treatments that may be delivered on computers in patient's homes (Hayes et al., 2016). Examples include computerised cognitive behaviour therapy (CBT) and mood monitoring apps (Hayes et al., 2016). We do not endeavour to reduce the value of these techniques, but assert that the belief that people can address all their mental health problems by following an interactive computerised algorithm flies in the face of the evidence presented in this book. In our view, technological advancements should be set in a social context. Our thesis is that meaningful social identities, belonging and engagement with communities are all fundamental to achieving and sustaining good mental health. We have learned in Chapter 3 that social isolation is a predictor of poor mental health and that belonging to multiple social groups can be protective against the potential mental health effects of significant life events, such as bereavement or physical health problems.

The ease of joining or leaving many online groups suggests that they might provide less-reliable support. Conversely, social networking sites could provide support for those people who find it hard to form or sustain other types of relationships by offering an opportunity to communicate with people who have similar experiences of life (Hayes et al., 2016). However, it remains unclear whether social networking sites, such as Facebook, can augment or replace offline and face-to-face social networks. However, Helliwell and Huang (2013) report a large Canadian survey that showed:

> First, the number of real-life friends is positively correlated with subjective well-being (SWB) even after controlling for income, demographic variables and personality differences. Doubling the number of friends in real life has an equivalent effect on well-being as a 50% increase in income. Second, the size of online networks is largely uncorrelated with subjective well-being. Third, we find that real-life friends are much more important for people who are single, divorced, separated or widowed than they are for people who are married or living with a partner.

Importantly, new services must be adapted for the digital era. Provision of healthcare is likely to be less successful if it lags behind the fast-paced changing face of technology, whether the intervention is for individuals or groups, using a computer or based in social settings. These technological issues all add complications when considering the practical policy implications of implementing the social identity approach to health in our current culture and context.

Funding of Public Health and Healthcare Services

A further obstacle to developing a social approach to health is the global issue of funding in healthcare. Data from the World Bank in 2014 (https://data.worldbank.org) suggest that health expenditure as a proportion of gross domestic product (GDP) has increased globally from 8.5 per cent in 1995 to 9.9 per cent in 2014. Spending in high-income countries has increased from 9.2 per cent to 12.3 per cent of GDP during these 20 years, while low- and middle-income countries have shown less of an increase (0.9 per cent in 20 years, to 5.8 per cent of GDP). This is, perhaps, unsurprising as costs of pharmaceuticals are increasing (Rockoff, 2016), people are living longer and there are increasing numbers of people who have complex comorbidities (NHS England, 2014). Financial constraints are likely to undermine efforts to develop any type of new service, particularly those which target social influences that require longer-term investment and support from different agencies to be successful. Further, in the context of tighter health budgets, these new services compete with existing healthcare services, some of which may be losing their funding in the current world financial climate. This makes it harder to present the case for developing such services.

Indeed, the gap between the current capacity and the potential capability (see Chapter 1) that exists in the National Health Services in the UK and in other healthcare systems is widening (Forster, 2017). Presently, the supply of professional practitioners is insufficient to meet the volume of demand. This not only undermines existing health and social care structures but it has a deleterious effect on the ability of service providers to respond to new policy directives. It is apparent that there are large challenges to be overcome in recruiting, retaining, supporting and ensuring the up-to-date training of all staff with a view to achieving closure of the capacity–capability gap while also managing better integration of health and social care sectors (Williams and Kerfoot, 2005).

The Ways in Which Governance of Health and Healthcare Services Have Been Implemented

The advent of corporate governance has also had an impact on the development of policy and practice (Williams & Kerfoot, 2005). In the UK over the past 20 years, the higher echelons of healthcare service management have become increasingly prescriptive about the direction and form of corporate governance. In 1997, for example, the UK governments outlined their programmes of National Health Services (NHS) quality reforms (Department of Health, 1997); agendas that created greater emphasis on organisational governance and performance management. They defined clinical governance as (Department of Health, 1998):

> . . . a framework through which NHS organisations are accountable for continuously improving the quality of their services and safeguarding high standards of care by creating an environment in which excellence in clinical care will flourish.

This approach has been accepted throughout the UK in the interval since then. In this system, quasi-autonomous agencies, external to state-funded agencies that commission and deliver healthcare, provide quality assurance at the corporate level. In parallel, clinical governance requires practitioners to continuously strive for quality improvement. overseen by these external agencies that license practitioners and their employers. International healthcare systems have undergone similar changes.

However, this model has been criticised as being overly controlling and not providing an adequate focus on improving models of healthcare (Miles et al., 2000). One particular concern about this strategy, which is led from top-down policies for governance, is that it emphasises monitoring and implementation. The external monitoring agencies publish detailed reports on healthcare organisations that are then incorporated into performance ratings. By contrast, we see in this book the importance of bottom-up appreciations of people's perceptions of their needs, and how it is vital to enable people to express their own agency (see Chapters 22–25) while the contents of Chapter 24 provide a framework for strategists to use when endeavouring to ensure that everyone's needs are considered.

Decisions about new policies and healthcare improvements are heavily influenced by these external monitoring bodies, and their reports often result in healthcare agencies being excessively wary of the requirements placed on them at the national level (Walshe, 2003). Walshe suggests that the effectiveness of external monitoring processes in achieving ongoing improvements to healthcare delivery (and design) is questionable, and that they likely bring other costs and adverse consequences alongside benefits (Walshe, 2002). Supporting this view, one study, which surveyed 100 different healthcare trusts in the UK (Freeman and Walshe, 2004), found that the structures and systems for clinical governance appear to have created more progress in quality assurance rather than quality improvement. The authors report that:

> The implementation of clinical governance has been shaped by an assurance focused performance management culture in the NHS in England that may not promote quality improvement, and can be argued to be antithetical towards it.

This illustrates how governance processes that insist on external procedures to ensure quality improvement are problematic. If practitioners and managers are to identify with their objectives and methods, a larger component of quality development should be internal and owned by the frontline services. One risk of the current approach in the UK is that institutions that attempt to achieve compliance with regulators can distort the goals of evidence-based policy. In this sense, practitioners, managers and researchers can be seen to have been robbed of their contributions to designing services that meet the particular needs of the communities they serve.

Finding the Way Forward

Finding the way forward with delivering effective services of a sufficient range of natures now requires knowledge and a series of skills if the services are to meet public expectations, offer interventions for a sufficient range of problems that impact on people's needs, while also ensuring that those interventions are coherent with the evidence about their effectiveness. Not only should leaders and managers recognise and work within the opportunities and constraints offered by the five main drivers mentioned earlier in this chapter. Plainly, development of policy, services and practice require a lead and funding from the top, but, in our opinion, they should also enable greater emphasis on bottom-up contributions that support the continuing agency of the staff.

It is important, therefore, that we are clear about what is required and how to achieve it, from both bottom-up and top-down perspectives. As we have just said, policy is essential to achieving this. So, here we review the policy landscape before considering the importance of the differing attitudes of stakeholders.

The Policy Landscape

One important way in which the context of public health and healthcare delivery can be managed is to recognise the importance of policy in creating agreed plans for services. But, successful synthesis of evidence into practice first requires awareness that there are multiple levels of policy that should be developed and that each should complement the others. Interestingly, this awareness also provides a mechanism for achieving a better balance.

Williams has noted previously that there are four levels of policy that require consideration (Williams et al., 2014). They are:

(1) Government policies;
(2) Strategic policies for service design;
(3) Service delivery policies; and
(4) Policies for good clinical practice.

More recently, Williams has added a fifth level to this list; that of recognising the importance of professional practice at the level of contact with patients and clients. in which practitioners come together with patients to develop personalised programmes of clinical care that enable unique sets of needs and people's social and relational circumstances to be included. In other words, while policies for good clinical practice may give rise to, or emerge from, evidence-based and evidence-informed protocols, every patient is different, has differing social identities, relationships and interdependencies, and protocols must be applied with awareness of each patient's circumstances and preferences, as Section 2 of this book shows.

So, while the first four levels of policy provide the context within which practice takes place, it is also clear that there are occasions when general policies and protocols may not provide sufficient or sensitively appropriate guidance. This is important when ascertaining the best way to assist people with their personal circumstances and individual experiences and, often, combinations of needs that arise from comorbidities. Indeed, this book highlights the significance of practitioners engaging sensitively with their patients in exercising sound clinical judgements and joint decision-making, which balance with the important guidance that protocolled approaches provide. If services are to deal effectively with local differences in populations' health needs and other contextual factors, it is crucial that the differences between these five levels of policy are recognised while alignment between them is achieved.

Problems can emerge when higher-level policies are misinterpreted, ignored or not known about at lower levels (Cabana et al., 1999) and vice versa. This is not always because of problems at service delivery level; comprehensive stakeholder engagement at a national level, alongside providing appropriate public information, can also be an issue. Rolling out any policy may meet some level of community resistance or low engagement that thwarts effective implementation (USAID, 2009). Early engagement of all stakeholders is essential to resolving this kind of barrier and, in Chapter 25, Haslam et al. show how the social identity approach can be used to this effect in the Actualizing Social and Personal Identity Resources (ASPIRe) framework.

However, our experience is that the most common missing link is that of creating strategic policies and designing services in a way that places the evidence alongside knowledge of the needs, experiences and preferences of people for whom the services are created. Arguably, the public morally owns tax-based, state-financed systems and should be treated as important stakeholders in the processes of designing, delivering and evaluating the care systems that are created for them. Coproduction is an important component of policy and practice at all five levels.

Attitudes of Stakeholders

An important matter to consider when attempting to agree and, then, implement policy is the triangle of differing attitudes and priorities of politicians, professionals and the public. Issues that affect political support are numerous, but financial concerns tend to predominate. One would expect professionals to support those interventions that have a sufficient evidence-base, but this is not always the case (Perkins & Slade, 2012). Public support is dependent on wide-ranging factors that include stigma, perceptions about personal safety, health literacy levels and the provision of ethical treatments (Jorm, 2000; Saraceno et al., 2007). Some treatments, including those offered in mental healthcare, are an ongoing source of controversy (Cooper, 2013). Electroconvulsive therapy (ECT) and community treatment orders (CTOs), for instance, have had strong public opposition from as far back as the asylum era through to the modern day (Cooper, 2013). There remain debates about the ethics of detaining people who have mental disorders, particularly children (Roberts, 2013), while, contrastingly, the media fuel the perception that psychiatrists do not do enough to protect society (Stout et al., 2004).

'Recovery Colleges' offer an example, drawn from the UK, of public and professional opinion affecting the growth of a new type of service. These colleges provide educational courses aimed at helping people who have mental ill health to achieve their goals and ambitions. Recovery Colleges have greatly increased in number over the past few years, despite a lack of evidence to support them (Phillips et al., 2013; Slade et al., 2012). People who suffer mental illness have been very supportive of them (Phillips et al., 2013), while mental health organisations have been very keen to develop them, with clinical staff independently volunteering to set up these services without a lead from governmental health policy or instruction from funders (Perkins and Slade, 2012). Recovery Colleges have gained support from these two powerful groups and it is likely that this support has led to their considerable growth, rather than an evidence-base, which is lacking. Research is key to developing services but it is not sufficient. Support is required from politicians, policy-makers, managers, professional practitioners and the public to create change. In other words, bottom-up and research-inspired developments require top-down support if they are to progress.

Research has demonstrated differences in attitudes between politicians, professionals and the public regarding prioritisation of health expenditure. One study of 2,000 people found that doctors are less inclined to consider a patient's economic status as a determinant of priority for treatment than politicians or the public, while both doctors and nurses were less punitive towards patients with self-induced diseases than the public and politicians (Myllykangas et al., 1996).

Another divide between these groups is that healthcare professionals have been sceptical about including patients in designing new healthcare models (Thompson et al., 2009). A report published in 1997 advocated developing what, today, would be called coproduction, and included a typology of ways in which service users, or patients, and their families and other carers, might be engaged in designing and delivering health service. Yet, its vision and recommendations remain only partially achieved more than 20 years later (Williams et al., 1997). There is also evidence to suggest that doctors may ignore new top-down guidelines from national policy agencies in response to either their feeling disempowered to change, or disagreeing with the policy (Cabana et al., 1999). This reinforces the importance of recognising and addressing the five levels of policy that we introduced at the beginning of this section. It is not sufficient to create a high-level policy and imagine that it will be implemented. In that regard, service design is the critical element that links top-down initiatives with bottom-up engagement.

These matters, which include attitudes to: policy; evidence; and involving patients, clients or service users, illustrate the importance of asserting a new balance between top-down and bottom-up approaches to planning and care. It should allow: the needs and opinions of the people (patients and practitioners) to be recognised; evidence as to effectiveness and cost to be weighed in the balance; and policymakers and politicians to ensure that the decisions made are just, inclusive and good value for the slender resources available.

Effective Implementation of Policy

As the ASPIRe framework, which is described in Chapter 25, implies, implementing policy at all five levels involves engaging relevant stakeholders and equipping them with the knowledge, skills and resources required to create and deliver the policy. Analysis of the drivers of change and the barriers to implementing new ideas is important when broad or complex changes in healthcare are being proposed. Here, we present a review of some of the matters that we should strive to get right when implementing the evidence from the social sciences. Fundamentally, this is about broadening our perceptions so we are able recognise better the power of groups and social approaches to healthcare. Our intention is to recognise the realistic challenges that are implied by the contents of this book.

One of the major challenges is that embedding the principles of social approaches to health involves reshaping health and social care services so that they become more group-oriented, with an explicit focus on creating belonging and social identities. As we have seen in Chapter 25, this process might be called social scaffolding. But the illustrations in that chapter show the complexity that this creates when developing policy, as the aim is not to add a particular intervention or service but to redesign and develop existing services alongside supporting provision of community groups. One of the dangers when developing a national policy for these types of changes is that broad and general language tends to be used when we try to encapsulate the principles of such an approach, and that can undermine the ability to create change (USAID, 2009). But, providing examples of models of care can help local services to develop in their respective areas.

Group treatments already exist, but, all too often, they are not driven by a framework that helps practitioners to understand how to make the most of the group ingredient to intervention. Thus, another matter is ensuring the availability of people who have the relevant skillsets: providing relevant training for staff is crucial. Appropriate training should be highlighted in the implementation plan for all policies and it must have relevance to the evidence-base for the social theories relating to health. Understanding the rationale for the changes enables staff to adapt the evidence to different contexts and, thereby, optimise the health benefits derived from membership of groups.

All too often, stigma, discrimination and gender issues are not considered in policy development, and yet they contribute significantly to the success or failure of policy implementation (USAID, 2009). This is likely to be the case with implementing the social identity theory for health because the issues involved in participating and feeling a sense of belonging to groups may be tied up with stigma and discrimination. People in different cultures may, for example, form groups in different ways and have different attitudes towards, for example, mixed-gender groups. Also, belonging to a group in which the uniting identity is that of illness could be viewed as stigmatising.

Social Prescribing

There is a tension between being overly prescriptive about using service specifications for interventions that have proved effective compared with allowing complete freedom for local services to develop models of care that have no evidence-base. In other words, should there be one size that fits all or should there be freedom to let many flowers bloom (NHS England, 2014)? Again, this reflects the tension between top-down and bottom-up approaches.

Let us illustrate this by referring to social prescribing, which is when practitioners prescribe people's attendance in community groups and activities (Branding & House, 2009). This practice recognises the role that social factors play in health (Kimberlee, 2013). But, in our experience, while social prescribing recognises the importance of social factors, there is often no framework to guide practitioners in using this approach. The social identity approach tells us that it is only those groups that give people's lives meaning and purpose and with whom they bond and connect, which have the power to change health outcomes. A one-size-fits-all approach is not particularly helpful in this context because of large differences between activities that are available locally and the motivations and interests of the people who are in receipt of social prescriptions (Kimberlee, 2013).

What has been found to be useful is using link workers to form a bridge between the healthcare system and community groups and activities (Maughan et al., 2015). The link workers develop an understanding of the local context and opportunities such that people who are referred can be signposted to the appropriate group or service. Nevertheless, what is currently missing in this practice is a framework from which to inform social prescribing so that it is optimally targeted, and this is where the social identity approach provides clear direction.

There are many other barriers to effective implementation that are dependent on the local context. Low motivation and commitment from service commissioners and provider agencies can serve to undermine successful implementation. Many factors can cause this, such as different priorities, a lack of incentives, limited resources and poor attention to agency. Financial incentives and ring-fenced budgeting can ensure that guidance or new standards provided nationally are delivered locally.

Practical Steps in Adopting an Approach to Healthcare as Informed by the Social Sciences

Successful implementation of approaches to intervention that are driven by awareness of people's needs for social connectedness, social support and agency requires us to contend with the current trend towards investing in technical or interventionist approaches, in a climate in which financial resources are increasingly constrained. Given this difficult context, this next section reviews how these developments could be driven and implemented.

As Chapter 25 shows, there are important steps involved in implementing the approaches to health, which are powered by awareness of social theories and evidence from the social sciences. Arguably, the evidence-base supporting this book justifies this approach. It presents evidence that belonging, attachment and helping people to sustain and develop their social identities can all lead to substantial health improvements. The analysis that we present in this chapter shows that 10 steps are required to embed this approach into services at local levels, in order to translate this evidence into policy. They are:

(1) Recognise the evidence-base for approaches to health and healthcare, which include theory and practice derived from the social sciences: it is presented in this book.

(2) Provide strategic support: use evidence-base for social intervention to assure all stakeholder groups.

(3) Set priorities for research: ensure funds are available to test new forms of service design that embody the principles presented in this book.

(4) Develop socially derived evidence-based interventions that involve conducting pilot and feasibility studies, and then evaluate their effectiveness (MRC, 2006) using appropriate mixed methodologies. Once these first four stages have occurred, evidence-based interventions can be promoted as examples of social interventions with clear health benefits for policymakers and funders.

(5) Develop national policy: developing a focus on approaches that are derived from the social sciences requires a shift in attitudes and balancing priorities in different ways, which take full account of technological and neuroscientific advances, alongside better recognition of social factors while not undermining existing interventions that are effective. Providing clear examples for policymakers would allow them to understand the necessary shift towards an approach that we call social scaffolding.

(6) Engage health funders: funders should be given appropriate advice and guidance in order for them to work with healthcare providers in developing new services. This could be in the form of a service framework. Local needs assessments are required to ensure that the appropriate strategy and service design are developed, according to the differing needs, provider organisations and cultural contexts of the populations in each area.

(7) Gain commitment from provider organisations: there are many competing demands for frontline services. Creating inter-agency pathways of care between the health and social care sectors can be a hard task for time-poor services. Appropriate support, targets, service standards and incentives are required to support these developments. Operationalising new services requires development of standard operating procedures, local policies and appropriate reporting structures. Ideally, funding should be matched to the identified target population, the levels of morbidity in the population and aims of the services.

(8) Deliver an appropriate mix of older and newer interventions: an important part of embedding approaches that are based on evidence from the social sciences is making sure that, when creating new interventions, pre-existing ones that are effective are not undermined. A map of existing local community groups, voluntary sector groups and health and social care groups should be developed first to ensure that pre-existing services that support social scaffolding are optimised before new ones are forged. Delivering augmented services is likely to depend heavily on local infrastructure, including, for example, whether healthcare facilities, community spaces or third-sector premises are used.

(9) Develop the workforce: training is required for existing staff to ensure that approaches which are based on evidence from the social sciences are embedded within new services. Questions should be asked about whether or not every group requires a trained facilitator, and the extent to which groups provide a meaningful basis for belonging and identification for those involved.

(10) Implement appropriate quality assurance: despite our critique of current approaches to quality assurance earlier in this chapter, it is clear that the present structures are well embedded in the culture of modern healthcare across different countries. Therefore, we take a realistic position in recommending that appropriate clinical governance structures are required to ensure ongoing improvements in safety and quality alongside a system of reporting to funders and external assessors. However, it would be antithetical to the science reported in this book if we did not take this opportunity to call for a better balance between bottom-up and top-down approaches to quality assurance, which mirrors the changes we recommend and which better reflects the needs of patients and populations for social connectedness, social support and engagement, through opportunities to express their agency and ownership of public services by coproduction.

Mapping the 'Five Ss' of social scaffolding, (schooling, scoping, sourcing, scaffolding and sustaining) onto these 10 steps, shows that all steps are relevant to schooling, which involves helping different stakeholders understand why social science matters in healthcare and to populations. Steps 1 and 2 are critical to scoping and Steps 3, 4, 5, 6 and 7 are important aspects of sourcing. Steps 5, 8, 9 and 10 are key components relating to scaffolding and sustaining.

Already, this chapter has discussed the complexities of, and complications and constraints within, the healthcare context, so, perhaps, it is unsurprising that schooling is the most crucial step in ensuring this approach is adopted. There are many different stakeholders in health and social care. Therefore, the process of getting support for this approach is multilayered and, because it involves gaining alignment from many influential people, also complex (Williams, 2002).

Fundamentally, the right level of evidence and support must be provided to convince each stakeholder group about the importance of adopting this approach. Specifically, it must be shown how the approach can provide added benefit, in terms of health outcomes, to the current health and social care context in each locality. Different stakeholder groups have different roles and responsibilities and, therefore, different levers are likely to be required for each group; see Table 26.1.

Knowledge into Action

Much evidence has been presented in this book about the benefits of applying the evidence available from the social sciences and public health in health service design. However, translating evidence into action is difficult and the reality is that research findings are still largely underutilised in decision-making about policy (Lomas, 2000). While the initial motivation for new service development might come from research evidence, such evidence may be neglected either when policy is written or when it is implemented. Limited use of research evidence can be partly attributed to the different cultures of the people who produce research and those who might be able to use the findings (Lomas, 2000). Many policymakers and researchers talk of 'the paradox of health services research' when discussing the issue of underuse of evidence while continuing to produce so much of it (Shulock, 1999).

Given this widespread issue, much work has been done around providing frameworks for ensuring that research evidence is used in policy, and to design services. This process of using evidence is called 'knowledge into action'. Despite a lot of work, there remains a lack of information about what works, in which settings, and for whom (Ward et al., 2009). Recent reviews have identified as many as 63 different theories or models of knowledge transfer, held by healthcare and social care practitioners and managers (Graham and Tetroe, 2007; Mitton et al., 2007). Of these models, some are more pertinent for technological innovations, while some have more relevance for agendas such as incorporating social approaches within healthcare.

One of the key challenges in embedding these approaches is the shift required for some stakeholders to understand that social interventions can bring about health benefits, i.e. that a person's social connectedness and activity have profound impacts on their physical and mental health. The models of knowledge transfer that best encapsulate this challenge are those that view the spread of knowledge as a social activity. In this circumstance, knowledge transfer involves the activities of many communities and is influenced by their belief systems and by the analytical or creative instincts of potential users (Rogers, 2010).

If we are to create change, realism tells us that we must address the triangle of relations between the public, politicians and the professions (Salter, 2001). Each of these groups must support the approach if it is to be wholly embedded and this is likely to require much communication and, sometimes, shifting attitudes. As one example, it is possible that members of the public might feel they are being short-changed if they are encouraged to accept social prescribing when, for example, they might prefer a biomedical intervention.

Table 26.1 Levers required to sustain change

Stakeholder group	Leverage to engage stakeholder group	Outputs supporting development of the social science approach
National strategic leaders (e.g. government health advisers, politicians)	Evidence of effects of social isolation Evidence of effect of groups Evidence of cost–benefit High profile public support Service example demonstrating the approach 'in-action'	Inclusion of approaches based on social science in governmental health policy Access to funding for new services
Research funding bodies	Political support Evidence supporting the social identity approach in terms of benefits for patients	Appropriate funds allocated to research projects in this field
Academics and universities	Ring-fenced research funding in this field Research collaborations Service providers which participate in research	Evidence of patient benefit/ cost-effectiveness/methods of service delivery
National and local policy developers	Political support Evidence of effects of social isolation Evidence of effect of groups Evidence of cost–benefit	Policy advocating approaches based on social science
Funders	National policy guidance National targets Ring-fenced funding	Specific funding arrangements for new services New service contracts for tender
Healthcare providers	Financial incentives for implementation or meeting the requirements of quality assurance	Provision of services that aim to support approaches based on social science
The public	Examples of benefit to patients Evidence of effect of groups Support from the media	Volunteers to run groups Supporting others to attend groups when needed Pressure groups to further support development of services

This presents a challenge to practitioners to find innovative ways to encourage people to accept evidence-based social interventions. It is important for practitioners to understand how these approaches are not pitted against each other but that they can be used synergistically and sequentially. Thus, social prescribing may optimise biomedical approaches. Practitioners who understand this point may be more successful in presenting the matter simply to patients so that the latter feel that they are receiving good advice. Those in professions might feel that they are over-stretched and have too few resources, and they are likely to need support, incentive and encouragement. The state is likely to require reassurance that these changes are likely to be successful and that there is an appetite in the public to engage within group settings.

An example of these tensions is offered by government action to reduce antibiotic prescribing. There are powerful arguments for this policy, but they alone are not sufficient to achieve success. In other words, there are limitations in cognitive approaches to change. They must be accompanied by sophisticated approaches to handling the pressures that are created by expectations of prescribing, even when it is unlikely to be effective, while emphasising the benefits of alternative activities.

Lavis et al. (2003) have proposed a framework for understanding knowledge transfer, which is widely accepted. They have identified five components of the knowledge-transfer process:

(1) Problem identification and communication;
(2) Knowledge and/or research development and selection;
(3) Analysis of context;
(4) Knowledge-transfer activities or interventions; and
(5) Knowledge and/or research utilisation.

The key component in this knowledge-transfer model is to promote close working relationships between the producers and users of research to ensure that research findings are used to improve health by highlighting, again, the importance of social connectedness. Researchers have an a-priori interest in engaging with people who develop services; the key, therefore, is to emphasise the importance of doing more to encourage the uptake of research (Department of Health, 2008). One aspect of research that could be improved is to provide cost-effectiveness studies, as evidence suggests that research continues to lack detail about the costs of developing and running new services (Innis et al., 2015). There is also a lack of research on how evidence-based practices may be sustained by organisations. Much of the research carried out to date has been cross-sectional. Longitudinal research would give insight into the relationship between organisational characteristics and the uptake, implementation and sustainability of evidence-based practice (Innis et al., 2015). Providing this information could encourage policymakers and healthcare commissioners to respond.

Conclusions

Fundamentally, there is a need for simplicity, clarity and consistency at all levels of work in healthcare. This is particularly important given the far-reaching effects and potentially revolutionary ideas of evidence-based social approaches to health and healthcare. Further research is needed, including feasibility studies, cost-effectiveness studies and, where possible and useful, RCTs into the effectiveness of social interventions, which focus on connectedness, social support and agency (see Chapter 22). It is also important for researchers, policymakers and service providers to engage in closer dialogue, alongside comprehensive stakeholder engagement and incentivisation through ring-fenced budgets.

On looking back through our chapter, we are struck by the focus that achieving system change places on the social connections and relationships, attitudes and social identities of the many people who are involved. Clearly, there is resonance between the task that we cover in this chapter, that of synthesising social science into healthcare, and the means by which any change is achieved. Successful implementation of approaches that are based on evidence for health and healthcare from the social sciences are likely to take time because a reshaping of both attitudes and services are required. Hopefully, the levers suggested in this chapter and the knowledge presented in this book will go some way to supporting this important change.

References

Branding, J. & House, W. (2009). Social prescribing in general practice: Adding meaning to medicine. British Journal of General Practice, **59**: 454–456; https://doi.org/10.3399/bjgp09x421085.

Cabana, M. D, Rand, C. S., Powe, N. R. et al. (1999). Why don't physicians follow clinical practice guidelines? Journal of the American Medical Association, **282**: 1458.

Chaudhry, B., Wang, J., Wu, S. et al. (2006). Systematic review: Impact of health information technology on quality, efficiency, and costs of medical care. Annals of Internal Medicine, **144**: 742.

Cooper, D. (2013). Psychiatry and Anti-Psychiatry. London: Routledge.

Croft, P., Malmivaara, A. & van Tulder, M. (2011). The pros and cons of evidence-based medicine. Spine, **36**: E1121–1125.

Department of Health (1997). The new NHS: modern, dependable. See http://webarchive.nationalarchives.gov.uk/+/http://www.dh.gov.uk/en/Publicationsandstatistics/Publications/PublicationsPolicyAndGuidance/DH_4008869.

Department of Health (1998). A first class service: Quality in the new NHS. See http://webarchive.nationalarchives.gov.uk/+tf_/http://www.dh.gov.uk/en/Publicationsandstatistics/Publications/PublicationsPolicyAndGuidance/DH_4006902.

Department of Health (2008). High quality care for all: NHS next stage review. See https://assets.publishing.service.gov.uk/government/uploads/system/uploads/attachment_data/file/228836/7432.pdf.

Forster, K. (2017). NHS faces "unprecedented workforce crisis" as vacancies rise 10% in last year. The Independent, 25 July. See www.independent.co.uk/news/health/nhs-staff-vacancies-rise-10-per-cent-2017–86000-nurses-midwives-doctors-recruitment-crisis-brexit-a7858961.html.

Freeman, T. & Walshe, K. (2004). Achieving progress through clinical governance? A national study of health care managers' perceptions in the NHS in England. Quality and Safety in Health Care, **13**: 335–343.

Graham, I. D. & Tetroe, J. (2007). Some theoretical underpinnings of knowledge translation. Academic Emergency Medicine, **14**: 936–941.

Grimshaw, J., Eccles, M., Thomas, R. et al. (2006). Toward evidence-based quality improvement. Evidence (and its limitations) of the effectiveness of guideline dissemination and implementation strategies 1966-1998. Journal of General Internal Medicine, **21**: S14-20.

Hayes, J. F., Maughan, D. L & Grant-Peterkin, H. (2016). Interconnected or disconnected? Promotion of mental health and prevention of mental disorder in the digital age. The British Journal of Psychiatry, **208**: 205–207.

Hedgecoe, A. (2004). The Politics of Personalised Medicine. Cambridge: Cambridge University Press.

Helliwell, J. F. & Huang, H. (2013). Comparing the happiness effects of real and on-line friends. PLoS One, **8**: e72754.

Innis, J., Dryden-Palmer, K., Perreira, T. & Berta, W. (2015). How do health care organizations take on best practices? A scoping literature review. International Journal of Evidence-Based Healthcare, **13**: 254–272.

Jorm, A. F. (2000). Mental health literacy: Public knowledge and beliefs about. The British Journal of Psychiatry, **177**: 396–401.

Kimberlee, R. (2013). Developing a social prescribing approach for Bristol. See http://eprints.uwe.ac.uk/23221/.

Lavis, J. N., Robertson, D., Woodside, J. M., Mcleod, C. B. & Abelson, J. (2003). How can research organizations more effectively transfer research knowledge to decision makers? The Milbank Quarterly, **81**: 221–248.

Lomas, J. (2000). Connecting research and policy. Canadian Journal of Policy Research, **1**: 140–144.

Maughan, D. L., Patel, A., Parveen, T. et al. (2015). Primary-care-based social prescribing for mental health: An analysis of financial and environmental sustainability. Primary Health Care Research and Development, **17**: 1–8.

Miles, A., Hurwitz, B. & Hampton, J. R. (2000). NICE, CHI and the NHS reforms: Enabling excellence. See https://kclpure.kcl.ac.uk/portal/en/publications/nice-chi-and-the-nhs-reforms–enabling-excellence-or-imposing-control(f1be1f0e-688e-4ea8-935f-aa63dd79ca0a)/export.html.

Mitton, C., Adair, C. E., Mckenzie, E., Patten, S. B. & Perry, B. W. (2007). Knowledge transfer and exchange: Review and synthesis of the literature. The Milbank Quarterly, **85**: 729–768.

MRC (2006). Developing and evaluating complex interventions: New guidance. See www.mrc.ac.uk/documents/pdf/complex-interventions-guidance/.

Myllykangas, M., Ryynänen, O. P., Kinnunen, J. & Takala, J. (1996). Comparison of doctors', nurses', politicians' and public attitudes to health care priorities. Journal of Health Services Research and Policy, **1**: 212–216.

NHS England (2014). Five year forward view. See www.england.nhs.uk/wp-content/uploads/2014/10/5yfv-web.pdf.

Perkins, R. & Slade, M. (2012). Recovery in England: Transforming statutory services? The International Review of Psychiatry, **24**: 29–39.

Phillips, P., Sandford, T. & Johnston, C. (2013). Working in Mental Health: Practice and Policy in a Changing Environment. London: Routledge.

Priebe, S., Burns, T. & Craig, T. K. J. (2013). The future of academic psychiatry may be social. The British Journal of Psychiatry, **202**: 319–320.

Roberts, M. N. (2013). The ethical implications of juvenile detention centers and the role of mental health and education in reducing recidivism. See https://repository.wlu.edu/handle/11021/24086.

Rockoff, J. D. (2016). How do we deal with rising drug costs? The Wall Street Journal, 10 April. See www.wsj.com/articles/how-do-we-deal-with-rising-drug-costs-1460340357.

Rogers, E. M. (2010). Diffusion of Innovations, 4th edition. New York, NY: Simon and Schuster.

Salter, B. (2001). Who rules? The new politics of medical regulation. Social Science and Medicine, **52**: 871–883.

Saraceno, B., van Ommeren, M., Batniji, R. et al. (2007). Barriers to improvement of mental health services in low-income and middle-income countries. The Lancet. **370**: 1164–1174.

Shulock, N. (1999). The paradox of policy analysis: If it is not used, why do we produce so much of it? Journal of Policy Analysis and Management, **18**: 226–244.

Slade, M., Williams, J., Bird, V. & Le Boutillier, C. (2012). Recovery grows up. Journal of Mental Health, **21**: 99–103.

Stout, P. A., Villegas, J. & Jennings, N. A. (2004). Images of mental illness in the media: Identifying gaps in the research. Schizophrenia Bulletin, **30**: 543-561.

Thompson, J., Barber, R., Ward, P. R. et al. (2009). Health researchers' attitudes towards public involvement in health research. Health Expectations, **10**: 129–220.

Tudor Hart, J. (2001). Commentary: Can health outputs of routine practice approach those of clinical trials? International Journal of Epidemiology, **30**: 1263–1267; doi.org/10.1093/ije/30.6.1263.

USAID (2009). Policy implementation barriers analysis: Conceptual framework and pilot test in three countries. See http://www.healthpolicyini

tiative.com/Publications/Documents/998_1_PIBA_FINAL_12_07_09_acc.pdf.

Walshe, K. (2002). The Evaluation of the Commission for Health Improvement's Performance and Impact on the NHS: A Scoping Review. London: Commission for Health Improvement.

Walshe, K. (2003). Regulating Healthcare. London: McGraw-Hill.

Ward, V., House, A. & Hamer, S. (2009). Developing a framework for transferring knowledge into action: A thematic analysis of the literature. Journal of Health Services Research and Policy, 14: 156–164.

Warner, M. & Williams, R. The nature of strategy and its application in statutory and non-statutory services. In: Williams R., Kerfoot M., editors. Child and Adolescent Mental Health Services: Strategy, Planning, Delivery and Evaluation. Oxford: Oxford University Press; 2005, pp. 39–62.

Williams, R. (2002). Complexity, uncertainty and decision-making in an evidence-based world. Current Opinion in Psychiatry, 15: 343–347; doi: 10.1097/00001504-200207000-00001.

Williams R. & Kerfoot, M. (2005). Setting the scene: Perspectives on the history of and policy for child and adolescent mental health services in the UK. In Williams, R. & Kerfoot, M., editors, Child and Adolescent Mental Health Services: Strategy, Planning, Delivery and Evaluation. Oxford: Oxford University Press, pp. 3–38

Williams, R., Bisson, J. & Kemp, V. (2014). OP 94. Principles for Responding to the Psychosocial and Mental Health Needs of People Affected by Disasters or Major Incidents. London: The Royal College of Psychiatrists.

Williams, R., Emerson, G. & Muth, Z., editors (1997). Voices in Partnership: Involving Users and Carers in Commissioning and Delivering Mental Health Services. London: The Stationery Office.

Chapter 27 Relationships, Groups, Teams and Long-Termism

Peter Aitken, John Drury and Richard Williams

Introduction

Speaking on the BBC Radio programme, Desert Island Discs, on 15 July 2018, Billie Jean King, a tennis star of the 70s and 80s and a campaigner for gender equality and social justice, summarised three quick things she says to students:

(1) Relationships are everything.
(2) Keep learning and keep learning how to learn.
(3) Be a problem-solver.

The focus of this book is on people and their relationships. Indeed, it covers many aspects of relationships that convey either strength or risk, or both, to variable degrees, upon people who work together, live together or who are drawn together by events. But, we now come to a series of chapters in which these matters come to the fore when we think about the staff of health and social care services.

This chapter focuses on the timeline that underpins all relationships between persons, groups, people within their workplaces and communities and between organisations and networks. Chapter 28 is about caring for staff who carry out hugely demanding jobs. It applies the principles in this book to them. Chapter 29 concerns leadership. In this chapter we refer to the National Health Services (NHS) in the UK to illustrate how our ideas might apply to healthcare agencies. We include a commentary, embedded in this chapter, which draws on the experiences of two of us (PA and RW) and which reflects our experiences and opinions in order to illustrate the points made. We do not reference all of those matters and, instead, allow readers to come to their own views about whether those experiences reflect their own or not. But, having offered that caveat, we note that some of the matters we raise are not solely those that impact on some organisations in one country's public sector healthcare system; there is some evidence that they may have a bearing on health and social care across more countries including, for example, the USA (Friedberg et al., 2013).

We, the authors of this chapter, argue that the quality of relationships is fundamental to the success of any group or organisation. Furthermore, although short-term relationships can work to people's benefit in some circumstances, short-termism can be very damaging. Our observation is that, generally, long-term relationships are more beneficial. In other words, one of the qualities that may define relationships turns on whether or not those relationships are sustained or not. Nonetheless, we have already summarised in this book some aspects of that timeline that may appear surprising at our first consideration. Emergent groups that may have evanescent lifetimes may be highly effective and important to our survival and the quality of our lives depending on the circumstances in which those groups form and dissolve.

Increasingly, we recognise the power and importance of people at all levels being enabled to contribute what they know, and their skills, to planning and delivering health and social care. Thereby, they influence the ways in which groups of people function at work to solve problems. Indeed, the contents of Chapter 26 address the challenges in changing and developing healthcare services.

Chapter 26 also describes the challenges to the ways in which we think, plan, communicate and practise, which stem from a number of sources and, not the least, the huge leap we are all making into the digital age. These will persist and in the main are things over which we have little choice. Rapid changes are affecting how we organise work in times of rapid communication, awe-inspiring technological advances, population development and a digital world that has speeded up our lives and is driving our expectations of services and one another. Society, therefore, must now actively explore new ways of construing relationships between people to better harness what they and groups can offer in pursuit of the common good. The construct of coproduction is, for example, now a much-used approach, in which hierarchies between people and organisations may be changed in order to benefit from both bottom-up as well as the much more traditional top-down approaches. This is useful in designing virtual organisations and uses people's skills more intuitively and democratically.

In other words, we should examine the advantages that short-term and long-term relationships offer with the intention of finding ways to achieve them in the modern world. Some features of previous styles in which staff relate to their employers in the health and social care sectors, such as job security, are important to sustain. Other aspects of our relationships might change, with advantage to both health service employees and employers. But, one thing is clear: we must not be tempted to construe information technology as replacing the importance of relationships and human creativity. Rather, we need to consider how we use it to build and sustain those relationships and achieve the results we require, albeit by different means. Our intention is to draw together various of these elements that have already been referred to and illustrated in this book in order to point up the practical, social aspects of what can make our relationships work well.

Timelines

Short-Termism and Long-Termism

We begin by focusing on the timelines that we have identified. In so doing, we are reminded of the oft-quoted statement, attributed to Gaius Petronius Arbiter (floreat 66 AD),

> We trained hard – but it seemed that every time we were beginning to form up into teams we would be reorganised; I was to learn later in life that we tend to meet any new situation by reorganising and I learned too what a wonderful method it can be for creating the illusion of progress whilst in reality producing confusion, inefficiency and demoralisation.

This quote summarises the not infrequent experiences of people who work in organisations of many natures and purposes, be they in industry, the caring and education services or military organisations, for example. Several of the authors have often had the kinds of experience about which Gaius Petronius comments. Indeed, public-sector services in the UK, as examples, have survived around four decades of reorganisation at increasing rates, such that changes are wrought, often for doctrinal, political or financial reasons, before previous ones have had time to bed in and be evaluated. This has brought a cynical view of change and resistance to it in the public and the workforce. The rapidly rising impacts of technological advance and growing limitations in the skilled labour market are happening in a setting where both inequity and inequality are rising between and within countries. These issues combine to indicate that we cannot and should not continue as we are. This is not solely a matter of practicality or of values, though it is both of these, but it is key to creating a platform for the future that is built on sharing our resources appropriately, and well.

Many of us will have experienced settings in which we set out to forge the relationships that appear vital to success in achieving good outcomes in our work and then have those relationships disrupted by, for example, a key person leaving or being switched to another job. This disruption forces us to start again and accept delay or accept a lower-quality or incomplete outcome. Frequently, we have struggled with circumstances in which relationships between organisations have deteriorated, for example, when arguments about priorities have emerged, or moves towards cost-shifting between the partners in multi-agency endeavours have arisen, following changes in key staff members who have led and signed off the arrangements. The impact may be to postpone our achieving previously agreed goals. By contrast, we have also seen circumstances in which key members of staff remain in post over substantial periods of time and are unable to stand aside from disagreements between organisations; in these circumstances, it is much more difficult for these perverse effects to arise. This gives rise to the opinion that success depends on having long-term relationships (between health and social care and education services, for example) that create and support partnerships. Our experience in working with statutory-sector health services in the aftermath of the arena bombing in Manchester, in May 2017, supports a view that cross-agency partnerships, in which trust and sharing of expertise are built up, provide advantages to rapid planning when major incidents occur. Thus, long-termism pays off and, in certain circumstances, senior managers may consider disrupting healthcare teams to be too great a risk.

However, there are other perspectives and experiences. Short-termism in working relationships could be a way of describing processes of emergent and situationally determined adaptive group relationships. Tierney describes how, during the attack on the World Trade Center (WTC) towers in 2001, the emergency services improvised a coordinated response (Tierney, 2001). The emergency services had had practice and preparation for such a coordinated multi-agency response. There was an attack on, and evacuation of, one of the WTC buildings in 1993 (Aguirre et al., 1998). And, in the following years, drills and improved emergency response procedures were introduced (Fahy & Proulx, 2002). However, the command and control centre for the emergency services in the 2001 attack was out of action because it was in one of the WTC towers; top-down command and control was lost. Therefore, the spontaneous self-organisation of the emergency services – that is, new emergent relationships – and bottom-up coordination were necessary.

In the context of emergencies, this positive version of short-termism is not limited to formal organisations. We conjecture that the shared understandings, shared training and previous experience of the emergency responders around agreed tasks, whether acknowledged or not, were such that they were able to rise to the occasion. But, we cannot base our planning on Micawber-like assumptions that effective practice will emerge, unless certain aspects of the work required are identified and people trained accordingly. What are these vital matters? As the authors of Chapter 17 discuss, under certain circumstances, crowds of people with no previous connections can coordinate and act together in a similar way in the very midst of an emergency. In the case of the survivors of the London bombings on 7 July 2005, for example, this meant providing emotional and practical support to strangers. In effect, survivors acted as the fourth emergency service (Drury et al., 2009). In a second example, a disaster was averted, in part, through such spontaneous cooperation in a large crowd gathered at a music event (Drury et al., 2015). The number of safety professionals available was too small for them to have a direct effect on the crowd at the venue. But, by working with, instead of against, the crowd's identity and values by, for example, asking the disc jockey, not the police, to request people to desist from climbing lighting rigs, they were able to contribute to a safe outcome.

These examples show that lessons learned by the emergency services about the relationships within crowds, and between crowds and the emergency services, should enable communities and organisations to carry forward into the longer term the benefits of people involved working together in informal and emergent groups around particular tasks. The UK Cabinet Office guidance on Community Resilience refers to 'communities of circumstance' that arise in emergencies and disasters, and suggests that members of these groups might provide support to each other after the acute period of the emergency (Cabinet Office, 2011). This points our thinking towards how we harness what groups can offer rather than seeing them as necessarily likely to thwart the top-down plans of people who hold responsibilities. In other words, we return to how we can achieve a creative and effective balance between top-down and bottom-up contributions to finding solutions to tough problems.

Also, under what conditions do short-term relationships become long-term ones? And how can the advantages of long-termism be achieved through prior evaluation of good practice, planning, training and support. Moreover, the suggestion that long-term relationships confer particular benefits carries within it the assumption that short-term relationships have certain disadvantages. So, we move on to review the problems of short-termism before outlining some of the conditions under which (a) useful short-term relationships arise and (b) such short-term relationship can be sustained and feed into longer-term ones.

Emergent Relationships

Here are the conditions that theory and research suggest are the ones in which people are more likely to see themselves as members of a group. They were developed to explain the circumstances when people's existing social identities become salient (e.g. when I see myself as a lecturer in contrast to my identity as a football fan). We summarise here how these conditions can be applied to explaining how people see themselves as members of emergent groups. First, there should be contextual affordances, or fit, that make it meaningful for each person to see their social world in terms of an 'us' (rather than in terms of a 'me' and disconnected others). An example would be when people see themselves as 'all in the same boat', because they are treated *as a group* by others. A case from research on crowds is offered by policing (Stott & Drury, 2000). Actions of the police that are experienced as indiscriminate in relation to a crowd often lead people in it to see themselves as a single, unitary group in relation to the police, thereby superseding previous divisions within the crowd.

Second, there are person variables. In the terms of *self-categorization theory* (Turner et al., 1994) there is a series of perceiver readiness factors. This refers to someone's history and knowledge, and includes factors such as their capacity to see the world in group terms, their track record of attachments, the strength of their social ties, and so on. The perceptions and actions of some people in a crowd may, for example, be shaped more by an existing commitment to a particular personal relationship of loyalty whereas others may be more open to new relationships of loyalty with fellow members of the crowd.

When these conditions hold, that is when there is both fit and readiness to understand the world in collective terms, group perception makes sense of the social environment, and so people construe themselves and others as part of a group, and emergent 'groupness' is possible. Then, once people see themselves as a group, a number of expectations and motivations arise (see Chapter 15). As well as seeking to support each other, group members now have the ability to do so because they are better able to anticipate each other's actions and needs.

A related question is about the conditions in which short-term relationships feed into and support long-term relationships. In brief, there are two answers to this question. The first is in terms of continuation of the situational affordances that made it meaningful, and indeed logical, for people to see themselves as members of a particular group. In other words, this answer translates the question into an enquiry about whether members of the group are still being treated as a group by others. After disasters, for example, most communities of circumstance do not sustain and most disaster communities eventually decline (Kaniasty & Norris, 1999).

The second answer to the question is that some people in a group may do things consciously to keep that group, and its benefits, alive. Thus it seems that the strategic actions of some members drive whether or not these emergent groups do develop into longer-term relationships. We have recently seen examples of the study by Ntontis et al (2017) of long-term responses among people who were affected by the 2015 floods in York, UK. Some interviewees said that the community spirit had soon disappeared, but others referred to activities that had served to keep it alive. They had commemorations. They met regularly and talked about shared experiences. They had a place to go to as a group. Through sustaining the community spirit, they sustained some of the emotional support that went with it.

Organisations and Networks

Next, we consider some of the features of organisations and networks that are key to promoting the benefits of sustained relationships and draw them into two collections, which concern organisations' values and cultures, and their practices that sustain effective teamwork and delivery of services.

Cultures and Values That Affect Productive Relationships

Our experiences are that organisations in which the values of transparency of negotiations and working processes, including honesty, integrity and honour, are evident and sustained are more likely to impact well on their employees, their working relationships and their productivity (see Chapter 24 by Montgomery and Williams regarding these values). In other words, there are reciprocal relationships between organisations' values, which are evident from their relationships with their employees and those with other organisations, and the values that their staff display in their work. These matters also arise in Chapter 28 where Neal et al. consider them as aspects of the moral architecture of organisations.

Transparency is important because it is easier to trust people and agencies if they are experienced as being open in their work and if they handle criticism well. Honesty is essential to the experience of openness, and integrity and honour are evident in the reliability that we learn to place on certain persons and organisations. In other words, it is important that employees and the organisations that employ them are seen as sticking to what they say they will do. Some aspects of these reciprocal relationships between employers and employees are covered by Neal et al. in Chapter 28. Perhaps another way of framing these observations is to say that shared identities between employees in organisations are more likely where there are shared values.

The Origins and Consequences of Good Relationships

Good relationships within and between organisations turn on a range of practical behaviours that emerge from the values on which we comment. So, it is important that staff of organisations are afforded opportunities to recognise, reflect on and discuss their own values and those of their employing organisations. Shared values are of critical importance to team members aligning themselves to the work of their organisation and the teams of which they are members within their employers' spheres of interest.

Trust is an important matter. At its most straightforward, it is a quality of relationships that is transactional and one in which people do as they say, and this might be reflected in people not needing to make formal agreements in writing about the matters on which they have agreed. However, it can be much more complicated than this because most people have multiple loyalties; they are members of many groups within and outwith their professions as well as the organisations that employ them. Also, it is taken as an essential feature of good practice that professional people and managers make notes. In part, this reflects the defensive nature of relationships into which many people feel forced in order that they can find the balance between defending themselves and their employer and the erosion of trust that can emerge, if this is not handled explicitly and well. This is an important matter in managing staff and is critical to their development within organisations.

A vital matter in developing the positive impacts of long-termism and sustaining relationships concerns members of teams spending time together. This matter must be reflected in people's job plans and it should not be seen as other than essential to strong performance. If this is supported by organisations' policies and practices and adequate time is afforded for people to develop trust in one another, behavioural consistency and reliability emerge and there is some evidence that fewer mistakes are made in organisations that feel psychologically safe to staff (Bleetman et al., 2012).

This also means that employers must take care to recognise and support the affiliations and multiple loyalties of their staff. Professional staff are required by law in the UK to identify clearly with defined professional values and practices that are attributable to the regulatory organisations while also working for and being loyal to the expectations and requirements of their employers. These multiple lines of accountability can cause tensions for staff if this circumstance is not well handled by staff and employers alike, and that may impact on their performance and wellbeing. But, where they are handled well and organisations take note of what kind of person each employee is, these organisations are more likely to reap the rewards of effective care, good external perceptions from other organisations and enhanced reputations.

Harnessing the Work of Groups, Teams and Firms

Teams and Firms

Over many years, practitioners who work in health and social care in the UK, for example, have found ways not just of grouping as tribes of varying kinds to protect themselves from the demands of the system, but also to set and maintain standards of practice. Thus, in the past, clinical firms in hospitals brought doctors in training into the hierarchical supervision of more senior medical colleagues, often under the watchful eye, day to day, of a senior nurse with a long-standing professional relationship with the senior consultant. This arrangement used to lie at the core of apprenticeship-based models of learning in healthcare.

More recent moves to shift work and multidisciplinary care planning have changed these arrangements hugely and have not been without difficulty. This is not least for doctors, for example, because the orientation of loyalty away from a medical firm within a common culture to a mixed professional group, with mixed culture and some historical antagonism, has been anxiety-provoking. In addition, moves to include and involve people with a lived experience of their ill health as experts within the context of coproduction has provoked a need for substantial cultural adjustment.

Working Together

Coproduction with the end users of systems is now recognised to be a key success factor in many creative and business enterprises. While welcome, its acceptance has taken time. The NHS Health Advisory Service published a thematic review of involving patients or users and their carers in designing, commissioning and delivering services in 1996, but its recommendations proved too ambitious at the time; though, most interestingly, many of them are now reflected in good practice (Williams et al., 1997). If the challenge of moving from single-discipline firms to multidisciplinary teams has been tricky, the idea that health services might improve if clinicians and managers worked with people who had a current or lived experience of the system under review has taken two decades to achieve currency in policy, and a foothold in practice.

Crucially, our experience is that coproduction results in very different ideas about who is included in groups of expert stakeholders with an interest in the outcome of any piece of work. Traditionally, health services called upon professional experts when planning change. Now, experts are qualified by their experience as well by their professional training and specialist expertise. Evidence in support of these developments comes not only from democratisation of services, but also from the six dimensions of the human condition covered by Smith in Chapter 2 and the findings of the work on horizontal epidemiology by Cieza and Bickenbach, which is reported in Chapter 7, and linked with other theoretical developments that are summarised by Williams et al. in Chapter 13.

Working Under Pressure

The airline industry has moved away from basing passengers' safety on consistent, long-standing cockpit crews, which were conceived in war-time; that is captains, first officers and navigators who worked regularly with one and other often in strict hierarchy. The industry has transformed to aircrew working with colleagues who may be relative strangers and, instead of familiarity, use Crew Resource Management, protocols and safety briefings

(Heimlich et al., 1999). This change has been very successful. It has similarities with the changes in working practices in healthcare in which long-standing 'firms' of professional experience have given way to multidisciplinary groups, working to protocols and procedures.

However, the experience of working under pressure in emergencies or unusual circumstances is different to working in ordinary circumstance that are just busy. Healthcare policies tend to adopt procedures and protocols that are often set for ordinary circumstances, but these practices may become obsolete or even a hindrance in the face of emergencies or other circumstances that demand innovation. So, the professions and managers now recognise the need for separate policies, procedures and protocols for emergency situations that come into play when an emergency is recognised and declared. The difficulty arises when a state of emergency goes unrecognised or undeclared when, for example, the business of ordinary services is disrupted by sudden loss of staff, resource or unexpected demand. In these circumstances, it is common for there to be fractious behaviour, helplessness and blame. It takes strong leadership to pull together clinical teams to meet the challenge and to alert responsible organisations to the emergency.

The Implications of Pressures on Modern Healthcare Practice: Harnessing Lessons from Social Science

The Nature of Groups

As we have seen throughout this book, there are many types of group and many definitions of groups in the literature. In the social identity approach, people are regarded as being a group when they see themselves as a group (Turner et al., 1994), though Reicher offers a caveat to that in Chapter 23 when he says that a group is only a group in social psychological terms when its members share a social identity. Often, the staff groups in healthcare services are populated with new faces, week on week. If so, they are not likely to satisfy the definition of teams as set out by Neal et al. in Chapter 28. But, if shared protocols were to speed the process of identity-sharing, these groups might satisfy the definition of groups set out by Reicher in Chapter 23.

However, there are other ways of being a group. First, there may be small groups in which all the members meet face-to-face, can see each other and can make decisions through direct discussion (as in team meetings, for example). Second, at the other end of the spectrum, the term may also cover social categories such as a nation or other dispersed groups, in which the sense of being a community together is not tangible but has to be imagined (Reicher & Hopkins, 2000).

A distinctive assumption of the social identity approach is the idea that the self is multiple, not unitary (we have many identities, not just our personal identity or personality); and, therefore, our self can also be collective as well as personal (Turner et al., 1994). Sharing social identity with others means seeing them as part of my group, as 'us' or 'we'. As Drury et al. discuss in Chapter 15, there are consequences for how we behave towards others when we and those other people with us share identity, and the boundaries of concern become extended from the personal self to these others. These changes facilitate co-action, communication, and the emotional qualities associated with group membership, including pride, empowerment and subjective wellbeing.

The context and nature of social relationships are key to the safe and effective operation of clinical services. So many of the things that go wrong in delivering healthcare can be attributed to human factors. In Chapter 28, Neal et al. cite a number of inquiries into services in which substantial problems have been found by way of service failures and far less than acceptable qualities of practice. In addition, there have been inquiries into the performance of the responding services after disasters (House of Commons, 2006; HM Government, 2012). Recurrently, inquiries of these kinds show that problems in communication top the list of human-factor violations (Leonard et al., 2004) and these communication failures are exacerbated by the stress and distress which are commonly experienced by people working in hard-pressed services, in which there is weak leadership and poor management. Here, we examine working patterns of doctors and medical students in the UK as a case in point.

The working hours for doctors in the UK have been reduced over a period of time to recognise the human-factor risks of tired doctors, who work long hours without adequate rest, making grievous errors and causing harm. These reductions have not been without debate because it is equally recognised that, in pursuing mastery, the number of hours on a task is important. Reducing hours has been achieved in part by the introduction of shift work. However, this has greatly increased the intensity of the work of the doctor during the shift. Nevertheless, the norm of long periods at work and on-call has given way, over the last 40 years, to shifts within highly regulated hours of work. Arguably, the result has both risks and rewards for practitioners and patients.

This pattern has, to some extent, been replicated in undergraduate medical education. It is no longer usual for students to spend lengthy periods of time attached to one group of doctors, and this reflects the fact that doctors no longer organise their work in this way. In some undergraduate medical school courses that are based on gathering experience and knowledge around key cases, students can find themselves in totally different clinical environments and relationships, week to week.

As the airlines have moved to manage aircrew as flexible teams using Crew Resource Management, rather than relying on the longevity and experience of cockpit crew (Heimlich et al., 1999), we have seen that there are similar trends in healthcare. The value of consistent and well-formed relationships as part of the structure seems to have given way to a system based on policy, procedure and protocol, which regards the contributions of humans as lying at individualised levels. This brings us back to the important matter of distinguishing personalised and individualised approaches that was first raised Montgomery et al. in Chapter 14, at the end of Section 2.

If policy sets the aims for, and the context of, the work done, then procedure sets out the principle of how the work ought to be done in the setting and context of the operator. When something should be done consistently in pursuit of quality and safety in many areas of life, protocols now prescribe precisely what is to be done. As a result, these forms of guidelines and prescription have become essential for people forming new relationships around a task. But, the importance of briefing cannot be understated. New people coming together must take time to brief and be briefed; that is, to talk to one another about the task in hand, the context and principles they are to follow and any precise actions that are required by protocol. Equally, it is imperative that groups come together at various points and at the end of tasks to check that the work is done and identify any learning arising as a result. These briefing and debriefing sessions allow for feedback and reflection and are also amenable to protocol or check-listing. Similarly, there is a risk of our failing to perceive the unique needs, circumstances and preferences of patients in protocol-dependent systems. We must find ways of restoring the balance with patients' perspectives and the changing, but, crucially, not less important, nature of judgement that practitioners require. Without developing judgement, in which practitioners align interventions offered, with each person's needs and preferences, the ability for them to innovate in challenging situations or create new learning may be reduced.

The knock-on effect is that this method or organisation, teaching and training reduces the contributions of longer-term relationships and teams that meet in person in providing resilience and emotional support. Another result could be that we develop and use protocols that achieve mediocrity, or care which is reasonably safe but which fails to support optimal, personalised rather than individualised care. We regret that, all too often, the importance of good relationships and the powerful influences of groups, whether they meet face-to-face or are virtual ones, has not been recognised or harnessed in healthcare systems as ways of filling the gaps left by moving away from firms and, even, moving to higher standards of care. This is the goal that is propelled by the social cure approach (Haslam et al., 2018).

Is it easier to give feedback in established teams or in new teams? In well-formed, well-functioning small groups, feedback and learning flows easily between people who are confident in their relational security. However, even well-established small-group culture can mitigate against safe challenge: 'Ginger has always got us home, he must have spotted that mountain he's about to fly into'; 'Surely our surgeon knows that's the wrong leg he's about to amputate.' And it can be less emotionally provocative to give negative feedback to relative strangers where there is little consequence. The well-known example is road rage. It might appear that feedback is easier in newly formed groups. But, this is a more complicated question than first appears to be the case. In a new group, time is often required to establish essential emotional relationships. The more confident and competent a person is, the more likely they are to solicit critical feedback and make use of it, while colleagues who have a negative experience of negative feedback, or who anticipate negativity, understandably, stop soliciting feedback.

With rising dissatisfaction among medical graduates and career burnout in doctors generally, nostalgia for some of the features of the firm model is leading to its re-evaluation by several of the medical Royal Colleges. How might the benefits of long-term, consistent team relationships be achieved in the context of reduced hours of work, the move to shifts and the shifting culture and context of healthcare? How might the advent of social media and digital health solutions help?

A balance must be struck between longer-term consistency in relationships and flexibility in working practice for the practitioners who contribute to different groups and teams. Clinical leaders and senior managers are important culture carriers for the groups they lead and manage, and ensuring consistency in these relationships makes sense. One of the advantages of the apprenticeship model of training was that the 'master' could judge when the 'apprentice' was ready to work at the next level. Their long-term relationship was key to that. But, the modern requirement that shift work and disarticulated teams present is the need to build team functioning quickly. If this is to be achieved successfully, leaders and managers must understand the psychology of groups and teams and be equipped with the coaching, mentoring and supervision skills to develop and manage not only the process and task but also, critically, the supporting human factors.

Data have a key part to play in this provided they are converted into useful, timely information that informs practice and progress. Otherwise, if practitioners cannot see the purpose and a helpful output, collecting data turns into a chore into which people are more likely to put minimal effort, and that feeds cynicism. Paper log books of clinical case material and comment have progressed to online electronic appraisal systems that capture an array of measures and feedback, which, when used well, can help to inform practitioners' development. What is of concern is that, often, human factors and character strengths and weaknesses are not well conveyed by these systems and they may turn out to be a poor substitute for the 'master's' eye on the practical and emotional readiness of 'apprentices' to take their next steps. Again, we need to use parallel processes in which we use digital systems for what they are good at, but also employ groups to assist us with the matters of practice, skill, quality etc. for which they provide good fora.

Thus, the revolution in digital technology and communication offers some opportunity. While no substitute for face-to-face meetings when making new relationships, social media and messaging platforms can strongly support existing relationships, and real-time video and telephone conferencing can enable remote working in virtual groups. Many clinical peer groups use social media for exactly these functions. In recent major incidents, some groups of doctors have used social messaging platforms to organise their emergency response far more quickly than conventional systems (Thomas, 2018). There is little that can't be found on platforms such as YouTube for learners. What helps is a complementary system of online peers, coaches and mentors who can discuss the material being viewed and guide learners in their acquiring knowledge, skills and, most importantly, judgement.

Lasting Lessons

In summary, long-termism matters in providing emotional resilience and support and is most important for clinical leaders and managers who are culture carriers for groups and teams. But short-termism is a reality for many team members who may work in different teams and groups in the course of a working week. Policy, procedures and protocols inform and guide the work of new groups. But leaders, managers and peers need skills in coaching, mentoring and supervising and, inevitably in the future, some of this work will be in the virtual digital environment. It is important that clinicians can feel an affiliation to great firms with which they have worked.

In this concluding section, we draw together and identify some of the key lessons that we identify from this chapter. The world has changed and will continue to change. We must recognise that, but also identify what is important in high-quality healthcare and seek ways to sustain and develop the skills of relating well, recognising people's needs and enabling the professions of the future to maintain and develop the quality of what they do, albeit in hugely changed environments.

We think that developing quality turns on recognising the importance of organisations:

(a) Identifying and 'living' their shared values and expectations deliberately through the relationships they foster;

(b) Developing their strength in depth;

(c) Engaging with the critical importance of great leadership;

(d) Being relentlessly reasonable; and

(e) Engaging well with what technology and emerging digital environments have to offer, in achieving creative coproductive relationships between patients and practitioners.

All of this requires us to harness learning about how groups function. But we must also come to terms with the risks that stem from poor and unsatisfactory relationships that can, all too easily, come back to bite. So, before closing, we summarise ideas about just three of these items: organisations' values and expectations; leadership; and being relentlessly reasonable.

Organisations' Values and Expectations

In Chapter 23, Reicher makes a number of concluding points. First, shared social identity in groups creates bonds between people and converts those bonds into social capital. In this chapter, we suggest exploiting this process to help us to replace the advantages of longer-term relationships in modern health and social care. In his second conclusion, Reicher asserts that the key to a new social model of mental and physical health lies in an understanding of how to support people in building and consolidating their own social groups. But, importantly, he points out that social identity can work for good outcomes but also for those that we see as less positive. In his opinion, projects with the objectives of supporting people to achieve positive outcomes can only be successful if they integrate a knowledge of psychological principles with a cultural understanding of the social, institutional and political contexts in which they are to be applied.

So, in Chapter 12, Montgomery considers the values reflected in tolerance and tolerating competing ideas. In Chapter 24, Montgomery and Williams consider the resources that can be drawn from public health ethics to understand how health can be sustained, and also recovered, in the face of challenges to wellbeing at community and national levels. This involves human systems in making values-laden choices about which preferences should be based on group identities and which not. Furthermore, there may be tensions between different groups for access to, and use of, the same resources for quite different objectives, and that takes us back to tolerance and our requirement for an ethical framework in making difficult decisions that everyone agrees are fair.

Thus, using social scaffolding, horizontal epidemiology and coproduction to improve the quality of health and social care services, and how we should choose between the different priorities proposed by different organisations or groups, raises their values and the requirement to make ethical choices. Montgomery and Williams explore these matters in Chapter 24. They consider the construct of public health ethics; this is a complex concept but they are able to identify a series of principles. They illustrate operationalising those principles in a commentary on the framework produced by the Committee on Ethical Aspects of Pandemic Influenza (CEAPI) to aid policymakers, practitioners and managers to make ethical decisions when planning for pandemics. The principles in that framework have much to offer in making ethical decisions when using the principles of social identity to develop the role of groups in delivering health and social care.

Leadership

Leadership is about enabling people to give of their best and is especially challenging when people are under pressure. This requires vision and strategic direction. Vision is the ability to identify, for groups of people, what is the common goal, and a strategic direction towards that goal. It describes the ability to paint a picture in the minds of colleagues of the steps required to achieve the goal. Too often, there is a temptation to confuse leadership with command, which is the function of legitimately making decisions according to delegated authority, and with management of resources. In truth, there are overlaps in the skills required to lead, command and manage and all three are transactional styles of required relationships. But it is important for members of teams to be clear about which roles fall legitimately to themselves and which to colleagues.

Leadership is an essential function in healthcare because if technical experts are to perform their tasks with success they need others to manage the mission and keep the whole care effort on track (Storey & Holti, 2013). Furthermore, leadership styles matter, and relationships are key. In the past, for example, the NHS in the UK has been criticised for fostering command and control over more engaging affiliation or delegation styles. Leaders need to be easy to follow and followers need to support their leaders to lead (The Hay Group, 2013). Readers can find two explicit presentations of leadership in this book. In the first, in Chapter 21, Alderdice looks at the kinds of leadership that are required to tackle intractable problems while the second is in Chapter 29, where Haslam et al. present a model of leadership that is based on the social identity approach.

Being Relentlessly Reasonable

While long-termism in close working relationships may no longer be the organisational form, the mobile, flexible nature of multidisciplinary and inter-agency working makes it more likely that we will work with people again. Memories of difficulties are longer than memories of routine. Bruised relationships inevitably impair effective working by impairing trust.

It is a reasonably safe assumption that most people come to work in health and social care to do a good job. Most, if not all, have an empathy for people in distress and few, if any, would consciously allow themselves to be angry or upset with a patient or their carers. Yet the same does not always seem apply to colleagues. Even the best of health and social care teams can have awkward moments internally and in their relationship with other teams. Blame and scapegoating of individual people and other teams are not uncommon. Therefore, it is important to consider how teams are built, led and managed, and nurtured in the longer-term. It is useful to anticipate these issues and prepare to manage them, with time and space together to address them.

Health and social care in emergencies are inherently stressful and upsetting, by the very nature of the human problems with which staff are asked to deal. They are asked to observe and listen to upsetting and troubling things. It is unsurprising, then, that the high level of emotion experienced needs to be expressed and that under pressure, this expression may be less than well considered. Circumstances in which debate and disagreement become personalised and accusative are deeply damaging to future working relationships. Rows are remembered, and for a long time.

It follows that it is of critical importance that we support the work of health and social care staff by fostering a group culture wherein we are relentlessly reasonable with one and other and seek to leave every encounter well. When moments of awkwardness arise, or if blame and scapegoating are apparent, leaders and managers must move to address these issues quickly. If we don't, the transitory nature of current multidisciplinary working means that offence taken often leaves groups without reconciliation, restitution or recovery.

References

Aguirre, B. E., Wenger, D. & Vigo, G. (1998). A test of the emergent norm theory of collective behavior. Social Forum **13**: 301–320.

Bleetman, A., Sanusi, S., Dale, T. & Brace, S. (2012). Human factors are error prevention in emergency medicine. Emergency Medical Journal, **29**: 389–393.

Cabinet Office (2011). Strategic National Framework on Community Resilience. London: Cabinet Office.

Drury, J., Cocking, C. & Reicher, S. (2009). The nature of collective resilience: Survivor reactions to the 2005 London bombings. International Journal of Mass Emergencies and Disasters, **27**: 66–95.

Drury, J., Novelli, D. & Stott, C. (2015). Managing to avert disaster: Explaining collective resilience at an outdoor music event. European Journal of Social Psychology, **45**: 533–547.

Fahy, R. F. & Proulx, G. (2002). A comparison of the 1993 and 2001 evacuations of the World Trade Center. Proceedings of the 2002 Fire Risk and Hazard Assessment Symposium, **24**: 111–117.

Friedberg, M. W., Chen, P. G., van Busum, K. R et al.(2013). Factors Affecting Physician Professional Satisfaction and Their Implications for Patient Care, Health Systems, and Health Policy. Santa Monica, CA: Rand Health and the American Medical Association.

Haslam, C., Jetten, J., Cruwys, T., Dingle, G. A. & Haslam, S. A. (2018). The New Psychology of Health: Unlocking the Social Cure. London: Routledge.

Heimlich, R. L., Merritt, A. C. & Wilhelm, J. A. (1999). The evolution of crew resource management training in commercial aviation. The International Journal of Aviation Psychology, **9**: 19–32; doi: 10.1207/s15327108ijap0901_2.

HM Government (2012). Coroner's inquests into the London bombings of 7 July 2005: Review of progress. See www.gov.uk/government/publications/coroners-inquests-into-the-london-bombings-of-7-july-2005-review-of-progress.

House of Commons (2006). Report of the Official Account of the Bombings in London on 7th July 2005 (HC Paper 1087). London: The Stationery Office.

Kaniasty, K. & Norris, F. (1999). The experience of disaster: Individuals and communities sharing trauma. In Gist, R. & Lubin, B., editors, Response to Disaster: Psychosocial, Community, and Ecological Approaches. Philadelphia, PA: Brunner Maze, pp. 25–61.

Leonard, M., Graham, S. & Bonacum, D. (2004). The human factor: The critical importance of effective teamwork and communication in providing safe care. Quality and Safety in Health Care, **13**(Suppl. 1): i85–i90; doi: 1136/qshc.2004.010033.

Ntontis, E., Drury, J., Amlôt, R., Rubin, G. R. & Williams, R. (2017). Developing community resilience through social identities. Paper presented at 18th General Meeting of the European Association of Social Psychology, Granada, Spain, July.

Reicher, S. & Hopkins, N. (2000). Self and Nation. London: Sage.

Storey, J & Holti, J. (2013). Towards a new model of leadership for the NHS. See www.leadershipacademy.nhs.uk/wp-content/uploads/2013/05/Towards-a-New-Model-of-Leadership-2013.pdf.

Stott, C. & Drury, J. (2000). Crowds, context and identity: Dynamic categorization processes in the 'poll tax riot'. Human Relations, **53**: 247–273.

The Hay Group (2013). Making clinical leadership work: Enabling clinicians to deliver better health outcomes. See www.kingsfund.org.uk/sites/default/files/media/kate-wilson-haygroup-making-clinical-leadership-work-kingsfund-may13_3.pdf.

Thomas, K. (2018). Whatapp Wanted: A WhatsApp alternative for clinicians. British Medical Journal, **360**: k622; https://doi.org/10.1136/bmj.k622.

Tierney, K. J. (2001). Strength of a city: A disaster research perspective on the World

Trade Center attack. See http://essays.ssrc.org/10yearsafter911/strength-of-a-city-a-disaster-research-perspective-on-the-world-trade-center-attack/.

Turner, J. C., Oakes, P. J., Haslam, S. A. & McGarty, C. (1994). Self and collective: Cognition and social context. Personality and Social Psychology Bulletin, **20**: 454–463.

Williams, R., Emerson, G. & Muth, Z., editors (1997). Voices in Partnership: Involving Users and Carers in Commissioning and Delivering Mental Health Services. London: The Stationery Office.

Chapter 28

Caring for the Carers

Adrian Neal, Verity Kemp and Richard Williams

Meeting the Challenges of Compassionate Healthcare

Setting the Scene

At the core of this book is the importance to people's wellbeing and health of their social connectedness, attachments and attachment capacities, and their social identities. It is clear that people crave society and that they gain support, meaning and a sense of control from their shared social identities that sustain them, day to day. Furthermore, their social connectedness and identities provide them with templates for how they respond, cope and are supported when they meet challenges and adversity.

But, turning the tables, what is it like to care for other people? While doing so may give much satisfaction and meaning to carers, that role is not without its own challenges. The focal matter in this chapter is that of how to encourage professional practitioners to engage fully in working compassionately for the people in their care while taking steps to reduce the potential burdens of so doing.

First though, we must recognise the common, though often unacknowledged, experience that providing compassionate care for another human being in distress is both physically and emotionally demanding. There is an abundance of evidence supporting this statement, particularly if care is focused on a single person – usually a relative or family member with whom the carer has a pre-existing relationship. Caring relationships are emotionally draining, physically demanding and can also impact on carers' financial security and social connectedness. In short, unless carefully managed, caring for people you know can be harmful to you despite all the best of intentions and whether or not it is a satisfying task. This applies to caring for relatives and friends, but also to care delivered by professional practitioners to their clients or patients.

Indeed, while providing high-quality, compassionate, professional care can be intensely rewarding, it may also be extremely challenging and requires a well-supported workforce. Perhaps, it is not surprising that there have been some very public, and many less public, failures in care. In recent years, taking the UK as just one example, there has been a number of high profile national enquiries across the UK into failures in professional care systems (e.g. the Mid Staffordshire National Health Service Foundation Trust Public Inquiry, Faculty of Intensive Care Medicine, 2016; Francis, 2013; Liverpool Care Pathway, Department of Health, 2013; Winterbourne View, Department of Health, 2012; Morecambe Bay, Kirkup, 2015; Southern Healthcare, Andrews & Butler, 2014, Richardson, 2015). In Australia, there have been some similar events in care services for older people, notably involving abuse and clinical failures. This has resulted in a national enquiry in the form of a Parliamentary review, focused on effectiveness of aged care frameworks in ensuring older Australians receive quality care and are protected from abuse (Parliament of Australia, 2018). Together, these inquiries identify a number of interrelated systemic factors that have contributed to these failures, including anti-therapeutic or toxic (macro- and micro-) cultures, fiscal over-control, rigid targets, staff shortages, collective denial and defensiveness, demoralisation and fear.

In addition, these inquiries identify that, in each case, staff have reported experiencing compassion fatigue, poor interpersonal relationships with their managers and leaders, high degrees of stress, and burnout. The organisations appear to have had leaders who displayed a marked poverty in their understanding of the psychosocial needs of their staff. Bhui et al. (2016) identified causes of work stress that they define as 'a harmful reaction that people have due to undue pressures and demands placed on them at work', including unrealistic demands, lack of support and effort–reward imbalance.

Williams et al. (2016) describe in a book chapter for psychiatrists how, despite the outrage expressed by the public about these failures, generally, the public remains supportive of healthcare systems and expect their staff to behave in professional and compassionate ways, even if their places of work are not optimal. Interestingly, failures in quality of care do not appear to have been eradicated by strengthened arrangements for corporate and clinical governance.

Surveys show that, as an example of a healthcare system, 'the public's pride in the NHS [National Health Services in the UK] is as strong as ever with . . . 78% agreeing . . . that it is one of the best healthcare systems in the world' (Ipsos MORI, 2016). However, as a result of its survey of health leaders in September 2016, the UK's Nuffield Trust was concerned that 'signs of poor morale and engagement are emerging in the NHS in recent years, leading to staff shortages and difficulties in recruiting'. Seventy-seven per cent of responders to the survey identified workload as being a key factor, as well as the negative aspects of the organisational culture and regulators and central bodies creating pressure.

Hacker Hughes et al. (2016) point to the effects on NHS staff of having to work to increasingly stringent performance targets. The effects quoted include increases in staff sickness days and the tragically high rates of suicide among healthcare professionals in England and Wales. They propose that organisations have a key role in staff wellbeing and the new Charter for Psychological Staff Wellbeing and Resilience in the NHS in 2016 states that 'those services which have good staff wellbeing will be more sustainable and make the most difference to those [people] they are helping'.

While science of organisational perspectives on understanding and meeting the needs of staff who are professional carers is in its infancy, there is material that shows the importance of caring for staff well. There are evidence-based recommendations in two reports and guidelines from the National Institute for Health and Care Excellence (NICE, 2009, 2013), but meaningful application of the evidence-base has had too little impact on the workforce in the UK.

We establish in Chapter 11 that psychosocial resilience is context-dependent and that the same staff may show differing levels of resilience depending on the circumstances in which they are working, the nature of their roles and the ways in which they, in turn, are supported and the care they receive. Thus, while resilience is related to certain personal attributes, knowledge and skills, an approach to supporting personal and professional carers that is based on coaching people on these matters risks missing out on the powerful influences on resilience that stem from social connectedness, attachment and shared social identities.

The business of health and social care exposes staff to primary stressors that are inherent and therefore inevitable, in the work they do. These stressors may cause distress to health and social care staff in the course of their work. They may arise from events and tasks that persist in the short and longer terms. Cumulatively, exposure to primary stress may bring about physical and psychosocial injury and disruption to lifestyles and, in more extreme circumstances, staff may require a significant period of recovery. The knock-on effects may affect not only the people who are directly involved but also their families, friends and wider communities.

Secondary stressors are not inherent in the events. Usually, they last longer than the primary stressors and they include, for example, failure of the infrastructure in working environments, gaps in provision of services, failures in developing services, and problems with personal and career development (Williams & Kemp, 2016).

Bhui et al. (2016) identify that effective organisational interventions include improving management styles, providing employees with time for planning their work tasks and breaks and for physical exercise. They compared management of stress in public, private and non-governmental organisations and found that public-sector organisations, notably the NHS in England, had more interventions in place to help employees manage stress.

Traditionally, workforce development and staff management is viewed through the prism of an industrial model in which staff are seen as resources, or parts of the organisation (or machine) that must be managed according to fiscal, strategic or structural demands. This metaphor holds some validity in highly mechanised industrial processes, but it quickly breaks down when the work involves complex human interaction, and when physical labour is largely exchanged for psychological labour and emotional resources.

Furthermore, our experience is that, when professional carers are offered supportive interventions, there is a tendency to focus our efforts at cognitive levels by encouraging reflexivity about personal knowledge and skill. But in addition, we emphasise in this book the importance of recognising the context-specific elements of coping, adapting and learning and the power of group-focused interventions. Deliberate system-focused interventions to promote reflection on the emotional impact of work such as Schwartz Rounds (Pepper et al., 2011) can help to support teams' growth of self-awareness and reflective working cultures. We offer these observations here because we see each of the parts as a component of a dynamic system rather than as separate.

The Contents of This Chapter

The chapter is organised into five main parts. They are:

(1) Intrapersonal relationships: relationships within oneself;
(2) Interpersonal relationships: relationships with colleagues and peers;
(3) Relationships between employees and their employers;
(4) Relationships within the work of professional caring; and
(5) A strategic approach to developing systems for caring for staff and responding to their needs.

This chapter posits that there is a *relational framework* underpinning the psychosocial wellbeing, coping, adaptation and learning of staff that can act to ameliorate the emotional demands that caring places on healthcare professional practitioners and managers in work environments that increasingly demand consistently high standards of care and uninterrupted compassion (Grandey, 2000). This relational framework links to a social evolutionary theory of human interaction, as well as psychological models that focus on the subtle, reciprocal nature of relationships, as well as wider models of relationship/emotional development such as adult attachment theory (Crittenden, 2006), models from organisational psychology (Daniels et al., 2017) and models from research on shared social identities. Therefore, we take an integrative approach in which learning from each of the five parts is brought together to design meaningful support for professional carers in their development, sustaining their wellbeing and mitigating the risks they face.

At intervals in this chapter, we call on evidence from our chapter in another book (Williams et al., 2016). We conclude by identifying what we think can be done in the short, medium and long terms to improve how organisations care for their professional carers.

Intrapersonal Relationships

The Self and Psychosocial Resources

A number of factors determine what psychosocial resources members of staff may have at their disposal (Bakker & Demerouti, 2007). They include: people's ego-protecting beliefs (e.g. self-serving biases); the adaptiveness of their dominant coping strategies; their capacity for self-compassion; their adaptive personality traits (e.g. optimism); and their emotional intelligence (to a large extent, the ability to manage one's emotional world). Conversely, the value of these psychological resources may well be limited by other psychological factors, such as each person's self-defeating coping strategies. Self-awareness, that is the ability to understand one's own internal or psychological world, is also an important resource. This section explores these factors and identifies what can be done to improve our intrapersonal relationships and resources. Taking a closer look at yourself can form an important part of personal as well as professional growth (Bailey et al., 2001). However, many professional carers only develop their self-awareness after a challenging experience.

Conservation of Resources

The conservation of resources model (Hobfoll, 1989) states that the function of much of our behaviour is to conserve and build precious emotional resources. Thus, without adequate self-awareness, we are likely to be drawn to use coping styles that only have short-term effectiveness, are ultimately self-defeating, undermine wellbeing and re-enforce psychological dysfunction.

In the extreme, Bandura (1997) posits that professional carers may start to morally disengage, which might lead to the increased permissibility of neglectful, or even overtly abusive, care. Recent research indicates that affect avoidance based coping styles in an acute medical setting actually maintains distress and is linked to burnout and compassion fatigue (Iglesias et al, 2010).

The emotional demands of life, including those posed by work, require us to utilise a wide range of psychological coping resources. Psychological therapies, including mindfulness (Brown et al., 2007), and the approaches outlined in the book *Intelligent Kindness* (Campling, 2015), have been shown to improve psychosocial resilience for some people. Self-compassion (SC) has been identified as essential to sustained wellbeing and also to the quality of relationships between colleagues, and with patients. Poor SC has clear associations with poor coping, depression (Allen & Leary, 2010), maladaptive psychological adjustment to trauma and reduced psychological adaptability and recovery (Thompson & Waltz, 2008).

Emotional intelligence (as measured by the Traits Emotional Intelligence Questionnaire (TEIQ)) has been acknowledged as important in good physical and psychological health (Tsaousis & Nikolaou, 2005). Currently one of the most empirically reliable and valid models of TEIQ is a trait model (Petrides & Furnham, 2003). This model considers TEIQ as a form of stable personality trait, dominated by factors that relate to emotional recognition and management of self. This suggests that a better understanding of our own TEIQ and that of the teams and managers with which we work may well offer helpful insights into how we recognise and regulate our own emotions and those of others.

Interpersonal Relationships

Psychosocial Resilience and Social Identity

We include this topic within the section on interpersonal relationships because research summarised in this book, and especially in Chapters 2, 11, 13 and 23 and 25, shows just how important to psychosocial resilience, coping and adapting are our interconnectedness and social identities.

Social connectedness is critical to how members of staff cope, adapt, recover from stressful challenges and behave. We concur with Norris et al. who define the kind of resilience we describe here as a process that links a set of adaptive capacities to a positive trajectory of functioning and adaptation after a disturbance (Kaniasty & Norris, 2004; Norris et al., 2009). The influences on our personal and collective psychosocial resilience are genetic, neurobiological, psychological, environmental and social. Importantly, the ability to make and develop relationships and to accept the support from these relationships are vital elements in people who demonstrate better psychosocial resilience. As well as practical and emotional help, social interaction also creates a network that can be drawn on when it is required (Haslam et al., 2012; Williams et al., 2014). Williams and Kemp provide a substantial overview of psychosocial resilience in Chapter 11.

Adult attachment patterns relate closely to secure and insecure attachment styles that are developed in childhood (Crittenden & Landini, 2011, p. 250). They influence our patterns of resilient behaviour. As we describe in Chapter 11, people's exposure to substantial stress appears to evoke established inner patterns for seeking the attachments that are developed from childhood onwards. In the absence of people with whom to have existing relationships, they are usually propelled to seek social connectedness with people around them who may be in similar circumstances. We may create connections rapidly with people who are available and these emergent relationships provide us with opportunities to gain social support, a sense of control, and personal and group agency. Research is ongoing in this domain, but there are sound theoretical psychosocial mechanisms to explain how past attachment styles and capabilities are projected into current social connections, including those at work, and especially so when that work is stressful.

This book shows how the concept of social identity is important in understanding how we connect with groups and build shared identities. Research has shown the significance of the social identity approach as a theory that explains how relationships at home and work as well as with strangers have positive impacts on how we deal with adversity and ill health. Chapters 4, 15, 23, 25 and 27 show how the positive effects of these identities support the adaptive capabilities that are core to psychosocial resilience.

Earlier in this book, we have drawn attention to research indicating that resilience may be context- and role-specific (Panter-Brick & Leckman, 2013). As we say in Chapter 11, people are not inherently resilient or vulnerable but, rather, are influenced by their contemporary circumstances and resources that affect the coping strategies they use to gain resilience (Southwick et al., 2014).

Relationships Between Team Members

Groups of people who work cooperatively within workplaces are often called teams. Teams should meet specific criteria and it is important to highlight that many teams do not meet the true definition (Carter et al., 2008). It is not uncommon for employers to fail to define at the outset what kind of team they are setting up. Shuffler et al. (2011) argue that to be labelled as a team, a group of people must have a shared and agreed set of aims and goals, as well as a shared identity (see Reicher's account in Chapter 23).

While we are highly evolved to connect and cooperate, as this book shows, we are also evolved to identify the potential for threat and danger. Teams can be powerful sources of psychosocial support to their members when relationships within teams are good and where rules, roles and purposes are agreed and aims and goals are clarified. But, all too often, organisations rely on groups to cooperate in this way without necessarily setting the conditions in which that can occur. As a result, staff are likely to be exposed to the stresses generated by the emotional labour of their caring roles without the protective potential of true teams.

It is not uncommon for a range of what Campling and Ballat (Ballat & Campling, 2011; Campling, 2015) describe as 'perverse dynamics' to be played out within teams and for relationships to be challenged and become a potent source of psychosocial threat. Reciprocally, defensive behaviours may be triggered, leading to escalation and conflict, and these interactions can become real challenges to the health of the social climate of the system in which people work. This may undermine corrosively both personal and team wellbeing and resilience, and, thereby, their members' ability to care for others.

Gilbert (2005) has argued that the largest source of psychosocial threat from within a team or with peers comes from the provocation of self-conscious emotions such as shame, humiliation and guilt, as can be seen after social rejection, and loss of rank. The chapters in this book that relate to social connectedness and identity show not only the power of these kinds of identities but also the mechanisms of relationships, which are supported by research.

Leadership

When considering what can be done by employing organisations, Williams et al. (2016) point to leadership as being one of the key factors in helping to keep staff well and performing effectively, with the importance of relationships between leaders and employees in maintaining staff wellbeing being well established (Black & Frost, 2011; NICE, 2013). Haslam et al. make this point in Chapter 29. The interesting question is why this might be so. At a very simple level, leaders who display qualities such as valuing and acknowledging staff, and being consistent and boundaried, appear to have better relationships with their staff. Leaders who create psychologically safe working environments are more likely to work with staff who feel safe and valued (Edmondson, 1999). Relationships between leaders and staff act as facilitators of wellbeing and resilience of staff and can be pivotal in creating and maintaining the psychological milieu in workplaces.

Our experience from clinical practice, leadership, managerial roles and research is that it is highly unusual to see teams that cope, adapt and sustain high-quality care in which these conditions are absent. Breakdowns in relationships between staff and leaders are often associated with higher sickness absence, complaints and poor quality of care. In turn, rates of sickness absences may be external indicators of organisational problems that should forewarn boards of problems that could be impacting on the quality of care they offer. The Department of Health asserts that, 'There is a strong relationship between healthcare sector staff wellbeing and performance outcomes and there is evidence of a causal link, however this will differ in different fields' (Department of Health, 2014).

Positively, Kuoppala et al. (2008) and Thomas et al. (2004) show the effect of good leadership on mental health and wellbeing for groups, including students and military personnel. However, it is important to point out that repairing a ruptured relationship rests upon both employees and employers accepting the reality, adopting adult positions (Berne, 1964) and correctly identifying and clarifying the problematic issues and their origins, and highlighting personal responsibility. In this approach, breaches and ruptures can be seen as an opportunity to strengthen a relationship, bolster staff wellbeing and promote their psychosocial resilience. However, before attempting to repair ruptured relationships, a competent, theoretically driven formulation is needed to understand how the rupture came about and how a better relationship is maintained. Later (see Box 28.1), we make suggestions for requirements of leaders to create psychologically safe and resilient teams (Williams et al., 2016).

Relationships between Employers and Employees

Relationships between employers and employees are partly governed by each employee's conscious implicit and explicit expectations of one other. The factors include: remuneration; agreed working conditions; perceived fairness; how employees expect to be treated; employees' personal agency; and the general demands of their jobs. Reciprocally, breaches in this informal relational contract can negatively affect the staff's morale, motivation and productivity.

Organisational psychology has identified that staff form a powerful though often unacknowledged relationship with their employing organisations, coined the 'psychological contract' (Rousseau, 1989). 'Good enough' psychological contracts and relationships are likely to bolster employees' motivation, and their willingness and capacity to cope with the challenges they face; but a poor relationship may well have the opposite effect. The concept of organisational justice (Adams, 1963; Barsky & Kaplin, 2007) is relevant to how good enough psychological contracts are maintained. Minimising unhelpful breaches to psychological contracts rests upon a broad web of factors, linked to organisational strategy.

We argue that these specific relational factors are the foundation stones of caring for professional carers whose roles are often highly emotional and demanding. Indeed, these factors may also be considered to be cultural foundation stones within each organisations' moral architecture (Williams et al., 2016). The power of interactions between persons and groups of people is highlighted by Williams et al. (2016), and this includes work colleagues. These interactions among healthcarers is valued and contributes to job satisfaction (Cicognani et al., 2009) and to their ability to respond positively to the effects of traumatic experiences.

All of these factors can be seen in effective individual human relationships, and are equally important in healthy organisational relationships. We argue that organisational cultures that avoid or deny problems are dangerous and can create and maintain toxic social climates wherein individual members of staff are increasingly blamed for what may be essentially systemic problems (Wilde, 2016). These systems also focus on solutions that are aimed at removing or curing 'bad' or 'sick' members of staff. Toxicity and attribution styles of this nature have been identified in all of the recent inquiries into failures of care.

It is vital to consider the emotional capability and capacity of managers and supervisors as they are pivotally important, and they can have positive impacts on the wellbeing of members of staff and teams. We advise that managers should consider the health and shared identity of each team for which they are responsible. They should determine if each group is a true team, and if it has the identified structural features and stability to achieve its purpose. This is especially important in a professional caring environment that appears to be in a constant state of flux, external scrutiny and criticism.

Relationships Within the Work of Professional Caring

Relationships with Caring

It is well known that many professional carers are intrinsically motivated by a desire to help others. Their drive to reduce distress, improve quality of life or be able to positively influence another, to make a difference, are all believed to be powerful intrinsic motivators.

What attracts people to the various types of, and specialisms and roles in, professional caring is less clear. In addition to the usual extrinsic motivators such as remuneration, associated social value, status and structure that most paid forms of work provide, we can assume that the balance of intrinsic factors that motivate people into chosen roles or careers includes how the work meets and interacts with their own underlying emotional needs. We also argue that their histories, personalities and attachment styles also influence their choices, as do their psychological resources, such as their ability to tolerate distress, capacity for empathy, sense of agency and self-worth.

Bion (1961) proposed that strong emotions can be supported or held within groups, without members realising it. Leaders should understand the potential of this social containment in developing organisations that provide compassionate care. Members of groups that offer social containment feel safer and better supported when exploring powerful emotions. The opposite is also true; group members feel exposed without containment.

There are two key factors in considering the potential emotional impacts of work. Emotional labour and psychosocial load are of particular significance as neither are commonly identified in job descriptions. Emotional labour describes the psychological demand placed on people by the effort required to show the 'right' emotions in spite of the emotions they might actually be experiencing. This requires staff to regulate their own emotional states as triggered by their role while maintaining a calm external appearance (Brotheridge & Grandey, 2002). Unsurprisingly, high emotional labour has been linked by the same authors to burnout and employee disengagement. At an extreme level, vicarious traumatisation in care workers has been linked to continued exposure to the distress of patients or recipients of care (Saakvitne et al., 2000).

The emotional labour and psychosocial load inherent in work varies significantly across the caring professions, but is rarely acknowledged in job design and planning. But, despite their greater knowledge and efforts to provide the right resources to offset the demand, a recent survey of psychological therapists in the UK (British Psychological Society, 2016) suggests that up to 46 per cent of them were experiencing significant symptoms of depression and burnout, and a motivation to leave their professions. This indicates that we must seriously consider the impact of emotional load and labour on professional carers when designing jobs and recruiting employees. Sustaining adequate performance, values congruence and wellbeing may well become impossible if these factors are not considered, by employees and employers.

A way forward may require employers to have a more psychosocially informed understanding of the complex demands of the jobs they require their employees to do, as well as what internal and external resources their employees need over time in order to do their jobs. Employees should show their willingness to better understand their own motivators and internal resources as well as the unique impact the work has on them as persons. This takes us on to the concept of moral architecture.

The Moral Architecture of Organisations

Williams et al. (2016) describe the construct of moral architecture as referring 'to the moral and human rights obligations that organisations acquire as employers and through their commitment to delivering high-quality services'. Implicit in this description is that employers have moral as well as legal responsibilities for their staff. 'The moral architecture of organisations includes how well employers discharge these implied responsibilities and recognising and attending to the implied psychological contract is one aspect'.

A Strategic Approach to Developing Systems for Caring for Staff and Responding to Their Needs

Now, as we conclude this chapter, we pull together the information and opinion we have offered in it to underpin an approach to developing coherent systems, practices and opportunities to turn research and theory into better systems to care for staff who face the emotional labour inherent in the stress created by their undertaking values-ridden and challenging jobs. We commend, for example, endeavours to create psychologically safe working environments that augment the skills and commitment of carers so that they can sustain the compassion that the people for whom they work, whether termed patients, clients or service users, require. Briefly put, attention to each organisation's moral architecture requires employers to offer staff the same compassion. Box 28.1 summarises some of the requirements that fall on leaders in so doing.

Organisations can demonstrate their commitment to creating moral architecture explicitly in their policies, their governance and how services are designed and delivered. The methods used by organisations to deliver services must be consistent with stated values, including the way staff are supported and cared for.

A Strategic, Stepped Model of Care for Health and Social Care Staff

We propose that employers should adopt a systematic and systemic approach to caring for carers, preparing themselves and their employees to cope with the emotional labour and psychosocial load of the particular work of caring. Such an approach would help ensure that

Box 28.1 Requirements of leaders to create psychologically safe and resilient teams (from Williams et al., 2016)

- Be accessible and supportive
- Acknowledge fallibility
- Balance empowering other people with managing the tendencies for certain people to dominate discussions
- Balance psychological safety with accountability, safety and other components of strategic and clinical governance
- Minimise exposure to shame, humiliation or guilt
- Guide team members through talking about learning from their uncertainties
- Balance opportunities for their teams' reflection with action
- Have the capacity for emotional containment/holding

Table 28.1 A strategic stepped model for responding to the needs of, and caring for staff (Copyright Williams R and Kemp V all rights reserved and reproduced with permission)

Step	Action levels	Purpose of action	Time scale
1	Preparedness: Strategic planning, leadership and management	Recognise the foundational value of clearly defining the roles of staff, their having accurate job descriptions, there being psychologically safe team cultures and the capability of leaders to understand and respond to the emotional needs of staff and the processes within teams	Before events and continuing afterwards
2	Mitigation: Developing the resilience of staff communities	Reduce the risks of staff becoming distressed or developing mental disorder through preparedness, prevention, risk communication and mitigation of risk and by increasing their familiarity with and confidence in plans through rehearsal and training before events occur	
3	Work community development: Day-to-day leadership and management	Deliver support for groups of staff through public welfare, public mental healthcare or psychosocial paradigms of response to their psychosocial needs that are based on the principles of psychological first aid	Immediate and continuing through events and afterwards
4	Universal and selective psychosocial interventions		
5	Surveillance and signposting staff in	Making available surveillance assessments to identify the needs	After 2 weeks and continuing into the

Table 28.1 (cont.)

Step	Action levels	Purpose of action	Time scale
	need to health and social care services	of: (a) staff whose distress is sustained by secondary stressors; and (b) staff who require more comprehensive personal assessment because they may have unmet mental health needs	medium and longer terms
6	Augmented primary health and social care for staff	Delivering personalised psychosocial, occupational health, primary healthcare and social care paradigms of assessment, indicated psychosocial interventions and treatments for people who need or may need primary mental healthcare or specialist mental healthcare	Medium and longer terms
7	Specialist mental healthcare		

professional carers are as well prepared as possible to cope with the demands of their work over a sustained period of time and that care is provided for carers in an appropriate manner.

The strategic stepped model of care we describe in Table 28.1 is intended as a conceptual and practical resource. The model has seven steps which describe the level of action and purpose of action required, and make proposals for the time scale for achieving those actions.

References

Adams, J. S. (1963). Towards an understanding of inequity. Journal of Abnormal and Social Psychology, **67**: 422–436.

Allen, A. B. & Leary, M. R. (2010). Self compassion, stress and coping. Social and Personality Compass, **4**: 107–118.

Andrews, J. & Butler, M. (2014). Trusted to Care: An independent review of the Princess of Wales Hospital and Neath Port Talbot Hospital at Abertawe Bro Morgannwg University Health Board. See http://wales.gov.uk/topics/health/publications/health/reports/care/?lang=e

Bailey, K. M. Curtis, A. & Numan, D. (2001). Pursuing Professional Development: The Self as Source. Boston, MA: Heinle & Heinle.

Bakker, A. & Demoerouti, E. (2007). The job demands–resources model: State of the art. Journal of Managerial Psychology, **22**: 309–328.

Ballatt, J. & Campling, P. (2011). Intelligent Kindness: Reforming the Culture of Healthcare. London: Royal College of Psychiatrists.

Bandura, A. (1997). Self Efficacy: The Exercise of Control. New York, NY: Freeman.

Barsky, A. & Kaplin, S. A. (2007). If you feel bad, it's unfair: A quantitative synthesis of affect and organisational justice perceptions. Journal of Applied Psychology, **92**: 286–295.

Berne, E. (1964). Games People Play: The Psychology of Human Relationships. Penguin; London (reprinted in 2010).

Bhui, K., Dinos, S., Galant-Miecznikowska, M., de Jongh, B. & Stansfeld, S. (2016). Perceptions of work stress causes and effective interventions in employees working in public, private and non-governmental organisations: A qualitative study. The British Journal of Psychiatry Bulletin, **40**, 318–325.

Bion, W. R. (1961). Experiences in Groups. London: Tavistock.

Black, D. C. & Frost, D. (2011). Health at Work: An Independent Review of Sickness Absence. London: Department of Work and Pensions.

British Psychological Society (2016). Psychological therapies staff in the NHS report alarming levels of depression and stress – their own. See https://www1.bps.org.uk/system/files/Public%20files/Comms-media/press_relea se_and_charter.pdf.

Brotheridge, C. M. & Grandey, A. (2002). Emotional labor and burnout: Comparing two perspectives of people at work. Journal of Vocational Behavior, **60**: 17–39.

Brown, K. W., Ryan, R. M. & Creswell, D. (2007). Mindfulness: Theoretical foundations and evidence for its salutary effects. Psychological Inquiry, **18**: 211–237.

Campling, P. (2015). Reforming the culture of healthcare: The case for intelligent kindness. BJPsych Bulletin, **39**: 1–5; doi: 10.1192/pb.bp.114.047449.

Carter, M., West, M., Dawson, J., Richardson, J. & Dunckley, M. (2008). Developing Team Based Working in the NHS. London: Department of Health.

Cicognani, E., Pietrani, L., Palestine, L. & Prati, G. (2009). Emergency workers' quality of life: The protective sense of community, efficacy beliefs and coping strategies. Social Indicators Research, **94**: 449–463.

Crittenden, P. (2006). A dynamic-maturational model of attachment. Journal of Family Therapy, **27**: 105–115.

Crittenden, P. & Landini, A. (2011). Assessing Adult Attachment: A Dynamic-Maturational Approach to Discourse Analysis. New York, NY: W.W. Norton.

Daniels, K., Watson, D. & Gediki, C. (2017). Wellbeing and the social environment of work: A systematic review of intervention studies. International Journal of Environmental Research and Public Health, **14**: Article No. 918.

Department of Health. (2012). Transforming Care: A National Response to Winterbourne View Hospital. London: Department of Health.

Department of Health (2013). More Care, Less Pathway: A Review of the Liverpool Care Pathway. London: Department of Health.

Department of Health (2014). Healthcare sector staff wellbeing, service delivery and health outcomes. See https://assets.publishing.service.gov.uk/government/uploads/system/uploads/attachment_data/file/277591/Staff_wellbeing__se rvice_delivery_and_health_outcomes.pdf.

Edmondson, A. (1999). Psychological safety and learning behaviour in work teams. Administrative Science Quarterly, **44**: 350–383.

Faculty of Intensive Care Medicine (2016). Regional workforce engagement report. See www.ficm.ac.uk/sites/default/files/ficm-workforce-regional-engagment-report-wales.pdf.

Francis, R. (2013). Report of the Mid Staffordshire NHS Foundation Trust Public Inquiry. Executive Summary (HC 947). London: The Stationery Office.

Gilbert, P., editor (2005). Compassion: Conceptualisations, Research, and Use in Psychotherapy. Abingdon: Routledge.

Grandey, A. A. (2000). Emotional regulation in the workplace: A new way forward to conceptualize emotional labor. Journal of Occupational Health Psychology, **5**: 95–110.

Hacker Hughes, J., Saleem Rao, A., Dosanjh, N. et al. (2016). Physician heal thyself (Luke 4:23). The British Journal of Psychiatry, **209**: 447–448; doi: 10.1192/bjp.bp.116.185355.

Haslam, S. A., Reicher, S. D. & Levine, M. (2012). When other people are heaven, when other people are hell: How social identity determines the nature and impact of social support. In Jetten, J., Haslam, C. & Haslam, S. A., editors, The Social Cure: Identity, Health and Well-Being. Hove: Psychology Press, pp. 157–174.

Hobfoll, S. E. (1989). Conservation of resources: A new attempt at conceptualising stress. American Psychologist, **44**: 513–524.

Iglesias, L., Vallejo, B. B. & Fuentes, S. (2010). The relationship between experiential avoidance and burnout syndrome in critical care nurses: A cross sectional questionnaire survey. International Journal of Nursing Studies, **47**: 30–7.

Ipsos MORI (2016). The mood in Britain: The context shaping the new agenda. See www.adviceuk.org.uk/wp-content/uploads/2016/02/Mood-in-Britain-Ipsos-Mori.pdf.

Kaniasty, K. & Norris, F. H. (2004). Social support in the aftermath of disasters, catastrophes, and acts of terrorism: Altruistic, overwhelmed, uncertain, antagonistic, and patriotic communities. In Ursano, R. J., Norwood, A. E. & Fullerton, C. S., editors, Bioterrorism: Psychological and Public

Health Interventions. Cambridge: Cambridge University Press, pp. 200–229.

Kirkup, B. (2015). The Report of the Morecambe Bay Investigation. Morecambe Bay Investigations. London: Department of Health.

Kuoppala, J., Lamminpää, A. & Husman, P. (2008). Work health promotion, job well-being, and sickness absence: A systemic review and meta-analysis. Journal of Occupational and Environmental Medicine, **50**: 1216–1227.

NICE (2009). Promoting Mental Wellbeing at Work. London: NICE.

NICE (2013). Policy and Management Practices to Improve Health and Wellbeing of Employees. London: NICE.

Norris, F. H., Tracy, M. & Galea, S. (2009). Looking for resilience: Understanding the longitudinal trajectories of responses to stress. Social Science and Medicine, **68**: 2190–2198.

Panter-Brick, C. & Leckman, J. F. (2013). Editorial commentary: Resilience in child development – interconnected pathways to wellbeing. Journal of Child Psychology and Psychiatry, **54**: 333–336.

Parliament of Australia (2018). Effectiveness of the aged care quality Assessment and accreditation framework for protecting residents from abuse and poor practices, and ensuring proper clinical and medical care standards are maintained and practised. See www.aph.gov.au/Parliamentary_Business/Committees/Senate/Community_Affairs/AgedCareQuality.

Pepper, J. R., Jaggar, S., Mason, M. J., Finney, S. J. & Dusmet, M. (2011). Schwartz Rounds: Reviving compassion in modern healthcare. Journal of the Royal Society of Medicine, **105**: 94–95.

Petrides, K. V. & Furnham, A. (2003). Trait emotional intelligence: Behavioural validation in two studies of emotional recognition and reactivity to mood induction. European Journal of Personality, **17**: 39–75; doi: 10.1002/per.466.

Richardson, A. (2015). Independent Review of Deaths of People with a Learning Disability or Mental Health Problem in Contact With Southern Health NHS Foundation Trust April 2011 to March 2015. London: NHS England.

Rousseau, D. M. (1989). Psychological and implied contracts in organizations. Employee Responsibilities and Rights Journal, **2**: 121–139.

Saakvitne, K. W., Gamble, S., Pearlman, L. & Lev, B. (2000). Risking Connection: A Training Curriculum for Working With Survivors of Childhood Abuse. Lutherville, MD: Sidran Press.

Shuffler, M. L, DiazGranados, D. & Salas, E. (2011). There's a science for that: Team development interventions in organizations. Current Directions in Psychological Science, **20**: 365–372; doi: 10.1177/0963721411422054.

Southwick, S. M., Bonanno, G. A., Masten, A. S., Panter-Brick, C. & Yehuda, R. (2014). Resilience definitions, theory, and challenges: Interdisciplinary perspectives. European Journal of Psychotraumatology, **5**: 25338; http://dx.doi.org/10.3402/ejpt.v.

Thomas, R., Mills, A. & Helms-Mills, J., editors (2004). Identity Politics at Work. London: Routledge.

Thompson, B. L. & Waltz, J. (2008). Self-compassion and PTSD symptom severity. Journal of Traumatic Stress, **21**: 556–558.

Tsaousis, I. & Nikolaou, I. (2005). Exploring the relationship between emotional intelligence with physical and psychological health functioning. Stress and Health, **21**: 77–86.

Wilde, J. (2016). The Social Psychology of Organisations. London: Routledge.

Williams, R. & Kemp, V. (2016). Psychosocial and mental health care before, during and after emergencies, disasters and major incidents. In Sellwood, C. & Wapling, A., editors. Health Emergency Preparedness and Response. Wallingford: CABI, pp. 82–98.

Williams, R., Kemp. V. & Alexander, D. A. (2014). The psychosocial and mental health of people who are affected by conflict, catastrophes, terrorism, adversity and displacement. In Ryan, J., Hopperus Buma, A., Beadling, C. et al., Conflict and Catastrophe Medicine. Berlin: Springer, pp. 805–849.

Williams, R., Kemp, V. & Neal, A. (2016). Compassionate care: Leading and caring for staff of mental health services and the moral architecture of healthcare organisations. In Bhugra, D., Bell, S. & Burns, A., editors. Management for Psychiatrists, 4th edition. London: Royal College of Psychiatrists, pp. 377–402.

Chapter 29

The Importance of Creating and Harnessing a Sense of 'Us': Social Identity as the Missing Link Between Leadership and Health

S. Alexander Haslam, Niklas K. Steffens and Kim Peters

Introduction

In the process of researching this chapter, the first author spent a crisp December day touring London's major bookshops in an attempt to discover what recent books on health might have to say about leadership and what those on leadership might have to say about health. It was a pleasant way to spend a day, but, as a research exercise, it was something of a failure. Of the books on health, not a single one had an index entry for leadership and most restricted their coverage of the topic to general discussions of team and patient management as aspects of effective healthcare. Conversely, very few of the books on leadership had much to say about health, although the biographies of influential leaders (e.g. Obama, Gillard, Thatcher) typically included significant sections devoted to the biographee's policy on health (e.g. democratisation, rationalisation, privatisation).

One notable exception was Nicklaus Thomas-Symonds' (2014) book, *Nye*, which offers an insightful treatment of the life of Aneurin Bevan, a pivotal figure in creating Britain's National Health Service. Bevan, Thomas-Symonds observes, saw health as one of the key things that leadership could, and should, promote. What is more, he devoted much of his political career to making this happen. On the leadership shelves, however, this worthy volume cuts a lone figure. Indeed, for the most part, one might be more likely to imagine that leadership generally involves *compromising* the health of others – by defeating them in sport, crushing them in elections, killing them in war. Certainly too, one could be forgiven for thinking that it is feats such as these that provide the warrant to call oneself a leader, and the right to occupy precious shelf space in Foyles and Waterstones.

In bringing the topics of leadership and health together, this chapter goes much against the grain of contemporary thought and practice. This is even more true because it argues that, far from being unnatural bedfellows, the psychology of these two processes is inescapably linked. More specifically, and in line with the major themes of this book, we argue that this linkage derives from the fact that both leadership and health are bolstered through cultivating and enacting *shared social identity* – a sense of 'we-ness'. Accordingly, our aim is to show not only why these things are bound together, but also how this understanding can be harnessed in order to promote both better leadership and better health.

The Importance of Social Identity for Health

One of the central ideas that is explored throughout this book is that groups have an important and distinctive role to play in promoting and maintaining our health. To be clear, this is not simply a restatement of the familiar observation that social contact, social connections and a rich social life are good for one's wellbeing, as demonstrated by, for example, House et al. (1988). Rather, it suggests that it is *particular forms* of social interaction that deliver these benefits. They are those that are grounded in, and promote, a sense of *social identity* – the sense that one is a member of a group and hence part of a bigger 'us'. We raised these points in Chapters 3 and 4 and Steve Reicher also comments on them in Chapter 23.

Why is social identity so important for health? As discussed in many places elsewhere in this book (including Chapters 1, 4, 17, 23 and 25) a core reason is that humans are social animals who live, and have evolved to live, in social groups. Accordingly, like hunger and thirst, physical and psychological isolation are inimical to our make-up and design. And in this regard, the fundamental significance of social identity is that it is *what makes group behaviour possible* (Turner, 1982).

Because this is such a pivotal point, it is worth pausing for a moment to flesh it out with an example, albeit a rather mundane one. Imagine that you wanted to engage in a relatively simple form of group behaviour as a member of a particular football team. Let us work with the example developed in Chapter 30 and call this team Smithtown United. What, psychologically, would allow you to do this? As John Turner first argued, the answer hinges on your having the capacity to define yourself, and hence to behave, as a team member. That is, rather than simply seeing yourself and other team members as individuals (i.e. in terms of *personal identities* as Alex, Bill, Cath, etc.), in order to have a meaningful game of football, you need to be able to see yourself and fellow team members as exemplars of, and united by, the same social category. In this instance, this means you have to have a sense of shared social identity as 'us Smithtown players'. Among other things, then, it is your sense of yourself (technically, your *self-categorization*) as a team member that would mean you passed the ball to a Smithtown player even if you didn't like them as a person, and wouldn't pass to Sam, a Jonesville (another fictitious town) Wanderers player, even if he were your best friend. Reicher offers empirical evidence about these sorts of identifications with sports teams in Chapter 23. At the same time, the fact that this identity is *context-sensitive and negotiated* would mean you *would* pass to Sam if you found yourself playing on the same team (e.g. if he got a transfer, or you were in a match where you were both playing for the same country). Importantly too, the internalisation of social identity provides the essential platform for a range of other psychological and behavioural phenomena. They include: (a) a sense of similarity and commonality (i.e. a sense that members of your team, the *ingroup*, are in some sense alike and 'in the same boat'); and (b) the ability to influence and coordinate the thinking and action of those ingroup members, but not of others, for example, Jonesville players.

In this relatively trivial example, we can see not only that social identity underpins group behaviour, but also that it is this that allows us to access whatever benefits a particular group activity affords. Accordingly, if it is the case that an activity, such as playing football, is good for you (e.g. for your self-confidence and physical fitness; Haskell et al., 2007), then it is also the case that social identity is a gateway to these benefits. More particularly, it is the fact that the team's members see themselves (i.e. they self-categorise) as being 'in the same team' in terms of a shared social identity that allows them to work together as a meaningful entity and that allows them to contribute to, and benefit from, their collective achievements. Moreover, the more that team members define themselves in this way – that is, the higher their *social identification* – the more true this is.

This point is confirmed by a large body of research that speaks to the fact that the benefits of various group interventions are contingent upon participants actually identifying with the groups in question (e.g. Cruwys et al., 2014b; Haslam et al., 2014; and see Chapter 25). It also follows that, because social identity is what allows us to fulfil our potential as humans, if the capacity to do this is compromised, for example, because we lose or lack social identifications, then this constitutes a major threat to our psychological, social and professional functioning (Cruwys et al., 2014a; Greenaway et al., 2016; Steffens et al., 2017a).

More generally, this example also allows us to see that social identity is a fundamental basis for a range of other psychological states that are critical to health and wellbeing. Among other things, this is because feeling that we are part of a team engenders a sense of trust and support, a sense of self-esteem, control and agency, and a sense of purpose, direction and meaning. Importantly too, as other chapters in this volume attest (e.g. Chapters 11, 15 and 17), in recent years each of these observations has been confirmed by empirical evidence, obtained from diverse populations, in multiple domains and across a range of clinical conditions (e.g. Haslam et al., 2009, 2018; Jetten et al., 2012, 2017).

The Importance of Social Identity for Leadership

Although the links between social identity and health have been a major focus for recent research, this is a relatively novel application of ideas in the social identity tradition. When the concept of social identity was originally fleshed out by Henri Tajfel at the University of Bristol, UK, in the 1970s, his primary concern was with its implications for intergroup processes such as conflict, prejudice and discrimination, as fleshed out in *social identity theory* (Tajfel & Turner, 1979). Indeed, it was only with the development of *self-categorization theory* in the 1980s and 1990s that researchers interested in social identity, notably John Turner, started to explore its relevance for group behaviour more generally (Turner, 1982; Turner et al., 1987, 1994).

One of the key insights here, which we have already touched upon, is that social identity is not only a basis for social perception, in which one sees oneself and others in terms of their group membership, but also for *social influence*. We can see this by reflecting again on our football example and by considering how social identity not only structures perception so that one reacts to other players as 'one of us', or 'one of them', but also how it determines behaviour and behavioural expectations. For example, it determines not only who you would pass the ball to and who you would expect to pass the ball to you, but also who you would discuss tactics with and who you would take instructions from. As Turner (1991) observed, the more general point is that social identity serves to determine both who we influence and who we are influenced by. More specifically, the capacity for another person to influence us depends critically upon their being seen to embody a social identity that we share, as does the capacity for us to influence them (Turner & Haslam, 2001).

The relevance of this point for a discussion of leadership is that it is classically defined as a process of influence that centres on the capacity for one or more people to motivate others to contribute to the achievement of group goals (e.g. Haslam, 2004a). What a social identity analysis suggests is that this capacity is fundamentally grounded in people's sense of shared social identity. In the case of our football team, for example, it's a fairly obvious, but routinely overlooked, point that the people who are likely to influence and motivate us –

that is, the people whose leadership we will respond to positively – need to be in our team. Moreover, the more they are seen to represent and promote the interests of that team, the more likely they are to be seen as a good leader.

Of course, the relevance of this point for this book as a whole is that, to be effective, leaders need to be seen by the targets of their leadership activity as working in their interests and on their side. This speaks to the problem that, all too often in organisations and institutions, the agents of change seem to people on the ground to be working for a different team – for Jonesville, if you will, rather than Smithtown. Not least, this is true of those people who design and implement health policy. Yet to the extent that this is the case, it is a major impediment to the followership that is needed to translate leaders' words and actions into the concerted and motivated forms of social action that are necessary to bring about meaningful and constructive change.

Again, there is a very large scientific literature that bears out these arguments. To give just one example that speaks to the significance of shared social identity for leadership, we found, in an archival analysis of the formal election speeches of prime ministerial candidates in Australia, that in 80 per cent of cases (34 out of the 43 elections that have been held since Federation in 1901) the election was won by the leader who referred to 'we' and 'us' most frequently in their speech (Steffens & Haslam, 2013). There are two significant dimensions to this finding. The first is that leaders who appeal to shared social identity, i.e. to a common sense of 'us-ness', are more likely to exert influence. The second is that feeling one is qualified to speak on behalf of a particular social identity is an important ingredient of leadership success.

More generally, what emerges from the broader corpus of social identity research on leadership is that the people we follow are those who are seen to *create, advance, represent* and *embed* (i.e. *care* about) the social identities that matter to us (Haslam et al., 2011; Steffens et al., 2014b). Indeed, just as shared social identity is what makes group behaviour possible, so too it is what makes leadership possible (Haslam, 2004b). Put another way, without social identity, leadership is rendered ineffective. Accordingly, a core task for would-be leaders is to mobilise this influence through what has been termed *identity entrepreneurship* (i.e. the creation of a sense of 'us'; Reicher et al., 2005) and *identity impresarioship* (i.e. translating a sense of 'us' into material reality; Haslam et al., 2011). In short, in order to succeed, leaders need to turn the idea of 'us' into a psychological and material force in the world.

Social Identity as the Missing Link between Leadership and Health

The ideas sketched out in the previous two sections provide a theoretical logic that shows how leadership is a basis for the development of social identity, and how social identity is a basis for leadership. In turn, these ideas show how health and wellbeing hinge upon people developing social identity. This set of relationships is represented schematically in Figure 29.1. As we have already intimated, two separate literatures speak to the robustness of each of these links. This separation owes much to the fact that the former link has been documented primarily by social and organisational psychologists (see Haslam et al., 2011) and the latter primarily by clinical and health psychologists (e.g. see Haslam et al., 2018).

A critical question, then, is whether there is any evidence of the two links co-occurring in the world at large. This is an issue that we have recently begun to explore in studies that

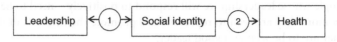

Figure 29.1 Social identity, leadership and health

examine the leadership and health dynamics of teams in organisational contexts. A first study involved surveying over 600 US employees, employed across a wide range of industries (Steffens et al., 2014a). In this project, we asked participants to report, among other things, on: (a) the extent to which their most proximal team leader engaged in identity entrepreneurship (i.e. by creating and advancing a shared sense of 'us'); and (b) their own subjective health and wellbeing, particularly in the form of greater work engagement and reduced burnout. As hypothesised, we found reliable relationships between these two elements. Importantly too, path analyses provided support for a mediational model in which the impact of leadership upon perceived group performance was partly explained by improved health. In other words, this suggests that one reason why groups perform well when their leaders strive to build social identity is that these actions help to promote the vitality and health of the group's members.

Nevertheless, one methodological problem with this study is that the cross-sectional nature of the data set makes it hard to draw causal inferences. This was a problem that we sought to address through a longitudinal study of 141 industrial workers in China (Steffens et al., 2017). In this research, we tracked employees' perceptions of leaders' identity entrepreneurship and their own burnout and work engagement, as well as their willingness to leave the organisation, over a 10-month period. Again, we found reliable relationships between these elements. Importantly, though, the longitudinal analysis indicated that the more leaders (at Time 1) worked to build team-based social identity the more this meant that employees (at Time 2) wanted to remain part of their organisation. At the same time, those employees were both more engaged in their work and had less burnout.

In reporting this finding, it is important to note that we are not the first researchers to observe the intimate association between leadership and health (see Skakon et al., 2010). However, where this link has previously been observed, it has largely been explained with reference to either strategic or stylistic factors. In particular, it has been noted that leaders can promote health by engaging in behaviours that directly support health (e.g. by building a gym; Wegge et al., 2014), or by dint of a transformational style (e.g. one that encourages followers to engage in worthy causes that move them beyond purely transactional concerns with 'what's in it for me'; Arnold & Connelly, 2013). Our analysis does not deny the importance of these processes but provides an explanatory framework that allows us to make sense of a literature that is otherwise largely descriptive (van Knippenberg & Sitkin, 2013). In particular, this is because shared social identity can be seen to underpin both the development of a particular leadership style (e.g. explaining why leaders typically adopt a transformational orientation towards ingroup members but not towards outgroup members) and the desire for particular forms of strategy.

Among other things, then, social identity theorising explains why leaders who identify with Smithtown might be more willing to build a gym for Smithtown residents than for the folk of Jonesville. It would also explain why they would put effort into ensuring that the gym was the facility that the people of Smithtown actually needed rather than, say, a civil development that suited their own commercial interests or those of the residents of onesville. Furthermore, it would also explain who was more likely to use that gym when it vas built – residents of Smithtown who wanted to spend time with other ingroup members, ut not those from Jonesville who, if the truth be told, found the users of the Smithtown gym little off-putting (Reicher et al., 2016). In short, what is novel about our analysis is that, by hedding light on the hitherto obscured role of social identity, it goes beyond a convincing lemonstration of the fact *that* leadership and health are linked, to explain *why*, and hence *vhen* and *how*, this is the case.

ractical Implications: Programmes to Improve Health and eadership by Promoting Social Identity Development

'et aside from the particular theoretical and empirical links that we want to make in this hapter, it is obviously the case that the topics of health and leadership are linked by the fact hat both represent end states that are seen to be highly desirable in the world at large. ndeed, just as billions of pounds, dollars and euros are spent each year on trying to promote ealth, so too enormous sums are invested in the task of training leaders. Moreover, in both lomains, a social identity approach leads us to question whether prevailing investment is as rudent as it might be (e.g. see Jetten et al., 2014). In both cases, this is because policymakers lisplay a strong preference for individualised interventions, whether in terms of medical or sychological treatments to tackle problems of health, or personality-based profiling to ddress deficiencies of leadership.

In contrast, the analysis presented in the previous sections suggests that far greater mphasis needs to be placed in both domains on the *group-specific* determinants of positive eadership and health outcomes. More particularly, we argue that policymakers who are nterested in fostering better health and better leadership should invest much more heavily han they have to date in the task of *developing social identities* in ways that promote roductive forms of interconnectedness. Working out exactly how this might be done is major challenge not only for social science but for society as a whole (e.g. Putnam, 2000). ecently too, this is an issue to which we have directed much of our own energy.

At one level, this has involved abstracting *general principles* that can help apply social dentity theorising to applied domains. A comprehensive review (Haslam, 2014) abstracted ive principles, most of which are anticipated and explained by the discussion above. They are:

1) *Groups and social identities matter* because they have a critical role to play in health and organisational outcomes.
2) *Self-categorizations matter* because it is people's self-understandings in a given context that shape their psychology and behaviour.
3) The power of groups is unlocked by working with social identities, not across or against them.
4) Social identities should be made to matter in deed, not just in word.
5) *Psychological intervention is always political* because it always involves some form of social identity management.

At a second level we have also endeavoured to translate these general principles into *nanualised programmes* that can be delivered to relevant participants in clinical or organiational contexts. In the clinical domain, this has led to development of the five-module GROUPS 4 HEALTH (G4H) programme that aims to tackle the challenges of social isolation

(Haslam et al., 2016; see Chapter 25 above). This has also led us to develop the 5R programme to tackle the challenges of leadership in organisational domains (Haslam et al., 2017). The latter builds on earlier work through which we sought to address the practicalities and challenges of identity entrepreneurship and identity impresarioship for leaders who manage multiple social identities on the ground in organisational settings (Haslam et al., 2003; Peters et al., 2013). These projects have also provided insights into the practice of identity leadership outlined by Haslam, Reicher and Platow in *The New Psychology of Leadership* (Haslam et al., 2011). The core modules of 5R involve: (1) *Readying* participants for the programme before engaging in collaborative strategies for: (2) *Reflecting* on the identities that matter for the groups one seeks to lead; (3) *Representing* those identities; and then (4) *Realizing* the goals and aspiration associated with those identities; prior to (5) *Reporting* back on its impact for both leaders and the group as a whole. Importantly, the 5R programme is not designed to be a one-off fix for ill health. Instead, it is more likely to contribute to sustainable health when its various components are embedded in ongoing practice – that is, the way leaders and their fellow group members relate to each other as a matter of course, so that the norms, values and goals that define 'who we are and who we want to be' can be continually aligned in ways that promote healthy forms of group life.

Given the distinct contexts, participants and objectives of G4H and 5R, there are obvious differences between the two programmes. Nevertheless, given the theoretical logic that is common to their design, and which is exposed by the earlier discussion in this chapter, there are very significant points of contact between them. In particular, both programmes have at their core the desire to understand, work with and advance social identities that matter both for participants and for significant others in their lives (e.g. family members or co-workers). This means that both programmes involve a process of social identity mapping, both are delivered in group contexts and both necessitate, and facilitate, interaction with other ingroup members.

As we have intimated, these features of the two programmes serve to differentiate them from many other health and leadership programmes (e.g. cognitive behaviour therapy, transformational leadership training) in which the target of intervention is primarily the *individual qua individual*. In seeking to target the *individual qua* (potential) *group member* they, therefore, provide an important alternative to, and corrective for, the deficiencies of prevailing approaches. Moreover, this conclusion is borne out by the results of recent programme trials in which developing social identity is shown to be a potent driver of both improved mental health (Haslam et al., 2016) and more effective leadership (Haslam et al., 2014; Slater & Barker, 2018).

Conclusion

The goal of this chapter has been to show that social identity is not only a determinant of health, but that it is also a determinant, and a product, of leadership. Putting these things together, we see that the links between social identity and health, which are a primary focus for this volume, are themselves tethered to matters of leadership. In particular, they are bound up with forms of identity leadership that serve to develop and advance social identity and which do so in ways that are sensitive to the needs and interests of the *multiple* groups that comprise the organisational and societal landscape at any time. Not only, then, is identity leadership a path to group efficacy, but so too, as a result of this, it is critical for health and wellbeing. Or, turning this around, we can see that it is hard to draw on a sense of shared social identity to deliver a social cure without the leadership that first helps to develop that shared identity. This is especially true in those, sadly quite common, circumstances in which social and organisational relations are characterised by group conflict and estrangement rather than by any sense of common ground.

This, we suspect, is a point that would not have been lost on Nye Bevan – someone who saw health as something that needed to be built upon a shared concern for the collective and who devoted his own energies as a leader to the challenges of creating structures that would instantiate this concern. Indeed, famously, he saw this not simply as a cornerstone of leadership and health, but as a benchmark for civilised society. So do we.

Acknowledgements

We are grateful to Vanessa Cameron and Richard Mills for their comments on an earlier draft of this chapter.

Work on this chapter was supported by fellowships from the Australian Research Council to the first two authors (FL110100199; DE180100676)

References

Arnold, K. A. & Connelly, C. E. (2013). Transformational leadership and psychological well-being. In Leonard, H. S., Lewis, R., Freedman, A. M. & Passmore, J. editors, The Wiley-Blackwell Handbook of the Psychology of Leadership, Change, and Organizational Development. Chichester: John Wiley & Sons, pp. 175–194.

Cruwys, T., Haslam, S. A., Dingle, G. A., Haslam, C. & Jetten, J. (2014a). Depression and social identity: An integrative review. Personality and Social Psychology Review, 18: 215–238.

Cruwys, T., Haslam, S. A., Dingle, G. A. et al. (2014b). Feeling connected again: Interventions that increase social identification reduce depression symptoms in community and clinical settings. Journal of Affective Disorders, 159: 139–146.

Greenaway, K. H., Cruwys, T., Haslam, S. A. & Jetten, J. (2016). Social identities promote well-being because they satisfy global psychological needs. European Journal of Social Psychology, 46: 294–307.

Haskell, W. L., Lee, I. M., Pate, R. R. et al. (2007). Physical activity and public health: Updated recommendation for adults from the American College of Sports Medicine and the American Heart Association. Circulation, 116, 1081–1093.

Haslam, C., Cruwys, T., Haslam, S. A., Dingle, G. & Chang, M. X.-L. (2016). Groups 4 Health: Evidence that a social-identity intervention that builds and strengthens social group membership improves mental health. Journal of Affective Disorders, 194, 188–195.

Haslam, C., Haslam, S. A., Ysseldyk, R. et al. (2014). Collective cognition in aging: Social identification moderates cognitive health and well-being following story- and song-based reminiscence. Aging and Mental Health, 18, 425–434.

Haslam, C., Jetten, J., Cruwys, T., Dingle, G. & Haslam, S. A. (2018). The New Psychology of Health: Unlocking the Social Cure. London: Routledge.

Haslam, S. A. (2004a). Leadership. In Kuper, A. & Kuper, J., editors, The Social Science Encyclopedia, 3rd edition. New York: Routledge, pp. 566–568.

Haslam, S. A. (2004b). Psychology in Organizations: The Social Identity Approach, 2nd edition. London: Sage.

Haslam, S. A. (2014). Making good theory practical: Five lessons for an Applied Social Identity Approach to challenges of organizational, health, and clinical psychology. British Journal of Social Psychology, 53: 1–20.

Haslam, S. A., Eggins, R. A. & Reynolds, K. J. (2003). The ASPIRe model: Actualizing social and personal identity resources to enhance organizational outcomes. Journal of Occupational and Organizational Psychology, **76**: 83–113.

Haslam, S. A., Jetten, J., Postmes, T. & Haslam, C. (2009). Social identity, health and well-being: An emerging agenda for applied psychology. Applied Psychology, **58**: 1–23.

Haslam, S. A., Reicher, S. D. & Platow, M. J. (2011). The New Psychology of Leadership: Identity, Influence and Power. Hove: Psychology Press.

Haslam, S. A., Steffens, N. K., Peters, K. et al. (2017). A social identity approach to leadership development: The 5R program. Journal of Personnel Psychology, **16**: 113–124.

House, J. S., Landis, K. R. & Umberson, D. (1988). Social relationships and health. Science, **241**: 540–545.

Jetten, J. Haslam, C. & Haslam, S. A., editors (2012). The Social Cure: Identity, Health and Well-Being. Hove: Psychology Press.

Jetten, J., Haslam, C., Haslam, S. A., Dingle, G. & Jones, J. M. (2014). How groups affect our health and well-being: The path from theory to policy. Social Issues and Policy Review, **8**: 103–130.

Jetten, J., Haslam, S. A., Cruwys, T. et al. (2017). Advancing the social identity approach to health and well-being: Progressing the social cure research agenda. European Journal of Social Psychology; doi: 10.1002/ejsp.2333

Peters, K. O., Haslam, S. A., Ryan, M. K. & Fonseca, M. (2013). Working with subgroup identities to build organizational identification and support for organizational strategy: A test of the ASPIRe model. Group and Organization Management, **38**: 128–144.

Putnam, R. (2000) Bowling Alone: The Collapse and Revival of American Community. New York, NY: Simon and Schuster.

Reicher, S. D., Haslam, S. A. & Hopkins, N. (2005). Social identity and the dynamics of leadership: Leaders and followers as collaborative agents in the transformation of social reality. The Leadership Quarterly, **16**, 547–568.

Reicher, S. D., Templeton, A., Neville, F., Ferrari, L. & Drury, J. (2016). Core disgust is attenuated by ingroup relations. Proceedings of the National Academy of Sciences, **113**: 2631–2635.

Skakon, J., Nielsen, K., Borg, V. & Guzman, J. (2010). Are leaders' well-being, behaviours and style associated with the affective well-being of their employees? A systematic review of three decades of research. Work and Stress, **24**: 107–139.

Slater, M. J. & Barker, J. B. (2018). Doing social identity leadership: Exploring the efficacy of an identity leadership intervention on perceived leadership and mobilization in elite disability soccer. Journal of Applied Sport Psychology; https://doi.org/10.1080/10413200.2017.1410255.

Steffens, N. K. & Haslam, S. A. (2013). Power through 'us': Leaders' use of we-referencing language predicts election victory. PLoS One, **8**: e77952.

Steffens, N. K., Haslam, S. A., Kerschreiter, R., Schuh, S. C. & van Dick, R. (2014a). Leaders enhance group members' work engagement and reduce their burnout by crafting social identity. Zeitschrift für Personalforschung (German Journal of Research in Human Resource Management), **28**: 173–194.

Steffens, N. K., Haslam, S. A., Reicher, S. D. et al (2014b). Leadership as social identity management: Introducing the Identity Leadership Inventory (ILI) to assess and validate a four-dimensional model. The Leadership Quarterly, **25**: 1004–1025.

Steffens, N. K., Haslam, S. A., Schuh, S., Jetten, J. & van Dick, R. (2017a). A meta-analytic review of social identification and health in organizational contexts. Personality and Social Psychology Review, **21**: 303–335.

Steffens, N. K., Yang, J., Jetten, J., Haslam, S. A. & Lipponen, J. (2017b). The unfolding impact of leader identity entrepreneurship on burnout, work engagement, and turnover intentions. Journal of Occupational Health Psychology; doi: 10.1037/ocp0000090.

Tajfel, H. & Turner, J. C. (1979). An integrative theory of intergroup conflict. In Austin, W. G. & Worchel, S., editors, The Social Psychology of Intergroup Relations. Monterey, CA: Brooks/Cole, pp. 33–47.

Thomas-Symonds, N. (2014). Nye: The Political Life of Aneurin Bevan. London: Tauris & Co.

Turner, J. C. (1982). Towards a redefinition of the social group. In Tajfel, H., editor, Social Identity and Intergroup Relations. Cambridge: Cambridge University Press, pp. 15–40.

Turner, J. C. (1991). Social Influence. Milton Keynes: Open University Press.

Turner, J. C. & Haslam, S. A. (2001). Social identity, organizations, and leadership. In Turner, M. E., editor, Groups at Work: Theory and Research. Mahwah, NJ: Lawrence Erlbaum Associates Publishers, pp. 25–65.

Turner, J. C., Hogg, M. A., Oakes, P. J., Reicher, S. D. & Wetherell, M. S. (1987). Rediscovering the Social Group: A Self-Categorization Theory. Cambridge, MA: Basil Blackwell.

Turner, J. C., Oakes, P. J., Haslam, S. A. & McGarty, C. (1994). Self and collective: Cognition and social context. Personality and Social Psychology Bulletin, 20: 454–463.

van Knippenberg, D. & Sitkin, S. B. (2013). A critical assessment of charismatic–transformational leadership research: Back to the drawing board? The Academy of Management Annals, 7: 1–60.

Wegge, J., Shemla, M. & Haslam, S. A. (2014). Leader behavior as a determinant of health at work: Specification and evidence of five key pathways. Zeitschrift für Personalforschung (German Journal of Research in Human Resource Management), 28: 6–23.

Chapter 30

Smithtown as Society

Verity Kemp, Daniel Maughan, Richard Williams, Richard Mills and Tim Healing

Background

We developed a fictional town, Smithtown, to support the exercises we undertook during the seminars that gave rise to this book. The town, and a small selection of its inhabitants, were presented to the seminars in 2014, in order to ground the ideas we discussed and focus our conversations about what approaches and actions might assist the population generally and, particularly, following a disastrous flood. We have included a summarised version of it in the book because we thought that readers might wish to think about the implications of the contents of this book for how responsible authorities might approach the challenge of planning for the population of Smithtown. Also, the nature of this fictional town and its recent narrative raises questions for theory, research and practice. Although the town and its inhabitants are entirely fictional, the problems faced by its inhabitants are not. When we created the narrative, we drew on information from publicly available data sets for several real towns in England though they are not included here. Attendees at the conversations were presented with a much more detailed description of Smithtown and its inhabitants than is given here.

We start this chapter by setting the scene; we outline the demography of Smithtown, describe a selection of its people and summarise some of the challenges they face in their community. Then, we identify principles for strategy development (Warner & Williams, 2005). We also draw attention to a selection of approaches in this book to embed social factors in planning changes to health and social care services. They include matters outlined in Chapter 26 and we indicate how the process of social scaffolding might assist planners, the town and its people. We intend this chapter to illustrate an approach that is based on established frameworks to which are added the frameworks offered by authors of various chapters in this book. But we do not develop or offer a detailed plan.

Smithtown

A General Description of Smithtown

Smithtown is in northeast England and lies about one mile inland from the sea.

A Brief History and Background

Historically, Smithtown was a small market town and fishing port that grew considerably during the Industrial Revolution as heavy industries were developed. A thriving chemical industry developed in the area towards the end of the nineteenth century. Smithtown is well connected by road and rail.

Smithtown now has a population of over 240,000 people. The town has a higher proportion of rented housing than the national average and nearly 9 per cent of its population are in receipt of state welfare benefits. The largest minority ethnic grouping is families of Pakistani cultural origin. In the latest census data, the city had a high proportion of people of working age who were unemployed, ranking in the bottom 18 of the 376 local authorities within England and Wales.

During the second half of the twentieth century, many of Smithtown's traditional industries declined and its local economy waned. The chemical industry has remained an important but not a large-scale employer.

Health, Wellbeing and the Health Services in Smithtown

Smithtown was a notoriously unhealthy town in the past due to serious industrial pollution and high levels of poverty. Even now, the health of the people in the town is generally worse than the average for England. Over 18,000 people live in poverty. Life expectancy for both men and women is lower than the average for England.

The health services in Smithtown include the usual array of primary and secondary care facilities and services. As in all parts of England, the numbers of people seeking to use health services has increased rapidly while their funding is under huge pressure. It has proved increasingly difficult to recruit general practitioners (GPs) and there are long waiting times for hospital appointments.

Some of the People of Smithtown

We created some fictional inhabitants for Smithtown to provide the seminars with a means of exploring the concepts we discussed during the conversations in a more practical manner. They include the Green Family: mother, father, four children aged from 10 to 19 years. They own their house. Father has been made redundant and has had difficulty finding a new job. Mother works at the local school. Eldest son joined the army having been unable to find employment locally. Also living with them are the mother's brother, whose marriage has broken down, and a grandmother who has problems with mobility and recently received a diagnosis of dementia.

There is also the Hamilton Family, long-standing residents of the town. Father retired from teaching because of chronic ill health. His wife is a community nurse. Their adult daughter lives with them, is in work and is saving to buy a home of her own.

Neighbours include a former soldier, a native of the town but with no family left living there. He served in Afghanistan and is affected by distressing events in which he was involved while deployed. He has not managed to hold on to a job, is currently unemployed and occasionally indulges in bouts of binge drinking.

There is another former soldier who left the army with specialist skills and who has found well-paid employment locally.

Other households in the neighbourhood include: multi-generational households of people of Pakistani heritage; Portuguese migrant workers; people publicly espousing racist views; older people with no social networks and at least one family whose behaviour is viewed by residents and the authorities as antisocial.

The small neighbourhood shopping centre and pub are closed and boarded up. The community centre is about to close. The local Christian church runs a food bank, a mother and toddler group and a lunch group for older people but struggles to find volunteers to assist its endeavours.

Smithtown: The Continuing Story

There was an unusually severe storm in the early hours of one morning in December of the previous year and large areas of Smithtown were flooded. The worst flooding occurred near where our families live. People were evacuated to a relief centre that the Council opened in a local sports hall. Other more affluent areas were also flooded. Many of those residents chose to book into hotels or go to stay with families elsewhere rather than use the relief centre.

The local church, the church hall, the community centre and the schools were flooded and were not available to provide shelter and support, but church facilities in unflooded areas throughout the town were opened to provide shelter and emergency meals. The local mosque established a welfare centre, open to all, where people could drop off items that might be helpful such as food, clothing and toys. It also became the focus for getting help from the Council.

The local news initially reported many acts of kindness and bravery, including descriptions of the heroic actions of the two former soldiers, and helping people to move possessions and themselves to safety. In addition, the news included stories of families helping one another and about the community spirit of the area.

Communications from the flooded areas to the people in the relief centre were poor. There were unsubstantiated reports of looting of empty homes and of people who had not been seen since the flooding started. The local Council was criticised for not doing enough and for providing services to suit them and not the people in need. Areas of the town were left devastated and contaminated once the flood waters receded.

At the same time, social media, local radio and television reported from a neighbouring town, Jonesville, which was unaffected by the flooding, that, at the end of a football match, a van was driven into a group of people who were leaving the ground. Police confirmed there had been an incident and several people had been injured but they were not prepared to state whether this might have been a terrorist attack or an accident but confirmed that they had arrested two people at the scene.

The headlines on the Smithtown newspaper website over the coming days and weeks include:

23 December: Local residents praise the work of the emergency services, 'our blue light heroes'.

26 December: Rescuing Christmas: Faith groups and local restaurants join together in effort to bring seasonal cheer to flood victims. 'Celebrations are a testimony to the strength of our multicultural community, local Imam says'.

28 December: 'Former Soldier Is a Local Hero – helping local old folk escape the floods'.

29 December: Residents of Jonesville accused of racially motivated attack at football match. Police appeal for calm.

23 January the following year: Flood victims meet local Council, 'Demand to know why response so slow'; 'Council not interested in us'.

1 April the following year: ex-soldier, hailed as local hero, arrested for being drunk and disorderly. 'He is a changed man since the floods, neighbours say'.

30 April the following year: Local action group calls for inquiry into Council's handling of flood response. 'Too many families have still not been rehomed, spokesperson says'.

'Blatant discrimination against poorer families alleged'; 'This will happen again unless something changes at the civic centre'.

A Strategic Approach to Designing and Delivering Responses to the Needs of Communities in Smithtown

The Requirement for a Strategic Plan for Responding to the Needs of the Population of Smithtown

One of the challenges in the seminars was for attendees to develop the outline of a health and social care strategy for the people and communities in Smithtown. Attendees were asked to come to a view about what this strategy would look like and how would it be different from existing models. Then, they were asked to reflect on the principles and actions for developing a plan that flows from the kinds of information that this book presents.

Chapter 11, for example, describes the cumulative risk model whereby long-term adverse effects are better predicted by the number of risk exposures rather than by the specific nature of those exposures. Certainly, the population of Smithtown has illustrated this cumulative risk model (Zeanah & Sonuga-Barke, 2016, p. 1099).

It is clear that the scenario presented by Smithtown to planners and practitioners of a wide variety of professions and roles is both complicated and complex (see Chapter 31). It is complicated because there are so many coincident problems for the population. They include the impact of: the continuing social determinants of ill health and especially the low levels of earnings and affluence; the disaster leaving parts of the town devastated; the van incident; and the longer-term cultural and political differences. They are also complex because each of these problems involves people with their differing perceptions, aspirations, expectations and priorities. Furthermore, it is evident that the financial resources are extremely limited. This mix of problems appears to have left people in intractable positions because many communities feel humiliated and that there is deep unfairness, and the democratically elected bodies have yet to agree on how to change the situation overall (see Chapter 21).

Some of the problems are of long-standing, others are of shorter-term development. The latter, necessarily, captured our attention. Now that the flooding has receded, our immediate priority is to develop a plan to respond in the recovery phase by considering the civil, health, social, financial and security contingencies of recent events while recognising that the background problems have become worse as a consequence of the disaster.

But, once recovery is in hand, we should not decide on longer-term actions without recognising and considering the background evolution of the challenges faced by the population of Smithtown. That is because, at the very least, they frame the cultural context of the situation, define the resources that can be brought to bear and influence the ability of the public to accept and support what is done. Importantly, the scenario overall heavily impacts the expectations of the public and their contributions to resolving the problems.

Clearly, too, there are important choices to be made. Resources are finite and there are practical realities that must be faced in determining the way forward. Therefore, we begin by identifying some of the guiding principles that impact on decision-making. The best approach, as we have indicated, is to take immediate actions to save life and then slow down to consider the next steps in a more strategic way so that decisions and actions taken in haste are not allowed to imperil good decision-making. Furthermore, the best and most

Table 30.1 Ten core principles for designing and delivering services for communities (copyright Williams R & Kemp V, 2018, all rights reserved and reproduced with permission)

1	Agree values, ethics and approaches to human rights
2	Agree definitions
3	Orientate services to families and communities in the cultures in which they live, relate and work
4	Recognise that social integration, social support and shared social identities are key
5	Translate lessons from evidence and experience into plans and frameworks for designing and delivering care
6	Adopt a balanced approach to designing and delivering services
7	Ensure that communications are effective
8	Ensure ease of access to health and social care for people who intervene
9	Work to agreed standards
10	Ensure that review, evaluation and research are promoted for each step taken

fair use of slender resources should be made to tackle a very wide range of matters of deprivation in coherent ways

Core Principles for Designing and Delivering Services for Communities

The purpose of this section is to identify principles that are important if the responsible authorities and the regional and national agencies are to respond to Smithtown's entrenched problems and the major incident that now superimposes on them. A key matter in all strategic approaches to developing communities and responding to the impacts of disasters is for the agencies to come together to agree a vision, an intent, a direction and priorities for development, which are inclusive of all communities in Smithtown (Warner & Williams, 2005).

There are principles that can be derived from established strategic approaches for developing communities (Warner & Williams, 2005) and responding to disasters (Sellwood and Wapling, 2016; Williams et al., 2017). We have found clear support for them and gleaned others from the chapters in this book. Thus, Table 30.1 summarises 10 core principles. As a minimum, we think that it is important that relevant agencies come together to agree the core matters that are described by these principles, whether in this format or any other.

Next, we expand, briefly, on each of these principles.

Principle 1: Agree Values, Ethics and Approaches to Human Rights

(a) The Purposes of Services

The core principles draw on work by others, including the Bevan Commission (2015), which states that values, ethics and human rights must be central to states', civil administrations', responsible authorities' and communities' design and delivery of services. Identifying values should be the starting point for defining the purposes of services and the principles that underpin them.

The Department of Health for England (2007) upholds that well-designed responses to people's health needs should be based on and promote awareness of human rights and ethical principles for good decision-making. Evidence about the effectiveness and efficiency of interventions should be used to determine the means by which these values-based purposes are best achieved, and how the principles are enacted.

In Chapter 12, we see that there can be a positive, constructivist angle to community bonds and that it is important to foster communities to support the resilience of their people. Sustaining communities of value where difference is tolerated, and understanding why this does not always happen, is important. Underpinning all services should be a regard for human rights and equality. We think that a response based on the framework from the Committee on Ethical Aspects of Pandemic Influenza (CEAPI) (Department of Health, 2007), which is presented in Chapter 24, could provide the basis for ensuring that Smithtown has an acceptable approach to meeting its human rights commitments.

(b) A Values Framework for Developing Services for the Population of Smithtown

We commend the framework developed by CEAPI as the starting point for Smithtown's development of its ethical approach to the immediate and longer-term needs of its population. This recognises one fundamental principle, which includes five values that inform delivering the fundamental principle and three process values.

The fundamental principle is *equal concern and respect for everyone*. It means that:

- Everyone matters.
- Everyone matters equally – but this does not mean that everyone is treated the same.
- The interests of each person are the concern of us all, and of society.
- The harm that might be suffered by every person matters, and so minimising the harm that the societal demography and narrative causes is a central concern.

As we have seen in Chapter 24, the values in the framework are of two types: ethical orientations and process values. The ethical orientations are: respect, harm minimisation, fairness, reciprocity and proportionality. The process values in the CEAPI framework emphasise: flexibility, good decision-making and working together.

Such an approach for the people of Smithtown would be embodied in a transparent and equitable response that clearly reflects an understanding of the different needs of the various communities in the town. Therefore, it is important that all agencies agree to follow the same ethical and decision-making process and to use it to resolve disagreements between groups about the priorities for using resources that are scarce.

Principle 2: Agree Definitions

It is important that actions are taken to agree definitions of terms across the agencies involved and then to disseminate and use those definitions. Our common experience is that failure to agree terms and definitions contributes to uncertainty, poor communication, confusion and diffusion of interventions.

Principle 3: Orientate Services to Families and Communities in the Cultures in Which They Live, Relate and Work

It follows from the concepts covered in Sections 1 and 2 of this book that all aspects of health and social care should be planned, designed and provided with full consideration for people's social environments, their cultures and the needs of their families and the communities in which they live and work.

In Chapter 10, Elder reminds us that it is incumbent on practitioners and policymakers to take account of the effects on families and communities. Furthermore, the communities we refer to are increasingly ethnically diverse. There are two important corollaries. The first is taking account of meeting the risk factors impacting on, and the needs of, people of all ages. The second is the importance of ascertaining and including awareness of the preferences of people and their families in designing and developing services.

Chapters 2 and 22 explore agency. They emphasise the need to plan from the ground up and to see events and circumstances through the eyes of people who have been affected. Distress and mental disorder are shown to be linked to lack of agency. The corollary is that restoring and sustaining group membership restores agency and wellbeing. People are likely to seek other forms of identity and agency when they feel rejected by a group or if it does not meet their needs.

Principle 4: Recognise that Social Integration, Social Support and Shared Social Identities are Key

This book posits an approach to improving the equity, equality and effectiveness of health and mental health services, based on adopting a values framework and on social connectedness, social identity and agency. The authors of Chapter 5 suggest that time for reflective thinking would enable adoption of a values-based approach to equitably delivered healthcare that could work together across agencies, ages and geography. The challenge is to build the link between people and groups, and that is a key aspect of social scaffolding.

In this context, social support '. . . consists of social interactions that provide actual assistance, but also embed people in a web of relationships that they perceive to be caring and readily available in times of need' (Haslam et al., 2012; Williams et al., 2014a, 2014b). There are informational, emotional and operational components of social support that are important in disasters and in engaging the public in civil planning and developments. Recent research sheds light on the conditions in which social support is more likely to be offered and be effective and they are covered in some depth in Section 3. See Chapters 15, 17 and 22, in particular, and Drury et al. (2015) and Carter et al. (2014).

If these conditions were applied in Smithtown, they would enable planners to respond around already formed groups, such as faith communities, as well as forming new groups and social identities by, for example, setting up a FLood Action Group (FLAG) basing it on communities and the initiatives of local people.

Thus, in Smithtown, the flood has disrupted their community. Initially, some members, including the former soldiers, grew as a result of their experience of rescuing neighbours, and they established a new social identity that was, unfortunately, lost as the waters receded. A key matter is to sustain the emergent social identities that arise in disasters. Also, faith groups provided for certain needs and filled a void in the statutory agencies' services.

Principle 5: Translate Lessons from Evidence and Experience into Plans and Frameworks for Designing and Delivering Care

Chapter 6 states the definition of public health and identifies factors that have an impact on it, such as the social determinants of health, including mental and physical health, wellness

Table 30.2 Translating lessons into effective policies, plans and service delivery (copyright Williams R & Kemp V, 2018, all rights reserved and reproduced with permission)

Policy level	Nature of the level	The intention of action at each level
1	National and provincial civil administrations set policies that determine the strategic requirements for services.	Policies at this level set the overall aims and objectives for responses to social need and disasters.
2	Responsible authorities design frameworks for services.	Government and state policies should require and enable the responsible authorities to create strategic plans for, and design services by bringing together evidence from research, past experience and knowledge of their populations and their risk profiles.
3	Responsible authorities create and deliver services nationally, provincially and locally.	Plans should be based on the best evidence available and awareness of the preferences of people who are likely to use them. The authorities should test delivery of services through projects and exercises that are based on coproduction.
4	Responsible authorities create plans for supporting, training and caring for staff in order to support good, effective professional practice and make the best use of slender resources.	Plans for good practice concern how staff take account of the needs and preferences of people in the areas they cover, and deploy their skills and work with people to agree how guidelines, care pathways and protocols are interpreted in individual cases. They should also include plans for sustaining and intervening with staff.
5	Civil administrations and the responsible authorities evaluate the performance of services.	Civil administrations and the authorities are responsible for evaluating and managing the performance of services against their identified purposes.

and wellbeing. The authors of this chapter believe it is unhelpful to make distinctions between healthy minds and healthy bodies as if they were separate. Translating lessons learned through research and experience into ethical and effective plans for delivering comprehensive programmes of all kinds requires action at a number of levels, which are illustrated in Table 30.2. An important matter is that top-down plans should enable people in the population to express agency by contributing from the bottom up, and to evaluate their perceptions of their needs and what they can contribute.

Principle 6: Adopt a Balanced Approach to Designing and Delivering Services

(a) Balance Top-Down with Bottom-Up Approaches

Healthcare provision should be titrated against awareness of the needs of the people in the population. Top-down approaches may be essential where, for example, there is great devastation after disasters. But, so as not to contradict the need for bottom-up planning, the responsible authorities should plan all top-down interventions in conjunction with leaders of affected communities to ensure that the population's priorities are recognised and respected and that the people receive the kinds of assistance that they value and need. This advice also reflects people's common preferences for receiving social support from their families and within their communities.

Restoring people's agency reduces the duration of their distress and so the initiative should be returned to local communities as soon as is reasonably possible. However, communities may require material and financial support for substantial periods in order to avoid 'resource gaps' that are created after the supporting agencies start to withdraw because this often occurs well before recovery is complete (Whittle et al., 2010). This emphasises taking actions that actively maximise participation of local, affected populations, whatever the degree of devastation in each area.

(b) Build on Existing Services and Skills to Develop and Deliver Effective Responses

Health and social care programmes should be capable of responding to a variety of types or causes of challenge, including disasters. Many of the lower-level psychosocial interventions required in the aftermath of disasters, for example, can be delivered by lay people and non-specialist practitioners, provided they have sufficient training, supervision and support. Specialist practitioners should avoid replacing existing community mental health resources.

(c) Shared, Cross-Agency Approaches to Planning and Delivering Responses are Vital to Harnessing Communities' Assets in Smithtown

The need to engage people, families and communities in planning and delivering responses is vital. The requirement is for a bottom-up approach that genuinely includes the people and communities that might be affected by change. Coproduction and co-design are techniques increasingly being used to ensure engagement. For example, coproduction is a 'way of working whereby citizens and decision-makers, for people who use services, family carers and service providers work together to create a decision or service which works for them all, the approach is value driven and built on the principle that those who use a service are best placed to help design it' (SCIE, 2015).

The values-based approach, which we have outlined under Principle 1, acknowledges the different values that are rooted in different communities in Smithtown. Applying a framework developed from the CEAPI framework would allow the agencies to use public health ethics in making good decisions, by engaging with the differing groups and choosing between their differing views of the priorities in ways that are fair, equitable and transparent. A framework of this kind would also assist the differing authorities to consider and resolve their different views of the priorities.

Table 30.3 Reasons for focusing on effective communications (Copyright Williams R & Kemp V, 2016, all rights reserved and reproduced with permission)

1	Ensuring the public receives information that is intended to: • reduce public apprehension • align the public to wise courses of action • align the public to evidence-informed interventions • avoid the corrosive effects of rumour
2	Keeping people well by sustaining and building the resilience of persons and communities
3	Promoting agency through community and personal self-efficacy
4	Providing information as part of intervention programmes for everyone
5	Meeting a 'right' (e.g. for freedom of information)
6	Recognising the importance of taking positive, cooperative stances to responding well to media enquiries

Principle 7: Ensure That Communications Are Effective

Good communications with persons and with the public are fundamental to sustaining their resilience, building the opinions of the public about authorities' legitimacy and, thereby, leading to public cooperation with advice provided by authorities (Carter et al., 2014; Welton-Mitchell, 2013). Successful responses in ordinary circumstances, and in emergencies, are underpinned by good communication within and between agencies, teams of responders, and the people and communities affected.

A core theme in this book is that of the importance of people and agencies that are responsible for healthcare responses working closely and adhering to a coordinated communications strategy. Advice about communications with the public about risks is available in the literature, including the work of Bish et al. (2011). Good communications help groups and communities to build trust in the authorities and, thereby, develop a willingness to cooperate with advice given by them (Carter et al., 2014). Table 30.3 summarises reasons for focusing on communications in Smithtown. As Katona and Brady point out in Chapter 18, inter-agency communication, joint working and sign-posting are crucial to caring for people who have many forms of complicated and complex needs.

Principle 8: Ensure Ease of Access to Health and Social Care for People Who Intervene

The extent and frequency of the psychosocial impacts of disasters, as well as more routine events, on rescuers and the staff of health and social care agencies that respond, are similar in their impact as those experienced by people who were directly involved and those affecting people who were not involved (Williams et al., 2017).

Similarly, Neal et al. remind us, in Chapter 28, that the staff of services that respond in the long term to the needs of the people of Smithtown are likely to require supporting interventions to assist them to cope with what may be substantial distress, consequent on their work. Many of them may be psychosocially resilient despite their distress. But, ensuring staff receive early psychosocial interventions can reduce the risks of their

Table 30.4 Advantages of adopting agreed standards for services and programmes for information-gathering, research and evaluation (copyright Williams R & Kemp V, 2016, all rights reserved and reproduced with permission)

Adopting standards contributes powerfully to risk reduction by inspiring well-designed and well-conducted mechanisms for information-gathering, research and evaluation that:	
1	Clarify the intentions, design, and effective conduct of specific programmes
2	Provide important information for, and about, the communities served
3	Promote effective practice by the staff of programmes
4	Reinforce fidelity of programme delivery with what is required by the populations involved and the intentions of the programmes' designers
5	Identify factors that contribute to success or failure of particular types of service, their organisation and delivery, and particular interventions
6	Include longitudinal and follow-up studies, designed to learn about the long-term psychosocial and mental health impacts of disasters and intervention programmes

developing problems later. Therefore, plans for psychosocial care to support healthcare staff should be developed, managed and monitored as an integral part of business continuity planning.

Principle 9: Work to Agreed Standards

Plans should include the minimum standards to be adopted in a range of circumstances. Situations should be anticipated in which there are challenges of such extent and short-term impact that high standards may not be achievable temporarily. Everyone who is involved in planning and delivering health and social care should agree to work to a common set of standards (Williams et al., 2008).

The standards adopted have substantial implications for training, information-gathering, evaluation and research because all of these capabilities should be core parts of disaster responses. Requirements for them must be anticipated and standards for these functions should be developed before disasters occur. Table 30.4 identifies some of the particular advantages of adopting agreed standards.

Principle 10: Ensure that Review, Evaluation and Research are Promoted for Each Step Taken

Well-designed and well-conducted information-gathering, research and evaluation should be conducted according to overt, transparent, acceptable and agreed ethical standards. Ethical procedures and standards should not be compromised. It is important to:

- Start designing information-gathering, research and evaluation programmes from the time when each plan is designed, developed, tested, rehearsed and revised; and
- Base the process of designing and implementing evaluation on agreed guidance.

The experiences and findings gained by everyone who is involved in conducting evaluation and research should be used to develop curricula for training relevant people in the skills of designing and delivering services and of interpreting the findings of evaluations of services, and adapting them to local situations.

Strategic Actions in Smithtown

Strategic Leadership

Responding to the many needs of the population of Smithtown presents huge strategic and operational challenges for all of the statutory agencies and for the non-statutory sector. There are background challenges that are exacerbated by the flooding. We do not diminish the background challenges onto which are superimposed the necessity of the communities and people who comprise the population of Smithtown also dealing with a large-scale disaster. Dückers (2017) reminds us that it is important to establish a multilayered resilience framework that conceptualises and connects capacities at individual, community and society levels.

Thus far, we have identified principles for planning and delivering services that are drawn from across this book. Chapter 26, for example, proposes that, in the difficult context of constrained financial resources, rethinking is required in how we design, deliver and prioritise care in order to capitalise on the substantial health benefits that could be derived from assisting people to develop their social connectivity. A 10-step approach is described by Maughan and Williams to embed an approach at local level that translates evidence into policy, and knowledge into action. Those 10 steps are:

(1) Recognise the evidence-base for approaches to health, healthcare and social care;
(2) Provide strategic support;
(3) Set priorities for research;
(4) Develop socially derived evidence-based interventions as well as those derived from biomedical evidence;
(5) Develop national policy;
(6) Engage health and social care funders;
(7) Gain commitment from provider organisations;
(8) Deliver an appropriate mix of older and newer interventions;
(9) Develop the workforce; and
(10) Implement appropriate quality assurance.

While this list was not designed for dealing with a mixture of emergent problems superimposed on long-term problems faced by the population of Smithtown, there are reminders in it that resonate with the principles that we extracted earlier in this chapter. Furthermore, there is also a great advantage in applying the processes of social scaffolding in tackling the evident problems.

Social Scaffolding

In Chapter 3, we see how the social identity framework fills a gap in theory about why social connectedness succeeds and fails. We then posed the question about how these theories might work in practice. Our particular focus here is on applying the concept of social scaffolding, as described in more detail in Chapter 25.

Social Scaffolding: The Definition

In Chapter 3, Haslam et al. define social scaffolding as 'the process through which practitioners work to promote health and wellbeing with community groups through structured activities that enable them to develop a positive shared social (community) identity from which to harness ongoing support'. There are models proposing how this statement can be put into effect in Chapters 3 and 25.

This approach could be used in Smithtown to sustain and support existing social groups and to enable local people to form new ones that reflect their locality and needs. Chapter 25 suggests that the benefits for health include aligning existing social identities with the overarching community identity, with the intention that groups work together rather than against each other, and this might lead to a new and broader community.

Social Scaffolding: Theory into Practice

Chapter 16 emphasises that planning, preparation and practice are essential in responses to disasters. It presents a 12-point table enumerating social principles for humanitarian aid, derived mainly from the authors' experience as well as from science. These lessons, while focused on disasters, employ principles of social identity and social networking. One example is that of involving local people, leaders and authorities in planning, with the objective of building capacity. It is entirely consistent with the aim of this book to promote sustainable forms of social connectedness.

In Chapter 23, Reicher describes how analysis and our knowledge of the social bases of mental and physical health can be applied in practice. He goes on to describe conditions for success in applying the power of groups. These conditions should inform how the responsible authorities set out to work with and empower groups of people in the communities that comprise Smithtown.

Chapter 3 introduces Groups 4 Health (Haslam et al., 2016), a recent social identity-derived intervention that aims to help people who are suffering from the effects of social isolation by providing them with the knowledge and skills to manage social group membership and the underpinning identities. It is a model that is available to people and communities as well as to practitioners who work with people and communities in need. Table 30.5 makes suggestions about how the Groups 4 Health model from Chapter 3 might apply to the people and communities of Smithtown.

Chapter 25 directs us to think about how to make the process of social scaffolding concrete and practical. It proposes that this be achieved by using the Actualising Social and Personal Identity Resources (ASPIRe) framework as a mechanism for acting on the principles of social scaffolding (Haslam et al., 2003). We see this as breaking the processes that comprise social scaffolding into components that inform the timeline as well as a means for achieving the conditions described by Reicher in Chapter 23.

The ASPIRe framework is used as the basis for understanding how effective group- or teamwork depends on a collective sense of identity and is developed through a bottom-up participatory process. ASPIRe gives a structured approach to helping practitioners work with communities to build social scaffolding in a similar process to Groups 4 Health.

We think that the application of these and similar models would work well with putting our 10 principles into effect. It indicates a progressive process for working with people to enable their agency and contributions to the plans that are made and to influence how the finance that is available is spent. Also, we suggest that these phases conform to the RITE process, which is also identified in Chapter 25, because it focuses on plans being Realistic, Implementable, Timely and Engaging.

Table 30.5 Modules in GROUPS 4 HEALTH applied to Smithtown

Phase in social scaffolding	Purpose and content of the phase	Examples of applying the phase in Smithtown
Schooling	Understanding why groups matter	Groups provide knowledge of local conditions (e.g. health and employment status of neighbourhoods) and awareness of people's needs and preferences.
Scoping	Mapping group ties	It is important to sustain extant groups. Therefore, mapping the groups that exist is vital. This means actively identifying social networks (e.g. the faith groups in Smithtown).
Sourcing	Mobilising existing group ties	It is important to recognise identified groups and their role in the community (e.g. the Muslim Welfare Centre).
Scaffolding	Building new group ties	It is important to inspire new groups that focus on particular needs of the communities in Smithtown and their people (e.g. people who need rehousing or who have been displaced and are disconnected from their families and the health and social care services they require). The councils, health service officials and community leaders might, for example, set up a special review board to address key challenges.
Sustaining	Embedding group ties	For example, the Flood Action Group should be sustained and supported in its work by the responsible authorities.

Social Scaffolding: The Benefits

Applying the models based on social processes offers the benefits of a framework within which the authorities and non-governmental organisations (NGOs) operate. These frameworks are available for all to use, including practitioners, responders, the responsible authorities, NGOs, people and the communities and groups to which those people belong, and they are based on grounded, participatory processes. The ASPIRe model identifies benefits that include awareness of people's social identities as well as building psychological capital. All the models point to the advantages of knowing people, their networks and their colleagues as a means of increasing the effectiveness of any interventions and responses.

Social Scaffolding: Resources

Applying the ASPIRe framework requires considerable investment on the part of practitioners, activists and community members. As Reicher observes in Chapter 23, adequate resources need to be available to enable the process and, thereby, move communities forward. It is not enough to rely solely on the emergence of social capital without ensuring that its development and sustainability is appropriately resourced.

Social Scaffolding: System Change

Chapter 26 reminds us that achieving system change places a huge focus on social connections and relationships, attitudes and social identities of everyone who is involved. We also need to remember the importance of basing change on evidence from a wide array of sciences, including the social sciences, about health and health and social care.

Social Scaffolding: The Role of Carers and Professionals

Chapters 27 and 28 emphasise the role of carers and professional health and social care staff, and the inherent impacts on them from the challenges they face in the context of circumstances such as those in Smithtown. In Chapter 27, clinical leaders and managers are described as culture carriers for groups and teams, their role being to enable people to give of their best whatever the challenge presented by circumstances. Chapter 28 is important for bringing us back to considering ordinary situations and making us think about how to make practical these theories and concepts. When we arrive at Chapter 29, we are ready to consider leadership and its different components and approaches and, particularly, how social identity influences leadership as well as health and group efficacy.

Leadership

Chapter 29 shows us that social identity is not only a determinant of health, but that it is also a determinant, and a product, of leadership. Sustaining the efficacy of staff and providing care for them frames a vital challenge for leaders. Leadership stands as one of the most important factors that are vital to keeping staff healthy and their work effective, as Healing et al. argue in Chapter 16. Good leadership raises the wellbeing of staff and reduces their rates of anxiety, depression, job stress and sick leave. It is based on a complex array of values, attitudes, qualities, perceptive skills and transactional and translational capabilities that create and communicate a vision of tasks.

Leaders play important roles in fostering environments that contain their staff's emotions in ways that are realistic and psychologically safe, which leave clients' and patients' care enhanced and staff ready for new challenges. This requires team leaders to be acutely aware of team members' psychosocial capabilities and training needs and to ensure that they receive professional supervision, effective management and psychosocial support.

Creating and running psychologically safe teams and sustaining the resilience of healthcare staff requires leaders to (Williams & Kemp, 2016):

- Be accessible and supportive;
- Acknowledge fallibility;
- Balance empowering other people with managing the tendencies for certain people to dominate discussions;
- Balance psychological safety with accountability, physical safety and professionally safe practice and other components of strategic and clinical governance;
- Guide team members through learning from their uncertainties;
- Balance opportunities for their teams' reflection with action; and
- Have the capacity for emotional containment.

Conclusion

What do all these theories and concepts described in this book mean to the people of Smithtown? If they are only theories and concepts that have life in print, then they are of no use. The contents of this book tell us that it is important that people and agencies that are responsible for developing the health and social care services in Smithtown work closely and adhere to an agreed values framework, good decision-making and a coordinated communications strategy. They should set out to:

- Provide effective community leadership that encourages people to become involved in expressing their opinions and foster a bottom-up, inclusive approach to confronting and resolving all the evident problems in a prioritised, strategic manner;
- Restore community groups;
- Work through and with existing community groups;
- Support new and emergent groups;
- Work with teachers and the children in schools;
- Enable people to sustain and, where necessary, regain their agency and perceptions of themselves as effective persons; and
- Restore work opportunities, if possible.

Elder shows how certain of these matters might be taken forward in Chapter 10. In addition, that work should be based on:

- Keeping in sight the people who are affected/being helped;
- Using evidence-informed and values-based guidance and policy;
- Taking regard of existing social identities and networks;
- Working with existing community and other leaders;
- Learning about what works with selected groups of people and applying the lessons to other groups; and
- Speaking a common language.

What we intend to show in this chapter is that the concepts and theories in this book do inform how the responsible authorities might set out to engage with the population of Smithtown and find solutions to long-standing, more recent and immediate problems. It is important that the focus is on supporting people, improving their lives and developing their communities. In addition, the staff who do the work must also be consulted and supported in ways that reflect the values that the authorities wish to see applied in the services they provide for the people of Smithtown. As Chapter 28 opines, this is an important component of the moral architecture of Smithtown. We do not diminish the huge challenges that the long-term financial, employment problems and other forms of deprivation pose. But, we believe that it is imperative to use what resources are available in ways that command the confidence of the population, and the staff who engage with people in need, and enable them to be more empowered than they were.

References

Bish, A., Michie, S. & Yardley, L. (2011). Principles of effective communication: Scientific evidence base review. London: Department of Health. See https://assets.publishing.service.gov.uk/government/uploads/system/uploads/attachment_data/file/215678/dh_125431.pdf.

Carter, H., Drury, J., Amlôt, R., Rubin, G. J. & Williams, R. (2014). Effective responder communication improves efficiency and psychological outcomes in a mass decontamination field experiment: Implications for public behaviour in the event of a chemical incident. PLoS One, 4 March; https://doi.org/10.1371/journal.pone.0089846.

Department of Health (2007). Committee on Ethical Aspects of Pandemic Influenza (CEAPI): Responding to Pandemic Influenza: The Ethical Framework for Policy and Planning. London: Department of Health.

Drury, J., Novelli, D. & Stott, C. (2015). Managing to avert disaster: Explaining collective resilience at an outdoor music event. European Journal of Social Psychology, **4**: 533–547.

Dückers, M. L. A. (2017). A multi-layered psychosocial resilience framework and its implications for community-focused crisis management. Journal of Contingencies and Crisis Management, **25**: 182–187.

Haslam, C., Cruwys, T., Haslam, S. A., Dingle, G. & Chang, M. X.-L. (2016). GROUPS 4 HEALTH : Evidence that a social-identity intervention that builds and strengthens social group membership improves mental health. Journal of Affective Disorders, **194**: 188–195.

Haslam, S. A., Eggins, R. A., & Reynolds, K. J. (2003). The ASPIRe model: Actualizing Social and Personal Identity Resources to enhance organizational outcomes. Journal of Occupational and Organizational Psychology, **76**: 83–113.

Haslam, S. A., Reicher, S. D. & Levine, M. (2012). When other people are heaven, when other people are hell: How social identity determines the nature and impact of social support. In Jetten, J., Haslam, C. & Haslam, S. A., editors, The Social Cure: Identity, Health and Well-Being. Hove: Psychology Press, pp. 157–174.

SCIE (2015). SCIE Guide 51: Coproduction in social care. See www.scie.org.uk/publications/guides/guide51/.

Sellwood, C. & Wapling, A., editors (2016). Health Emergency Preparedness and Response. Wallingford: CABI.

The Bevan Commission (2015). Prudent healthcare: Setting out prudent principles. See www.prudenthealthcare.org.uk/principles/.

Warner, M. & Williams, R. (2005). The nature of strategy and its application in statutory and non-statutory services. In Williams, R. & Kerfoot, M., editors, Child and Adolescent Mental Health Services: Strategy, Planning, Delivery and Evaluation. Oxford: Oxford University Press, pp. 39–62.

Welton-Mitchell, C. E. (2013). UNHCR's mental health & psychosocial support for staff. See www.unhcr.org/51f67bdc9.pdf.

Whittle, R., Medd, W., Deeming, H. et al. (2010). After the Rain – Learning the Lessons from Flood Recovery in Hull. Final Project Report for Flood, Vulnerability and Urban Resilience: A Real-Time Study of Local Recovery Following the Floods of June 2007 in Hull. Lancaster: Lancaster University.

Williams, R. & Kemp, V. (2016). Psychosocial and mental health before, during and after emergencies, disasters and major incidents. In Sellwood, C. & Wapling, A, editors, Health Emergency Preparedness and Response. Wallingford: CABI, pp. 83–98.

Williams, R., Bisson, J. & Kemp, V. (2014a). OP 94. Principles for Responding to the Psychosocial and Mental Health Needs of People Affected by Disasters or Major Incidents. London: The Royal College of Psychiatrists.

Williams, R., Kemp. V. & Alexander, D. A. (2014b). The psychosocial and mental health of people who are affected by conflict, catastrophes, terrorism, adversity and displacement. In Ryan, J., Hopperus Buma, A., Beadling, C. et al., Conflict and Catastrophe Medicine. Berlin: Springer, pp. 805–849.

Williams, R., Bisson, J. & Kemp, V. (2017). Health care planning for community disaster care. In Ursano, R. J., Fullerton, C. S., Weisaeth, L. & Raphael, B., editors, Textbook of Disaster Psychiatry, 2nd edition. Cambridge: Cambridge University Press, pp. 244–260.

Williams, R., Kos, A. M., Ajdukovic, D. et al. (2008). Recommendations on evaluating community based psychosocial programmes. Intervention, **6**: 12–21.

Zeanah, C. H. and Sonuga-Barke, J. S. (2016). The effects of early trauma and deprivation on human development: From measuring cumulative risk to characterizing specific mechanisms. Journal of Child Psychology and Psychiatry, 57: 1099–1102.

Section 5 **Sustaining**

Chapter 31

Suit the Action to the Word, the Word to the Action

Richard Williams

Introduction

This chapter pulls together key matters in this book. Its title is a quote from a line given to one of the characters in Hamlet by Shakespeare. That sentence perfectly outlines the intention of Section 5 of this book and the function of this final chapter in which I endeavour to align theory, research and the practical impacts of the topics covered by this book with the circumstances in which we find health services as we near the close of the second decade of the twenty-first century. But, first, I return to Chapter 1, to recapture some of those circumstances. Then, I look at the matters on which I think we should focus in order to sustain healthcare services and incorporate the social agenda identified in this book.

Returning to Chapter 1

In Chapter 1, I said that the roots of this book '. . . are in an impactful seminar series hosted by the Royal College of Psychiatrists in which practitioners and scientists from a wide array of disciplines came together in 2014 to explore the social influences on our health and recovery from ill health.' In it, we look '. . . at the impacts on our health and healthcare services of the social worlds in which we live.'

'[But] the editors do not pretend that taking the social sciences into account will fill the gaps or answer the questions relating to values and funding public services.' Rather, we embarked on our task of writing this book in the hope that its contents would, '. . . illustrate the importance of our including research from the social sciences in the evidence that we consider when we plan and deliver health and social care services and think about their patients and clients as human beings. They have many needs, preferences and expectations that interconnect with the physical and brain sciences, the nature of their problems, and their outcomes' In other words, as Smith shows in Chapter 2, we *are* our health, but we are also much more than finite and embodied people. Our sociability and agency are vital aspects of us too, as are our cognitive abilities and capacities for evaluation. Thus, this book substantiates the importance of taking all aspects of being human into health and social care and focuses especially on sociability and agency. The science shows that our health is improved when all our needs are considered in a coordinated, collaborative manner that maintains our agency. When we perceive ourselves to be considered as persons by our relatives, friends, acquaintances, the public and the organisations that provide our services, we are likely to feel and function at our best.

Thus, readers should find running throughout in this book a focus on how people experience their health and needs whether in ordinary day-to-day circumstances or in less common but potentially devastating contexts. Thus, we *are* also our social relationships and our contexts as well as our health, but also more than that. We hope that this book enables readers to see that social influences on our health are huge. Despite the extremely rapid advances in the neurosciences that have already had an undeniable impact and promise much, much more in the future for designing preventative interventions and treatments for ill health, we often present to practitioners the outcomes we desire from our treatment in social and functional terms as frequently as in requests for symptom relief.

Furthermore, we are aware of the interchange between people's distress and their physical symptoms. Research conducted in the aftermath of the terrorist attacks in Paris in 2015, for example, has shown the high rates of first responders, (47 or 20 per cent) who reported seeking healthcare for a non-psychological health problem since the attacks (overwork, fatigue, physical injuries, dermatological, osteoarticular or respiratory problems) that were statistically significantly related to differences in level of exposure (Vandentorren et al., 2018). In not dissimilar terms, Katona and Brady recognise, in Chapter 18, the high levels of interrelationships between mental and physical symptoms and suffering and the particular importance of chronic pain in their clients, who are survivors of human rights abuses including torture, human trafficking, domestic abuse and violence relating to gender or sexual orientation.

But, we go further than noting these associations in extreme circumstances and hypothesise that the gains from the neurosciences are likely to be limited if we do not take these social matters into account when producing interventions for people rather than organ systems. Thus, we include in our endeavour both people's physical and mental health because we see them as intimately related rather than as representing separate matters. In other words, throughout this book, we stand away from the body–mind dualism on which so many practitioners have been reared; we see that approach as having done more harm than good.

The Contents

We lay out certain background values- and evidence-based concepts in Section 1 in which we cover the *schooling* aspect of social scaffolding. In Section 2, on *scoping*, we introduce the fields of: the social determinants of health; horizontal epidemiology; attachment and belonging; the importance of families, communities and culture; psychosocial resilience; and the values, ethics and rights involved in these matters, before looking at overlaps between the concepts and the importance of partnerships. Next, in Section 3, on *sourcing*, we look into many challenging world circumstances of the twenty-first century and find that the concepts covered in Section 1 and 2 recur even in the most troubling and adverse situations. What is striking about the topics our authors cover in Section 3 is that each of the scenarios they touch on is uncommon though, cumulatively, they form the content of most national news bulletins! The editors' intention in selecting those topics was to present readers with stimuli to their own thinking about the wide array of people's experiences and novel approaches to problem-solving.

We lay out, in Section 4, some approaches to modern and future healthcare for readers' consideration. Thus, we begin to identify practical aspects of *social scaffolding*. In Chapter 25, Haslam et al. consider social scaffolding as an important way forward in describing a process that encapsulates the theses in this book by using relationships to develop better and more effective and acceptable services. Thus, we see that frameworks for thinking, planning and acting are very helpful, but that it is vital that we attend to the human aspects of care and do not minimise the challenges of developing services in a cash-strapped environment. We recognise the difficult challenge of allocating limited resources to different tasks and finding our way between different groups' and organisations' preferences; thus, we introduce the important field of public health ethics. All of this requires leadership, and Chapter 29, by Haslam et al., applies social identity theory to this most vital matter.

There is synchrony between the processes advocated and the outcomes that are desired. Maughan and Williams look in more depth at synthesising social science in developing healthcare services, in Chapter 26. But, as Aitken et al. show in Chapter 27, the culture, organisation and functioning of healthcare services have all shifted under huge pressures of rapidly rising demand and limited resources in the early twenty-first century. While they use the National Health Services in the UK as a case study, their findings apply on a much wider compass. This reminds us that we must apply solutions to the real, rather than our preferred, world circumstances. But, critically, we must also recognise the risks to their health that the staff who work in health and social care services experience as a consequence of their engaging directly and indirectly with clients and patients. Research on disasters shows the realities in high profile, but the emotional labour inherent in health and social care are omnipresent, including in less challenging circumstances. Thus, in Chapter 28, we deal with the imperative of applying the lessons from this book to sustaining and promoting the health of staff.

Now, as we arrive at this single chapter in Section 5, on *Sustaining*, I return to the huge implicit challenge that the editors set themselves in drawing together the body of evidence-based and evidence-informed knowledge in Sections 1 to 4, with an emphasis on lessons from research and experience for changing healthcare in much the ways for which Heath (2016) calls. That challenge might be summarised as how can we use all the knowledge gathered in this book – about the social determinants of health, the power of social connectedness and social support and the mediating influences of groups and shared social identity – to improve people's health and, especially, people's experiences of living and of using and/or working in the health and social care services. Therefore, we draw on the theories and hypotheses that spring from the work of so many able practitioners, academics and thinkers, who have a vast collective experience, to summarise the key ideas and approaches.

But, before we step forward, we should remind ourselves of the challenges, implicit and explicit, in changing how services function. That is, after all, what we are seeking through the medium of this book. It is no less than a change in the ways in which we conceive of, design and deliver health and social care, and this challenges the cultures of the organisations that do those important jobs. As I say, we do not minimise the challenges involved in propelling change, either in what services deliver or in the ways in which people in them deliver care for people. We must also do so in ways that are sustainable. Therefore, we review the challenges and the realities.

Complexity and Healthcare

Implementing Sustainable Development and Change in Healthcare Services

I have lost count of the number of schemes for improving, reforming or redesigning healthcare services that have reached out to find me or which I have tried to inspire.

I have played a variety of roles in them from highly engaged leader, through project driver to supporter, or I have been a passive observer. What is clear to me from these perspectives and looking back over more than 40 years is that a select few of these schemes has achieved real success and delivered on stakeholders' ambitions; others have delivered positively but not in ways that were originally anticipated; and many have flourished for a while and then stagnated, with goals being met partially. Often the latter has occurred when the circumstances have changed, or key people have moved on. Others have fizzled out and, fortunately, a tiny number has risked making matters worse.

But, what makes the difference between initiatives being successful, making moderate or unanticipated impacts or failing? There are powerful factors and, in my opinion, they include: the quality of the leaders, their approaches to the people with whom they work and on whom they depend and their commitment to what is being done; adequate resourcing; realising that embedding change in systems requires long-term support and nurturing; and everyone who is affected being engaged and their contributions valued and supported. Thus, personal and group relationships, the circumstances in which initiatives were made, and the resources available, emerge from my memory as key factors for success. Sheard et al. (2017) found not dissimilar opinions held by the 15 people with whom they conducted in-depth interviews. They say (p. 1):

> Four themes emerged from the data: personal determination, the ability to broker relationships and make connections, the ways in which innovators were able to navigate organisational culture to their advantage and their ability to use evidence to influence others. Determination, focus and persistence were important personal characteristics of innovators as were skills in being able to challenge the status quo. Innovators were able to connect sometimes disparate teams and people, being the broker between them in negotiating collaborative working. The culture of the organisation . . . was important . . . .

Next, I raise the topic of additions to governance mechanisms that are usually proposed alongside the projects on which I have worked. My observation is that these mechanisms are intended as chocks behind the wheels of change, to promote adoption of new practices, to prevent developmental gains being lost and to assist in sustaining forward momentum. Similarly, targets may be created away from the frontline of delivering change, mainly, in my experience, to allow senior stakeholders to reassure themselves about progress. While these objectives are all entirely legitimate, there is a risk that these distant approaches can create perverse incentives. Consequently, I have become disillusioned by the nature and impacts of the, mainly top-down, governance systems that have been introduced into health and social care services. Too often, I have noted that preoccupations with aspects of performance do not include, in my opinion, adequate engagement with the potential users of the services, attention to qualitative and values-orientated methods, engagement with people who deliver the services in the frontline and actions to sustain the people who deliver services. Curiously, the word frontline conjures a military metaphor that invokes the notion of healthcare being a battlefield on which there are friendly forces, danger in the face of opposition, chaos and enemies of achieving the intended objective. However, the ubiquity of use of this language does suggest to me that some elements of this notion may describe how some staff feel besieged.

Should anyone think that I am pessimistic about change, I assert that, while I have become sanguine, my only intention is to identify what propels and sustains desirable changes. I am still an enthusiast. But, let us face the realities rather than work with a web of assumptions! What is also clear is that, often, I have been engaging in complex systems. Perhaps, then, some of the projects in which I have been involved did not allow us to appreciate the true complexity of seemingly straightforward changes and work with them sufficiently? This threatens to make complex systems even more complex.

I looked at some of these matters in an editorial published in 2002 (Williams, 2002). It is interesting to read that paper again after an interval of 16 years. In that paper, I referred to an article by the editor of the *British Medical Journal* in which he asks why doctors are so unhappy (Smith, 2001). My editorial also drew on a paper from Ham and Alberti who had provided an analysis of the breakdown of the old compact between doctors, patients and society though they caution that '. . . current discontents are not unique to the UK or to the medical profession' (Ham & Alberti, 2002, p. 841). It is clear that that unhappiness persists and has, probably, grown in the UK, with substantial numbers of graduates no longer seeing their future in the health services (General Medical Council, 2018). In the two decades running up to the 70th birthday of the National Health Services in the UK, we have re-examined what kind of compact the UK desires between patients, healthcare practitioners and society. So, this is a good time to engage in discussing change and sustainability.

While there is, appropriately, a huge focus on adequately financing healthcare systems, it is clear that this is by no means the only matter with which we must engage. The cultures of modern organisations have shifted and service change and developments are only likely to be sustainable if we engage with that reality too. Some aspects of this matter are considered by Aitken et al., in Chapter 27. Certainly, as Neal et al. opine in Chapter 28, we cannot stand away from the challenge of making healthcare services more able to support their staff and recognise their wider emotional and social needs. All of this requires leadership and, as I have said, Haslam et al., deal with that challenge on the basis of applying social identity theory in Chapter 29. In addition, Alderdice has an important commentary on leadership in Chapter 21, where he covers lessons from dealing with intractable conflict.

In one way, I am relieved to know that the experiences and opinions that I summarise here are not solely my own. Braithwaite (2018), for example, says that, 'We need to understand why system-wide progress has been so elusive and to identify the kinds of initiatives that have made positive contributions to date' (p. 2). Braithwaite offers five key messages:

- The key messages of health system performance have been frozen for decades – 60 per cent of care is based on evidence or guidelines; the system wastes about 30 per cent of whole health expenditure; and some 10 per cent of patients experience an adverse event.
- Proponents of change too often use top down tools, such as issuing more policy, prescribing more regulation, restructuring, and introducing more stringent performance indicators.
- We must move instead towards a learning system that applies more nuanced systems thinking and provides stronger feedback loops to nudge systems behaviour out of equilibrium, thereby building momentum for change.
- Effective change should factor in knowledge about the systems' complexity rather than perpetuate the current improvement paradigms, which applies linear thinking in blunt ways.
- Yet we should recognise how truly hard this is in the messy, real world of complex care.

Braithwaite's opinions are hard-hitting. He challenges his readers to change their collective mindset. In his opinion (p. 2), we need to recognise three problems (my bold type):

(1) Implementing and securing acceptance of new solutions is difficult, even when armed with . . . persuasive evidence – this is the **take-up problem.**

(2) Disseminating knowledge of an intervention's benefits across the entire system is hard – this is the **diffusion problem.**

(3) Even if a new model of care, technology, or practice is successfully taken up and widely spread, its shelf life will be short – this is the **sustainability problem.**

Certainly, the editors recognise each one of these matters and we suggest that knowing *what* to do is often easier to identify relative to getting systems to agree and then act. Similarly, the editors of this book are clear that *how* is the most challenging part of putting the agenda that this book creates into effect, but it is also vital to approach how to *sustain* development.

Brathwaite suggests that we should change what he styles 'the 'software' of the system by tackling the culture of work settings and the quality of leadership offered by managers and policymakers. We cover matters of organisational and professional culture and leadership in Chapters 24 and 26 to 29. We take a brief look at other aspects of these matters next.

Complexity, Uncertainty and Decision-Making

The notion of complexity science has a ring that is stimulating and fascinating in itself. While definitions are not fully agreed, complex systems have a number of features, which include:

- A multiplicity of many parts or contributors whose interaction produces emergent behaviour that is not observable in the parts alone;
- An absence of a central control element; and
- A responsiveness to an environment or context.

In these terms, the topics covered by this book are clearly complex matters and readers only need to return to the topics covered by Drury and his colleagues in Chapters 15 and 17 to see illustrations of the features I have listed.

I recall reading a series of four articles in the *British Medical Journal* in 2001 on complexity science (Fraser & Greenhalgh, 2001; Plsek & Greenhalgh, 2001; Plsek & Wilson, 2001; Wilson & Holt, 2001). In one of them, Plsek and Greenhalgh talk of a 'zone of complexity' in human systems that lies between areas in which decision-making is predictable, on one side, and circumstances, on the other, in which there is 'so much disagreement and uncertainty that the system is thrown into chaos' (Plsek & Greenhalgh, 2001, p. 627). They say that 'the development and application of clinical guidelines, the care of a patient with multiple clinical and social needs, and the coordination of educational and development initiatives throughout a service are all issues that lie in the zone of complexity'. They recommend that we should accept unpredictability, respect and utilise autonomy and creativity and respond flexibly to emerging patterns and opportunities if we are to cope with escalating complexity in healthcare. I contend that much of what constitutes health and social care services lies in the zone of complexity. Decisions about meeting people's needs are complicated because of the importance of balancing scientific evidence with the resources available, but they are also complex because we must incorporate people's, groups' and communities' preferences into decision-making about service design, resource allocation and personal assessment, care and treatment. Joint decision-making cannot and should not be avoided. Thus, we have to find ways of adapting clinical guidelines to the realities of people's differing circumstances.

One of the challenges that face healthcare practitioners, managers and policymakers is that of uncertainty. Knowledge, technology and communication systems have mushroomed in the last two decades, as Maughan and Williams show in Chapter 26, but much, much more remains to be learned in a world in which so much more is expected of practitioners than has ever been the case hitherto. So, another of the pressure points in practice, change and sustaining good practice lies in uncertainty.

Hall (2002) has reviewed the implications for doctors' education of intuition and uncertainty in decision-making. I imagine that Hall could, of course, talk in similar terms about other professions. While her paper is quite old now, its contents are still highly relevant. She talks of the explicit and implicit rules used by clinicians when making decisions, particularly in conditions of uncertainty, and she uses Beresford's categorisation of sources of uncertainty. They are technical, personal and conceptual (Beresford, 1991). The contents of this book challenge us to look at healthcare through each of these lenses. As I said in 2002 (Williams, 2002, p. 345):

> Technical sources relate to uncertainty about information that can often be reduced or eliminated through research and education. In Hall's view, personal and conceptual sources of uncertainty are likely to remain, despite factual education as they concern the nature of matters such as doctor–patient [or practitioner–client] relationships and organisational features of the services in which we work. For example, conceptual sources of uncertainty may 'arise from an inability to assess differing patients' needs competing for the same resources (incommensurability), and the application of general criteria, guidelines, for example, to individual patients. There is also the uncertainty arising from the applicability of past experiences to present-day patients' [Hall, 2002, p. 217].

This is one reason why we have included work on values and ethics in two chapters (12 and 24) in this book. Hall has said that, 'What makes Beresford's analysis particularly useful is that it shows that the management of uncertainty is more complicated than the simple provision of more information' (Hall, 2002, p. 217). There is, I think, much in common between Plsek and Greenhalgh's zone of complexity and Hall's conditions of uncertainty in decision-making. Both approaches '... suggest that the issues go beyond knowledge, and both suggest we require evidence on matters that relate directly to medical conditions and interventions, but, very importantly, not only those topics' (Williams, 2002, p. 345).

In 2002, I said, 'I believe that professional decision-making skills that are informed by patients' experiences and opinions should take their place alongside wise use of clinical guidelines, algorithms, and protocols in assisting practitioners to cope with contemporary issues of complexity and uncertainty in practice and the wider context of service delivery' (Williams, 2002, p. 346). Such a stance is still applicable though I might write now in much more emphatic terms about shared decision-making.

Let me illustrate this point by referring, first, to the contents of Chapter 24. Here, Montgomery and Williams extend ethics from the personal arena into those recognised in this book that consist of families, groups, workplaces, communities and nations. By way of example, we offer a framework developed for testing policy and practice relating to better managing pandemic flu. But, that framework has had rather wider application in the decade since its publication. The intentions of Chapter 24 are to reach into the ways in which humans tend to make difficult decisions about allocating resources to different groups of people who have differing needs, but to do so in ways in which the values-laden parameters involved are visible and open to review. The intention is to provide an approach to handling conceptual and personal sources of complexity that give rise to uncertainty.

Next, I turn to the information, in Chapter 6 in this book, from Bhui et al., about the social determinants of health. That information is intended to start readers on a line of exploration and, thereby, open up the task of finding answers to matters of technical and conceptual uncertainty. Certainly, that chapter is a primer rather than a full statement because to have written a substantial treatise could have occupied the entirety of this book. Lund et al. (2018), for example, develop this area of science into the realm of sustainability. They say that, 'The Sustainable Development Goals (SDGs), endorsed by all United Nations member states in 2015, represent an ambitious plan for sustainable human development by the year 2030' (Lund et al., 2018, p. 357). The authors of that paper say (p. 357):

> However, uncertainty exists about the extent to which the major social determinants of mental disorders are addressed by these goals [meaning the SDGs]. The aim of this study was to develop a conceptual framework for the social determinants of mental disorders that is aligned with the Sustainable Development Goals, to use this framework to systematically review evidence regarding these social determinants, and to identify potential mechanisms and targets for interventions.

In their paper, Lund et al. conclude that, 'This study sheds new light on how the Sustainable Development Goals are relevant for addressing the social determinants of mental disorders, and how these goals could be optimised to prevent mental disorders' (Lund et al., 2018, p. 357). On the basis of their systematic review of the literature, they offer a conceptual framework, and readers are recommended to consider this paper.

Finally, in this section, I refer to the material in this book that draws together research on all three fronts: technical, personal and conceptual. I refer to the contributions that relate to the culture of healthcare and the social identity approach to understanding the vital role that groups play in sustaining people and in improving their health. Chapter 22 draws on the content of Section 3 of this book to recognise the importance, when making right decisions, of respecting people's needs for agency as well as maintaining their social connections and social support. In Chapter 4, Haslam et al. point out that people derive the gains of meaning and control if they are engaged in and share an identity with other group members. Thus, including people, groups and communities in decision-making processes is key to change and to sustaining what is agreed. The construct of horizontal epidemiology provides a clear rationale for considering people as living in systems that are both complicated and complex, in which their social relationships are vital components. Therefore, people must not be considered as passive when decisions are made at all levels: from day-to-day health and social care practice: through managing delivery of services; to their design and funding; strategy; and government policymaking. These five areas for decision-making represent the five policy levels of which Maughan and Williams speak in Chapter 26.

More emphatically, many of the United Nations' SDGs will not be achieved unless the power of group membership is harnessed positively. So, it is clear that social scaffolding could contribute enormously to the decisions that must be made. Furthermore, books such as *The New Psychology of Health* apply the theory to a large number of domains in health and social care and provide explorations that take the theories covered in this book into their role in practice (Haslam et al., 2018). They reduce, thereby, the technical and conceptual gaps.

Alongside these contributions, frameworks that build on the work of the Committee on Ethical Aspects of Pandemic Influenza (CEAPI; see Chapter 24) have a great deal to contribute in working to resolve otherwise intractable values-laden arguments and are likely to contribute to better decision-making in challenging circumstances. Lund et al. say, 'Addressing the SDGs that are relevant for the social determinants of mental disorders requires a coordinated, truly global effort by governments, civil societies, and the private sector. The interruption of negative cycles of poverty, violence, environmental degradation, and mental disorders is possible, as is establishing virtuous cycles of mental health, well-being, and sustainable development.' (Lund et al., 2018, p. 365).

Contextual Sustainability

Recently, I have come across an operational, strategic and conceptual framework for understanding and responding to young people's experiences of significant harm, beyond their families (Firmin, 2017). Termed contextual safeguarding, it endeavours to provide a framework against which to design systems that address extra-familial risk faced by young people.

I think that there are lessons we might learn from this approach to a particular, very traumatic and damaging hazard, based on humans' behaviour. I think that a similar approach might be used more widely to apply the material in this book to integrated policymaking, service design and practice, in which the power of social factors for good and coproduction are brought together with strategy for developing services in bottom-up initiatives that are supported and endorsed from the top. The key matter is recognising the importance of the social contexts in which we all live, work and relate. Thus, I propose that we embark on generating a process of *contextual sustainability* for responding to the implications of our social contexts for our health. Social scaffolding is a process that sits as a tool in the engine room of this wide approach.

Braithwaite identifies six principles on which to build a new approach to change. He encourages us to (Braithwaite, 2018, pp. 2–3):

(1) 'Pay much more attention to how care is delivered at the coalface';
(2) Recognise that 'all meaningful improvement is local, centred on natural networks of clinicians and patients . . . We must encourage ideas from many sources; care processes and outcomes will vary whatever we do';
(3) 'Acknowledge that clinicians doing complex everyday work get things right far more than they get them wrong . . Understanding errors is critical, as is seeking to stop outmoded, wasteful or excessive care. But, if we also better appreciate how clinicians handle dynamic situations throughout the day, constantly adapting, and getting so much right, we can begin to identify the factors and conditions that underpin that success';
(4) 'Remember that the lone hero model does not work, and collaboration underpins all productive change; and always start with patients at the centre of any reform measure';
(5) 'Be more humble . . . [and] recognise that big, at-scale interventions sometimes have little or no effects and that small initiatives can sometimes yield unanticipated outcomes'; and
(6) 'Adopt a new mental model that appreciates the complexity of care systems and understands that change is always unpredictable, hard-won and takes time, is often tortuous, and always needs to be tailored to the setting.'

Social Scaffolding in Health and Social Care

These principles resonate with so many contributions in this book. Haslam et al. say in Chapter 25, 'we conceptualise social scaffolding as the process through which practitioners work to promote health and wellbeing with community groups through structured activities that enable them to develop a positive shared social (community) identity from which to harness ongoing support.' This appears to embody and exemplify Braithwaite's principles and, vice versa, his principles reflect those of social scaffolding that we endorse in this book.

In Chapter 30, we provide readers with a synopsis of the task that we created for the seminar series that gave rise to this book. We also offer some strategic principles for working towards a better way of responding to the problems that beset the population of our mythical town, Smithtown. Those principles are drawn from the material in this book. We also reprise the 10 steps that were identified in Chapter 26 to embed awareness of the social factors that influence health, in planning and developing services. Most importantly, we show that social scaffolding can be used as a process for drawing the population of Smithtown into designing future plans and delivering services that use the bottom-up approach to engaging with people that we espouse. We return to the Actualising Social and Personal Identity Resources (ASPIRe) framework, outlined in Chapter 25, to illustrate its utility for improving the services available to the population of Smithtown by better ensuring that their needs and opinions are reflected in planning processes.

Social scaffolding and Braithwaite's principles also resonate with another new approach, as detailed by Paul Thomas in his book, *Collaborating for Health* (Thomas, 2018). The author recognises that healthcare is increasingly under pressure. The cover of his book says, 'Budget crises are making collaboration and smart thinking essential, while increasing numbers of people with multiple long-term conditions make specialist models of health care increasingly inefficient – patients too often go from one specialist to another, duplicating effort and paying too little attention to the bigger picture of their health.' Thus, '*Collaborating for Health* outlines a solution: community-oriented, integrated care and health promotion. Designed to prevent problems of fragmented care, this approach focuses on building teams, networks and communities for health and care at local level, where it is easier to see the range of factors that affect people's health'. The author's intention is '. . . to develop community-oriented integrated care in a sustainable way, and [show] how to practise the skills in small ways before . . . [performing] on a big stage'.

Concluding Comments

This book set out to tackle big topics. The editors have striven to do so in ways that are evidence-based but also fully aware of and influenced by the values that are both explicit and implicit in any decisions we make. Abundantly, health and social care are complex matters that require both science and social science to find solutions to persisting and new problems.

We have been keen to blend theory with experience, and practice with scientific exploration. Indeed, we introduce a number of theoretical approaches and endeavour to identify their similarities and differences in Chapter 13. We have also been keen to allow our authors to offer their expertise alongside their opinions but also to create a narrative that runs through the book rather than collecting a series of chapters as separate exhibits. The editors have illustrated the complexities involved in making sustainable improvements in our health and healthcare. We think we have found a way forward in this book and we hope our readers have found this book thought-provoking.

The contents of this book pose significant challenges to the status quo; they call for ystem change in how we design, deliver and practice health and social care. We have said nuch about tackling sustainability, but, before we can get to that part of the agenda, we have et to tackle what Braithwaite calls the diffusion and take-up problems. We hope that this ook will contribute to readers acting on all three challenges.

Looking back through to Chapter 1, it is clear that the intervening chapters cover very wide range of circumstances in which people find themselves, and the work of so nany scientists. In Chapter 1, we recognise Heath's call for a new approach to designing nd delivering healthcare (Heath, 2016). She asks clinicians to bridge the rift between vidence and humanity to deliver more coherence. The editors hope that the contents of his book show how this might be done by developing closer relationships with our atients or clients and greater awareness of their opinions, preferences and family and ultural contexts. We recognise that enabling people to express agency in whatever ircumstances they find themselves is a key mechanism by which their social connectdness is such an asset. Thus, we also return to Smith's important commentary in Chapter 2 on six features of the human condition. But this is not an argument for the esponsible authorities doing little to support the people they serve and, thereby, nisconstruing the real nature of psychosocial resilience, covered in Chapter 11. n reality, the approach that we espouse demands investment by the authorities in rder to mobilise its advantages. This is worthwhile because, as Elder reminds us in Chapter 10, 'This approach … unlocks resources that may otherwise remain unrealised'. In these ways we hope that we may all move from theory into practice and align vords with action, as Shakespeare inspires one of his characters to say.

The approaches and activities on which we focus in this book outline the responibilities of the accountable and funding authorities, which include facilitating people to ngage in social scaffolding from the bottom up, by providing top-down frameworks nd opportunities within which people can develop their social connectivity, gain social upport and express agency. Essentially, life is about relationships. This book shows hat our experiences of social connectivity, social support and agency are sustaining and llow us to ascribe meaning to our social circumstances and events. These are the uilding blocks of social scaffolding. They apply to people and to the design and lelivery of services.

References

Beresford, H. B. (1991). Uncertainty and the haping of medical decisions. Hastings: Center Report, **21**: 6–11.

Braithwaite J. (2018). Changing how we think about healthcare improvement. British Medical Journal, **361**: k2014.

Firmin, C. (2017). Contextual Safeguarding: An Overview of the Operational, Strategic and Conceptual Framework. Bedford: The International Centre Researching Child Exploitation, Violence and Trafficking, University of Bedfordshire.

Fraser, S. W. & Greenhalgh, T. (2001). Coping with complexity: Educating for capability. British Medical Journal, **323**: 799–803.

General Medical Council (2018). The State of Medical Education and Practice in the UK. London: General Medical Council.

Hall, K. H. (2002). Reviewing intuitive decision-making and uncertainty: The implications for medical education. Medical Education, **36**: 216–224.

Ham, C. & Alberti, K. G. M. M. (2002). The medical profession, the public, and the government. British Medical Journal, **324**: 838–842.

Haslam, C., Jetten, J., Cruwys, T., Dingle, G. A. & Haslam, S. A. (2018). The New Psychology of Health: Unlocking the Social Cure. London: Routledge.

Heath, I. (2016). How medicine has exploited rationality at the expense of humanity. British Medical Journal, 355: i5705; doi: 10.1136/bmj.i5705.

Lund, C., Brooke-Sumner, C., Baingana, F. et al. (2018). Social determinants of mental disorders and the Sustainable Development Goals: A systematic review of papers. The Lancet, 5: 357–369.

Plsek, P. E. & Greenhalgh, T. (2001). The challenge of complexity in healthcare. British Medical Journal, 323: 625–628.

Plsek, P. E. & Wilson, T. (2001). Complexity, leadership, and management in healthcare organisations. British Medical Journal, 323: 746–749.

Sheard, L., Jackson, C. & Lawton, R. (2017). How is success achieved by individuals innovating for patient safety and quality in the NHS? BMC Health Services Research, 17640; doi 10.1186/s12913-017-2589-1.

Smith, R. (2001). Why are doctors so unhappy? British Medical Journal, 322: 1073–1074.

Thomas, P. (2018). Collaborating for Health. London: Routledge.

Vandentorren, S., Pirard, P., Sanna, A. et al. (2018). Healthcare provision and the psychological, somatic and social impact on people involved in the terror attacks in January 2015 in Paris: cohort study. The British Journal of Psychiatry, 212: 207–214.

Williams, R. (2002). Complexity, uncertainty and decision-making in an evidence-based world. Current Opinion in Psychiatry, 15: 343–347.

Wilson, T. & Holt, T. (2001). Complexity and clinical care. British Medical Journal, 323: 685–688.

Index

Bold type refers to tables; *italic* to figures